Monte Carlo Simulation Power Analysis
Using Mplus and R

Methodology in the Social Sciences

David A. Kenny, Founding Editor
Todd D. Little, Series Editor

This series provides applied researchers and students with analysis and research design books that emphasize the use of methods to answer research questions. Rather than emphasizing statistical theory, each volume in the series illustrates when a technique should (and should not) be used and how the output from available software programs should (and should not) be interpreted. Common pitfalls as well as areas of further development are clearly articulated.

RECENT VOLUMES

INTRODUCTION TO MEDIATION, MODERATION, AND CONDITIONAL PROCESS ANALYSIS: A REGRESSION-BASED APPROACH, THIRD EDITION
Andrew F. Hayes

THE THEORY AND PRACTICE OF ITEM RESPONSE THEORY, SECOND EDITION
R. J. de Ayala

APPLIED MISSING DATA ANALYSIS, SECOND EDITION
Craig K. Enders

PRINCIPLES AND PRACTICE OF STRUCTURAL EQUATION MODELING, FIFTH EDITION
Rex B. Kline

MACHINE LEARNING FOR SOCIAL AND BEHAVIORAL RESEARCH
Ross Jacobucci, Kevin J. Grimm, and Zhiyong Zhang

BAYESIAN STATISTICS FOR THE SOCIAL SCIENCES, SECOND EDITION
David Kaplan

LONGITUDINAL STRUCTURAL EQUATION MODELING, SECOND EDITION
Todd D. Little

COMPUTERIZED ADAPTIVE TESTING: FROM CONCEPT TO IMPLEMENTATION
David J. Weiss and Alper Şahin

STRUCTURAL EQUATION MODELING OF MULTIPLE RATER DATA
Michael Eid, Christian Geiser, and Tobias Koch

CATEGORICAL DATA WITH STRUCTURAL EQUATION MODELS: APPLICATIONS IN Mplus AND lavaan
Kevin J. Grimm

MONTE CARLO SIMULATION POWER ANALYSIS USING Mplus AND R
James Peugh and Kaylee Litson

Monte Carlo Simulation Power Analysis Using Mplus and R

James Peugh
Kaylee Litson

Series Editor's Note by Todd D. Little

THE GUILFORD PRESS
New York London

A Division of Guilford Publications, Inc.
www.guilford.com

Printed in the United States of America

This book is printed on acid-free paper.

For product and safety concerns within the EU, please contact *GPSR@taylorandfrancis.com,* Taylor & Francis Verlag GmbH, Kaufingerstraße 24, 80331 München, Germany.

Last digit is print number: 9 8 7 6 5 4 3 2 1

Library of Congress Cataloging-in-Publication Data is available from the publisher.

ISBN 978-1-4625-6284-8 (paperback)
ISBN 978-1-4625-6285-5 (cloth)

To my wife, Jennifer,
my daughter, Mary Catherine,
and my son, Gerard

—J. P.

To my late grandma, Helen

—K. L.

Series Editor's Note

The importance of the topic of power cannot be understated. The validity of statistical inference is predicated on having sufficient power to detect effects of interest. Simple designs can be addressed with formulaic methods to determine sufficient power, though Monte Carlo simulation is still preferred. Complex designs, on the other hand, are not as straightforward and necessitate a Monte Carlo approach. As James Peugh and Kaylee Litson clarify, Monte Carlo simulation is the only technique that can reliably produce power estimates for all designs, from cross-sectional designs, path models, to all manner of structural equation models. Peugh and Litson provide us with a wonderful and comprehensive resource to conduct Monte Carlo simulation power analysis. They offer thorough examples of conducting such analyses using the R platform as well as the Mplus software package.

Worthwhile, real-world data are decidedly complex and messy, with issues like attrition, nonresponse, and nestedness being ubiquitous. Peugh and Litson detail step-by-step instructions for navigating the complexity and messiness of data in the context of power analysis. The accessible examples are comprehensive in our massively multivariate world, including multiple groups, growth curves, mediation, moderation, using covariates (time varying and time invariant), randomized clinical trials, and categorical variables. Moving beyond simple models and cross-sectional data, they cover numerous longitudinal models, survival models (both discrete time and continuous time), two-level models, and moderated mediation.

Conducting an appropriate power analysis is a necessary element of any quantitative grant proposal. A key element of Peugh and Liston's book is the clear explication of how to write up each type of power analysis that they present. Moreover, the topics are self-contained such that users can go directly to the example that is most relevant to the analysis needed to address the research question. The write-up examples are perfect models for convincing grant reviewers that the study is properly powered to accurately address the aims and goals of the proposed study. This book will have a lasting impact on the conduct of science across the social, behavioral, and health sciences. The costs and losses incurred by underpowered studies will be eliminated and resources will be realistically allocated toward the sweet spot of a properly powered project that will effectively inform policy and practice.

As always, enjoy!

TODD D. LITTLE, PhD
At my "Wits End" in Lakeside, Montana

Preface

So, why write a Monte Carlo simulation power analysis book? Why *now*? Two things still surprise us even after putting this book together: (1) the fact that the research that comprises the bulk of Chapter 1 shows sample sizes and statistical power levels really haven't changed much in 60 years, and (2) the fact that there hasn't been a Monte Carlo simulation power analysis book written in well over 20 years. The truly surprising part is that, during this same time span, there have been massive changes in the entire quantitative methodology landscape, far too many to mention. This book has been a work in progress for a very long time, but it all started with a "memorable" incident from way back in graduate school . . .

In the spring of 2004, the first author was in a Structural Equation Modeling class at the University of Nebraska–Lincoln taught by my dissertation chair (more on him in a minute . . .). One of the first topic lectures of that course introduced Sewall Wright's (1921, 1934) path tracing concepts and rules. I can recall we were all frantically drawing, labeling, and taking notes (or, maybe I should speak for myself) when suddenly, from the back of the room, we heard the unbelievable: "WHY ARE WE STUDYING THIS?!?!? THIS IS ARCHAIC!! DOES ANYONE EVEN **USE** THIS ANYMORE?!?!" While half the class sat motionless in stunned horror, the other half rubber-necked, if for no other reason, to catch a rare, live glimpse of graduate student verbal *seppuku*. My dissertation chair's immediate response was just as memorable: "Yeah, . . . I had a feeling I should have kept this class small . . ." That graduate student never returned to class and dropped the course a short time later. For me, the result of that spring day in 2004 was that Sewall Wright's path tracing rules were memorably stuck in my brain, but at that time, I had no idea when, why, or how to apply it.

The key to writing this book (20+ years later) was realizing three themes. The first theme arose from finally realizing that (quite opinionated) graduate student back in 2004 could not have been more wrong: Wright's rules enable the power analysis mission-critical calculation of residual variances even in the most complicated (see Chapter 11) research designs and data analytic models. The second theme came from a Special Topics class taught by my dissertation chair in graduate school a year later (eligibility for attendance was severely restricted this time): *standardization simplifies*. The third theme, the ability to use the linear model algebra equations for longitudinal models offered by both Bollen and Curran (2006) and Grimm, Ram, and Estabrook (2017), is the key to obtaining Monte Carlo simulation power estimates as longitudinal designs increase in complexity (see Chapters 9–11). A global COVID-19 pandemic and lockdown provided the opportunity to write a 12-chapter plus four-appendix Monte Carlo simulation power analysis book we hope researchers worldwide will find helpful.

About This Book

The layout of this book moves from the simple to the more complex. The first six chapters describe cross-sectional power analyses; the next five chapters describe longitudinal power analyses. Within both sections of the book, examples begin with simpler analysis examples to illustrate foundational techniques such as Wright's path tracing rules (e.g., *t*-test and bivariate regression examples in Chapter 1, an unconditional growth model in Chapter 7) and move to the more complex analyses (SEMs in Chapter 4 and complex longitudinal mediation in Chapter 11). More importantly, although it appears to be a digressive tangent, incorporating missing data into a power analysis is shown in Chapter 6 immediately after logistic regression power analyses in Chapter 5 because logistic regression principles are used in Mplus and R to specify and control the amount of missing data incorporated into power estimates. In our opinion, incorporating missing data into power analysis estimates is a highlight of this book.

Researchers unfamiliar with Wright's path tracing rules, missing data specification, and incorporation, or both, would likely find the first six chapters of this book beneficial. With a firm grasp of both concepts, researchers can then choose from the longitudinal power analyses in Chapters 7–11 or the power analyses in Appendices A–D that best meet their needs. Although the supplemental power analyses shown in Appendices A–D could not be included in the book (it would have exceeded 800 pages), it is important to note those power analysis examples are available at the companion website:

- Appendix A. Statistical Power for Latent Variable Moderation Power Analysis
- Appendix B. Part I: Statistical Power for Survival Analysis
- Appendix C. Monte Carlo Simulation Power for Two-Level Models (Based on Arend & Schafer, 2019)
- Appendix D. Statistical Power for Moderated Mediation

Mplus and R syntax scripts and supplemental materials for Chapters 1–11, as well as text narrative, Mplus, and R syntax scripts, and supplemental materials for Appendices A–D mentioned above, are all available online at the following address: *www.guilford.com/peugh-materials*.

An Important Caveat

This book was originally intended to be a Monte Carlo simulation power analysis book that featured Mplus syntax examples only. Book proposal feedback from several anonymous reviewers was unanimous on one point: R syntax needed to be included. Again, special thanks to Kaylee Litson for doing a fantastic job following up the Mplus examples with equivalent R syntax specifications. It is important to note that for many of the chapters in the book, the Mplus and R sample size estimates are identical or reasonably close and the models are essentially equivalent. However, readers will see a notation that states for four of the chapters, equivalent R syntax for the Mplus example was not possible. In the second half of Chapter 8, as well as in Chapters 9 and 11, it was not possible in the R package simsem to covary the binary covariate (which is how the binary predictor variable needed to be simulated) with a continuous covariate in the presence of a complex SEM model. In Chapters 5 and 11, the inclusion of both a binary predictor and binary outcome was not possible to model in either lavaan or simsem. Readers will find the R code we were able to specify for these chapters in the supplemental online materials, but sample size estimates between that code and the Mplus code for the same example will not match because they reflect different underlying population and/or analysis models. When reading these chapters (and later conducting your own power analyses), it is important to note that even minor differences in the population and/or sample model, such as the inclusion or exclusion of a correlation among predictor variables, can *drastically* impact statistical power estimates.

Acknowledgments

From JP: I owe an enormous debt of gratitude, first and foremost, to my former mentoring professor and dissertation chair, Craig Enders. Your guidance and patience have made a huge difference in my professional development and this book would not have been possible without everything you've taught me. All I can say is that I will continue to try my best to pay it forward. You've shown me the difference one person can make.

I also would like to extend a big thank you to my good friend and colleague, David Feldon. Collaborations with you have always been enjoyable and productive, and the large dividends that resulted in the end have always been a very rewarding bonus. Most importantly, I am grateful that you allowed me to recruit (your then postdoctoral fellow) Kaylee Litson to provide the R syntax for all the power analyses in this book (more on that below).

Belated and long overdue thanks go to my University of Nebraska doctoral dissertation committee members (and a special thank you to both Rafael de Ayala, the department chair in my PhD program, and Calvin Garbin from the Psychology Department), all my former professors in the Quantitative PhD program in the Teacher's College, as well as to my postdoctoral fellowship supervisors from the Psychology Department: David DiLillo and Mario Scalora. I will always look back at graduate school and my postdoctoral fellowship with enormous personal satisfaction; my training was top-notch and I am grateful to you all.

In addition to the faculty members in the Behavioral Medicine Clinical Psychology division of the Cincinnati Children's Hospital Medical Center, I need to extend much thanks to several more individuals within my division and outside the hospital for allowing the use of their quotable comments, power analyses, and pilot data for the contents included in this book: Scott Powers (Chater 1), Kevin Hommel (Chapter 2), Zarina Vakhitova (Chapter 5), Julia Carmody (Chapter 7), Nina M. Tauber and Rosalie Corona (Chapter 8), Stephen Becker (Chapter 10), Sarah Beal (Chapter 11), Pin-Lun Kuo, Judd Walson, and my two trusted colleagues and friends Michael Toland and David Dueber (Appendix B, Parts 1 and 2), Matthias Arend and Thomas Schafer (Appendix C), and Nurit Tal-Or (Appendix D).

I must give a very big and well overdue thank you to the Mplus support group. I have tested your patience for decades. Thank you.

Thank you also to C. Deborah Laughton, Katherine Sommer, Jared Greenberg, and all at The Guilford Press for your help and support. Thank you also to Chia-Lin Tsai, Statistics Department, University of North Colorado; Fred L. Oswald, Psychology Department, Rice University; and Guilford's other anonymous reviewers willing to give their time and offer their suggestions to make this book the best product it could be. Special thanks also to Ryne Estabrook for his excellent answers to all of my linear model equation questions.

Finally, and most importantly, I want to dedicate this book to my wife, Jennifer (who challenged me to write this book), my daughter, Mary Catherine, who keeps me company at times in my new post-COVID-19 office in the basement of my home, and my infant son, Gerard. Everything I do is always for the three of you.

From KL: Although I came to this book much later in the game, I have had an incredible, educational, experience writing it. First and foremost, thank you to my good friend and colleague David Feldon, who connected me with James and helped me see that the translation of quantitative work into practice is where my passion lies. Second, I want to thank the many, many scholars and programmers who have contributed to and continue contributing to open-source SEM software packages, such as lavaan and simsem. I hope these packages continue to be developed and receive funding to make them more accessible to researchers as well as more robust to different research designs and applications. I also would like to thank those who have fielded my questions in online forums, particularly Terrence Jorgensen, whose email responses to my questions about simsem and lavaan have been immensely helpful as I grappled with how to translate Mplus syntax to R across some more complex research designs.

Thank you also to C. Deborah Laughton and all at The Guilford Press for your support and advice as I've navigated writing this book. Although I feel I should have heeded your warning about not taking on a book project so early in my career, I couldn't have had a better first book writing experience. And finally, a huge thank you to James Peugh, for trusting me and bringing me on to this project. It has been an uphill battle at times, and I couldn't have done it without your support and continued collaboration.

On a personal note, I'd like to thank my mom, my siblings, and my grandma (who has since passed away). All of these individuals listened to me talk, complain, and rejoice as I worked through some of the more difficult parts of this book. You all got to see moments where I was frustrated because R froze or I had a minor error in code that led to unexpected problematic results. Each of you also saw joyful moments when I finally figured out the solution to my problem or came to the realization that I wasn't in the position to solve the problem I had encountered. My grandma was one who was very excited for me having this opportunity, and I spent many nights working on this book while spending time with her in her last years. For this reason, I dedicate the work I did in this book to her.

Contents

Mplus and R syntax scripts and supplemental materials for Chapters 1–11, as well as text narrative, Mplus, and R syntax scripts, and supplemental materials for Appendices A–D are all available online at the following address: *www.guilford.com/peugh-materials.*

Part I

Cross-Sectional Power Analyses

1

Introduction

Statistical power analysis can be defined as the answer to a scientific researcher's question: "How many participants do I need to recruit to detect the effect or phenomenon of interest?" "How many participants?" questions directly address the issue of sample size (N), and "detect the effect or phenomenon of interest?" questions directly address the issues of a researcher's ability to obtain $p < .05$, reject a null hypothesis of no effect, and publish the study results. Without question, sample size, $p < .05$, and statistical power analysis are *inextricably linked*, and these relationships are critically important to scientific researchers for two reasons. First, probability (p) values come directly from test statistics, and all test statistics (t, F, χ^2, Wald z, etc.) have the same generic formula: Test statistic = Effect/Standard error; where Standard error = Effect standard deviation/$\sqrt{N}$. All else being equal, larger (N) sample sizes produce smaller standard errors, larger test statistics, smaller probability (p) values, and a greater likelihood of rejecting the null hypothesis and obtaining results deemed publishable by most current journal standards. Smaller (N) sample sizes produce larger standard errors, smaller test statistics, larger probability (p) values, and a greater likelihood of retaining the null hypothesis, making results far less likely to be published or inform future research and practice.

Second, of the four influences on statistical power (sample size [N], size of the effect of interest [e.g., Cohen's d, R^2, odds ratio, etc.], dependent variable [DV] variance, and the nominal alpha [$\alpha < .05$] level), the only one completely under the researcher's control is *sample size* (for more details, see the Appendix at the end of this chapter). Taken together, the conclusion is a crucial one: A researcher's ability to publish significant, novel, and meaningful findings is contingent on an adequate sample size, and a power analysis is required to determine an adequate sample size. Given its importance, it would seem intuitive to assume that scientific researchers would place a premium on a rigorous and defensible power analysis for sample size determinations. However, the published empirical research that investigates statistical power levels across numerous fields of scientific inquiry shows this is not the case.

Statement of the Problem: Statistical Power in the Empirical Literature

Jacob Cohen's 1962 publication was a landmark across all fields of scientific inquiry because it was the first to examine publications in a specific research area, compute levels of statistical power, and answer a research question regarding an investigator's actual probability of rejecting a false null hypothesis in the population. Cohen (1962) computed statistical power estimates from 78 manuscripts published in the *Journal of Abnormal and Social Psychology* in 1960 and 1961. Results showed that the average sample size used in analyses to test the primary research hypothesis was $N = 68$. Cohen's results also showed average statistical power estimates of .18, .48, and .83 to detect small, medium, and large effect sizes, respectively. Cohen concluded by calling on all researchers to, ". . . increase sample sizes (p. 151)."

Cohen's (1962) publication spurred additional research both within and outside of psychology. Within psychology, several researchers later replicated Cohen's study to determine if his sample size recommendation was heeded. Researchers in other related fields began similar inquiries into statistical power levels. A summary of these studies, presented in chronological order, is shown in Table 1.1.

When these studies in Table 1.1 are summarized, an inescapable conclusion must be reached. With very few possible exceptions (see Gaskin & Happell, 2012; Maddock & Rossi, 2001; Shen et al., 2011), neither sample sizes (Holmes, 1979, 1983; Marszalek, Barber, Kohlhart, & Cooper, 2011) nor statistical power estimates (Schimmack, 2012; Smaldino & McElreath, 2016) have appreciably changed in the past 60 years.

Additional published research addressing the question of why statistical power has remained both unacceptably low and stagnant for six decades has identified three causes: a publication bias, Campbell's Law, and questionable research practices. Publications are required to obtain, maintain, and expand a scientific investigative career (e.g., Anderson, Kelley, & Maxwell, 2017; Higginson & Munafò, 2016). However, a publication bias has long been well-known to exist (e.g., Anderson, Kelley, & Maxwell, 2017; Ioannidis, 2008; Kuhberger, Fritz, & Scherndl, 2014). For example, research has shown that 96% of published psychology manuscripts contain statistically significant findings, but Monte Carlo probability testing shows a majority of these findings are more likely false discoveries instead of true effects (Bakker, vanDijk, & Wicherts, 2012). It has also been shown in the published scientific literature that false discoveries increase as perceptions of study novelty, use of data mining programs, outside financial stakeholders (Ioannidis, 2005), and journal impact factors (Fraley & Vazire, 2014; Szucs & Ioannidis, 2017a) all increase, and sample sizes decrease (Kuhberger, Fritz, & Scherndl, 2014).

Campbell's Law has been defined by Smaldino and McElreath (2016, p. 4) as follows:

> Campbell's Law, stated in this paper's epigraph, implies that if researchers are incentivized to increase the number of papers published, they will modify their methods to produce the largest possible number of publishable results rather than the most rigorous investigations.

There appears to be empirical support for Campbell's law. Using Monte Carlo simulations guided by optimality theory, Higginson and Munafò (2016) found that conducting multiple studies with inadequate statistical power is the most efficient way of quickly find-

TABLE 1.1. Power Estimate Studies

Field of study	Power estimate	Data	Source
Abnormal Psychology	.12, .37, and .86 for small, medium, and large effect sizes	56 published articles	Sedlmeier and Gigerenzer (1992)
Personality Psychology	.17, .57, and .83 for small, medium, and large effect sizes	6,155 analyses in 221 publications	Rossi (1990)
Rehabilitation	.26, .63, and .90 for small, medium, and large effect sizes	32 publications in 4 journals	Kosciulek and Szymanski (1993)
Organizational Psychology	37% had power >.80 for small or medium effect sizes	2,6471 analyses in 210 articles	Mone, Mueller, and Mauland (1996)
Psychology	.16, .59, and .82 for small, medium, and large effect sizes	54 publications in the United Kingdom	Clark-Carter (1997)
Neuropsychology	.45 for a meduim effect size	66 published articles	Bezeau and Graves (2001)
Neuroscience	.21	49 meta-analyses; 730 individual studies	Button et al. (2013)
Social Psychology	.43–.60	824 articles, 1,934 studies	Fraley and Vazire (2014)
Behavioral Sciences	.24	60-year meta-analysis	Smaldino and McElreath (2016)
Psychiatry, Neurology, and Somatic Disease	.09–.30	660 meta-analyses	Dumas-Mallet, Button, Boraud, Gonon, and Munafò (2017)
Cognitive Neuroscience and Psychology	.12, .44, and .73 for small, medium, and large effect sizes	26,841 statistical analyses from 3,801 publications	Szucs and Ioannidis (2017a)
Clinical Trials	.16–.23	136,212 clinical trials from 1975 to 2014	Lamberink et al. (2018)

ing and publishing statistically significant findings even if more than half are, in fact, false discoveries.

Further research shows that a convergence of publication bias and Campbell's law produces a systemic and self-sustaining phenomenon termed "questionable research practices." Consistent with Campbell's law and optimality theory, questionable research practices begin with researchers conducting multiple studies, each with inadequate statistical power to detect the effect of interest. Researchers then conduct multiple statistical analyses (see "The Curse of Multiplicity" in Maxwell, 2004; Wilkinson and the Task Force on Statistical Inference, 1999) within each of the studies to increase the likelihood of obtaining significance, but report and subsequently publish only the significant results. In reality, such results are more likely false discoveries that also produce inflated effect size estimates. Such publications increase the need for multiple statistical analyses to obtain statistically significant findings in subsequent studies (Anderson, Kelley, & Maxwell, 2017; Bakker, vanDijk, & Wicherts, 2012), especially if subsequent studies used the original publication's inadequate sample size and inflated effect size estimate (the "winner's curse"; Open Science Collaboration, 2015) as a basis for determining their sample size requirements (see Zickfeld & Schubert, 2019).

What Does This Mean?

If questionable research practices are responsible for keeping both sample sizes and statistical power at inadequately low levels, then a collision among three trends appears inevitable for a number of reasons. First, the current generation of scientific researchers, if influenced by Campbell's law and optimality theory, may be basing study sample size requirements on subjective intuition, convenient availability, or budget constraints rather than statistical analytics because if they received any statistical power analysis training, it was likely inadequate or viewed as unnecessary. By extension, this means that the current generation of scientific research trainees (e.g., graduate students, research lab interns and residents, and postdoctoral fellows), who are likely to become the next generation of scientific researchers, will also receive inadequate statistical power analysis training if they receive any training at all. Second, recent decades have shown an exponential growth in advanced statistical analysis techniques and a rapid increase in the sophistication and availability of advanced statistical analysis software packages capable of performing such analyses. Such availability has enabled researchers to pose more complex research questions that require both complex statistical analyses and complex power analyses to answer accurately. Without adequate statistical power analysis training for even comparably simple statistical analyses, evaluating statistical power for advanced statistical analyses will lag even further behind current statistical capabilities and methods. Third, the statistical power needed to detect the small and medium effect sizes that can be expected in many different areas of scientific inquiry can be increased only by increasing sample sizes. This will greatly increase the cost of conducting such studies (An anonymous reviewer of this chapter stated it best: "It takes *money* to do good science."), which will increase the need to acquire external grant funding and will require a rigorous and defensible power analysis. In addition, several scientific journals now require an a priori power analysis for manuscripts submitted for publication consideration, and it is reasonable to assume that more journals will follow that trend. Two conclusions can be drawn: (1) The ability to conduct sophisticated, rigorous, and defensible statistical power analyses has further increased in importance and (2) scientific researchers able to conduct such power analyses will find themselves in possession of a distinct professional advantage.

Why Monte Carlo Simulation Power Analyses?

More than a decade ago, Abraham and Russell (2008) advocated for the use of Monte Carlo simulation methods (described later) to determine estimates of statistical power but, by many indications, their suggestion has rarely been heeded. Part of the reason can be attributed to the increased training needs in power analysis techniques at all levels of professional development. However, a better explanation may be attributed to the amount of quantitative information that is required a priori as input data before Monte Carlo simulation methods can be used to estimate statistical power. One of the goals of this book, for all power analysis examples presented, is to clearly articulate the logical assumptions that can be invoked that will supply the input data required for a Monte Carlo simulation power calculation.

Possibly the greatest benefit for using Monte Carlo simulation methods to estimate statistical power is that the logic behind Monte Carlo simulations is consistent with central limit theorem, which is the foundation underlying all statistical inference. Central limit theorem states that if a researcher was able to draw a very large number of samples, each of size N, from the population of interest, each sample would differ slightly, and randomly, from the population from which it was drawn. However, if the researcher was able to perform the research study, collect and analyze the data to obtain the estimate of interest (such as the difference in means between a treatment group and a control group) from all samples of size N drawn from the population, a histogram of the accumulated results for the parameter estimate(s) of interest will always produce a normal distribution, the width of the normal distribution will be determined by variation in the estimate of interest and the sample size N from which it was obtained, and the mean of the normal distribution will be the true population value for the parameter estimate of interest.

Monte Carlo simulations follow this same logic. Specifically, after a researcher specifies: (1) an analysis model of interest, (2) a sample size N to be considered, (3) the magnitude of the effect of interest (e.g., a mean difference between the treatment and control groups), and (4) the number of sample dataset replications to be generated, statistical analysis software programs capable of performing Monte Carlo simulations will begin generating datasets of size N consistent with the analysis model specified. The software package will also add a random variation to each generated dataset to mimic the fact that samples will vary randomly from the population from which they were drawn consistent with the central limit theorem. The statistical analysis of interest is conducted on each sample replication, and the statistical analysis software package keeps track of the number of sample replications in which the null hypothesis for the effect of interest was rejected at $p < .05$ (two-tailed). The Monte Carlo simulation statistical power estimate is then obtained by dividing the number of sample dataset replications in which the null hypothesis was rejected by the total number of sample dataset replications requested. Assuming a properly specified and admissible analysis model, Monte Carlo simulation methods generate thousands of possible outcomes a researcher could obtain and compute statistical power in a way that reflects the probability of rejecting the null hypothesis for the one outcome a researcher will observe. In summary, Monte Carlo simulation methods are preferable for their ability to produce *precise* estimates of statistical power.

Software to Conduct Power Analyses

This book considers both Mplus and R as statistical software packages for evaluating Monte Carlo simulation statistical power analyses. Mplus offers a great deal of flexibility with relatively little prior coding knowledge, yet its functionality, yearly updates, and ease-of-use come with an annual price tag. R is a free, open-source program that contains many tools to conduct Monte Carlo simulation power analyses, yet requires a more in-depth knowledge of coding, takes a consistently longer time to run analyses when compared to Mplus, and has a steeper learning curve with regard to Monte Carlo simulation power analyses. Considering the numerous statistical software packages available that can perform power analyses available either as internet freeware or commercially for purchase, the question of why such an emphasis on statistical coding packages, such as Mplus and R could be reasonably posed. Internet freeware power analysis programs, such as G*Power (Faul, Erdfelder, Buchner, & Lang, 2007, 2009) and Optimal Design (Liu, Spybrook, Congdon, Martinez, & Raudenbush, 2006), suffer from two notable drawbacks that limit their utility. First, such freeware programs, based on analytic methods of power analysis, do afford the convenience of requiring relatively little a priori quantitative information, but researchers often must pay a steep price on the back-end in the form of sample size estimates for adequate statistical power that are larger than needed or even feasible in some instances. Second, such internet freeware programs can estimate statistical power for a relatively limited number of specific research design and data analysis scenarios. Schoemann, Boulton, and Short (2017) described well both these limitations (pp. 381–382, *italics added*):

> However, power analyses using analytic methods only cover a small portion of possible analyses (e.g., *t*-tests, analysis of variance, correlation, regression), and even in these cases, *researchers are often forced to make possibly unrealistic assumptions (e.g., equal group sizes, no missing data)*. When study designs or analyses are complex (e.g., mediation models with bootstrapping) *analytic models are often not available and a Monte Carlo simulation approach to power analysis is preferred.*

Furthermore, there are commercially for purchase (e.g., Stata, WinBUGS, LISREL, EQS, etc.) advanced statistical analysis software programs capable of performing Monte Carlo simulation power analyses, but few if any can match the myriad of response variable types and data analytic design options afforded by Mplus or the flexibility in coding afforded by R. Perhaps the greatest advantage of Mplus, as well as recent package advances in R, is the ability to easily specify and generate missing values for response variables measured on any scale to assess the impact of missing data on statistical power estimates. Most importantly, researchers that want to learn more about how to use Mplus can choose from a number of excellent published introductory resources (Byrne, 2013; Finch & Bolin,

2017; Geiser, 2012, 2020; Kelloway, 2014; Muthén, Muthén, & Asparouhov, 2017; Wang & Wang, 2019; Wickrama, Lee, O'Neal, & Lorenz, 2016), and those that want to learn more about how to use R can browse discussion boards and online R documentation that is readily available. For these reasons, we present Mplus and R code to conduct statistical power analyses throughout this book, noting key differences among the two programs and highlighting advantages and disadvantages to currently available versions and packages.

Why Use the Approach Shown in This Book?

Scientific researchers would appear to be at a crossroads at this point. On the one hand, advances in statistical analysis techniques and the availability of sophisticated statistical analysis software programs have enabled researchers to pose complex research questions. However, determination of the sample size needed to correctly answer these questions requires complex power analysis techniques. A wide gap currently exists between the complex research questions that can now be posed and the implementation of the power analysis techniques required to determine the acceptable sample size necessary to accurately answer those questions. A better method is needed for estimating statistical power that is: (1) capable of handling very complex analysis models that answer complex research questions, yet (2) straightforward enough so that researchers familiar with analysis of variance (ANOVA) and multiple regression terminology and techniques can implement it, and (3) presented in a manner that emphasizes "hands-on" application instead of conceptual theory.

This book will show how to obtain Monte Carlo simulation statistical power estimates from cross-sectional or longitudinal research designs that involve comparative-based or relationship-based research questions. This book takes a purely applied approach because, admittedly, one potential drawback to using Monte Carlo simulation techniques for estimating statistical power is the requirement that all estimated model parameters be assigned a priori values. This includes not only values for the parameter estimates representing the effects a researcher is interested in but also includes values for parameters such as residual variances and covariances that a researcher is not interested in and can be extremely difficult to obtain. This book also includes (1) discussions of the logical assumptions that can be invoked and the specific techniques needed to obtain all parameter estimates needed as Monte Carlo simulation input data, (2) syntax scripts that will assist researchers in checking their model specifications and values for admissibility, (3) demonstrations of how to convert model admissibility check information into Mplus Monte Carlo syntax specifications, and (4) instructions on how to specify and incorporate reasonable amounts of missing data into syntax specifications to obtain more rigorous and realistic statistical power estimates. Most of the power analysis example models and techniques shown in this book have been used in successfully funded federal grant applications, which means that the approach described in this book has been scrutinized at the national level and been shown to be both rigorous and effective. Finally, as shown in the following examples and in the chapters that follow, the techniques and procedures used in this book to obtain Monte Carlo simulation statistical power estimates, even for complex cross-sectional, longitudinal, or two-level models, are no more difficult than the computations needed to obtain a *correlation matrix*.

Proof of Concept: Why and How the Assumption of Standardization Simplifies

An assumption made throughout the book is that all analysis model variables for all power analysis examples are *standardized,* which is defined as converting variable scores from their original raw score (X_{raw}) metric to *z*-scores with Equation 1.1:

$$z - \text{score} = \frac{X_{\text{raw}} - \bar{X}}{SD} \tag{1.1}$$

Standardization is a crucial assumption because *standardization simplifies* the process of providing population values for all analysis model estimates that are required for Monte Carlo simulation statistical power calculations. As a simple example, consider the relationship between a covariance and a correlation. A covariance is an unstandardized quantification of the relationship between two variables. It is difficult to meaningfully interpret without additional information about the variances of the two variables in question. A quantification of the relationship between two standardized variables is one definition of a correlation. Correlations are bounded at ±1 and can be interpreted based on magnitude and sign. Two Monte Carlo simulation power analysis examples, one involving a relationship research question and another involving a comparative research question, can further illustrate how the standardization assumption simplifies the Monte Carlo simulation power calculation process.

A Relationship Research Question Power Analysis

A simple bivariate regression analysis model example involving two predictor variables (*X*1 and *X*2) and a response variable (*Y*) is shown (Figure 1.1).

The values on the rectangles (46.642 and 25.706) are the variances of the two predictor variables, respectively. The value for the curved double-headed arrow (21.429) represents the covariance, or unstandardized relationship, between *X*1 and *X*2. The values shown on the regression arrows ($b_1 = 1.25$; $b_2 = 2.55$) represent the unstandardized regression slope coefficients that quantify the relationships between *Y* and both *X*1 and *X*2, respectively. Finally, the circle above the response variable *Y* represents residual variance, or the amount of variance in *Y* not explained by *X*1 and *X*2. The question mark within the circle represents

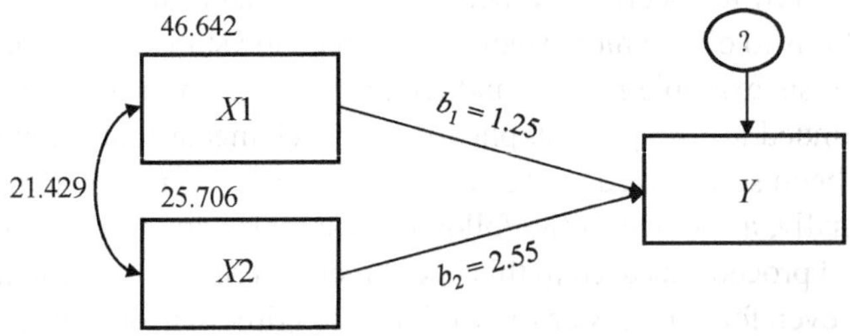

FIGURE 1.1. An unstandardized regression example.

the fact that residual variance is unknown but must be calculated prior to conducting a Monte Carlo simulation power analysis.

Although unlikely, let's further assume for illustration purposes that, in addition to the above information, a researcher was also able to obtain via a literature search the following covariance matrix quantifying possible unstandardized relationships among the three variables.

	Y	*X*1	*X*2
Y	65.033		
*X*1	24.218	46.642	
*X*2	19.972	21.429	25.706

If a researcher wanted to know the minimal sample size needed to reject the null hypotheses for both slope estimates (b_1 = 1.25; b_2 = 2.55) with statistical power ≥ .80, it would appear that plenty of information was available to compute the one unknown ("?") residual variance estimate and conduct a Monte Carlo simulation power analysis. In reality, without more information (which a researcher may not have) for the three analysis variables, computing the residual variance for the response variable *Y* can be extremely difficult. Unlike the bounded limits for an admissible correlation, the bounded limits for an admissible covariance can be difficult to determine.

To illustrate, consider the same relationship research analysis model scenario assuming standardization, where a researcher was able to specify the following values based on prior research but has no additional information regarding the three variables of interest (Figure 1.2).

Under standardization, (1) both predictor variables *X*1 and *X*2 have unit (1) variances, by definition, (2) the correlation between the two predictors ($r_{X1,X2}$ = .55) is known and is easily interpretable, and (3) the regression slope coefficients for *X*1 and *X*2 as predictors of *Y* are standardized (β_1 =.25; β_2 =.35). The question mark indicates that the residual variance for *Y* is still unknown but still needed prior to conducting a Monte Carlo simulation power analysis.

Here is where standardization simplifies the problem. First, the R_Y^2 statistic is defined as the proportion of variance in *Y* that is explained by both *X*1 and *X*2. Second, assuming standardization, the total variance of *Y* is also equal to 1. Third, if R_Y^2 quantifies the pro-

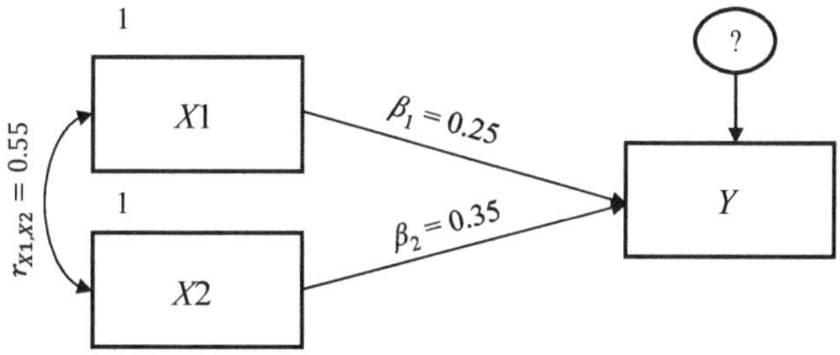

FIGURE 1.2. A standardized regression example.

portion of variance in Y explained by $X1$ and $X2$, then residual (or unexplained) variance ($\sigma^2_{\text{RESIDUAL}}$) in Y must equal $\sigma^2_{\text{RESIDUAL}} = 1 - R^2_Y$ by definition. Finally, because Y is predicted by both $X1$ and $X2$, then the total variance explained in Y (R^2_Y) must equal the proportion of variance in Y explained by $X1$ ($R^2_{Y|X1}$) *plus* the proportion of variance in Y explained by $X2$ ($R^2_{Y|X2}$), or $R^2_Y = R^2_{Y|X1} + R^2_{Y|X2}$.

More than 100 years ago, Sewall Wright (1921, 1934) proposed a set of *path tracing rules* that, combined with a general form equation, can be used to calculate the variance explained in a response variable. Wright's path tracing rules can be stated as follows:

1. A path cannot involve tracing through the same variable twice.
2. A path can involve only one correlation tracing (i.e., double-headed curved arrow).
3. A path can involve tracing both backward (from the arrowhead of a regression arrow back to its source) and forward (from the source of the regression arrow to its arrowhead), but once a forward tracing is made, additional backward tracings are prohibited.
4. A path can involve as many backward and forward tracings as are permissible.

Further, Wright has also shown that the general equation for computing the response variable (Y) variance explained by one or more predictor (Xn) variables can be expressed as a function of both the *direct paths* and *indirect paths*, as shown in Equation (1.2), in an analysis model.

$$R^2_{Y|X1} = \text{Direct path} * (\text{Direct path} + [\text{Indirect effect product}]) \quad (1.2)$$

For example, Wright's rules and the general form equation can be used to compute the variance in Y explained X1 ($R^2_{Y|X1}$). By definition, the direct path between $X1$ and Y is β_1, so, by substitution [Equation (1.3) below],

$$R^2_{Y|X1} = \beta_1 * (\beta_1 + [\text{Indirect effect product}])$$

or

$$R^2_{Y|X1} = 0.25 * (0.25 + [\text{Indirect effect product}]) \quad (1.3)$$

According to Wright's path tracing rules, there is only one possible indirect effect path tracing between $X1$ and Y: the combined path from Y to $X2$ to $X1$ (Figure 1.3; **bolded**).

So, by substitution [Equation (1.4)],

$$R^2_{Y|X1} = 0.25 * (0.25 + [Y \text{ to } X2 * X2 \text{ to } X1])$$
$$R^2_{Y|X1} = 0.25 * (0.25 + [0.35 * 0.55])$$
$$R^2_{Y|X1} = 0.110625 \quad (1.4)$$

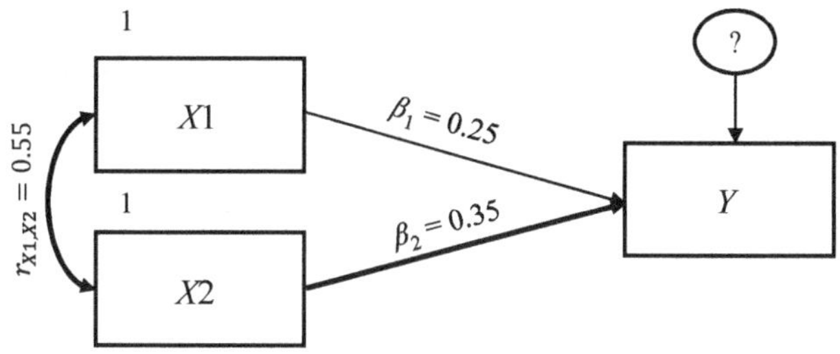

FIGURE 1.3. Indirect path from *Y* to *X*1.

The same procedure can be used to compute the variance in *Y* explained by *X*2, as shown in Equation (1.5):

$$R^2_{Y|X2} = \text{Direct path} * (\text{Direct path} + [\text{Indirect effect product}])$$
$$R^2_{Y|X2} = \beta_2 * (\beta_2 + [\text{Indirect effect product}])$$
$$R^2_{Y|X2} = 0.35 * (0.35 + [\text{Indirect effect product}]) \tag{1.5}$$

Again, there is only one possible indirect effect path tracing between *Y* and *X*2: the path from *Y* to *X*1 to *X*2, as shown in Figure 1.4 and Equation (1.6):

$$R^2_{Y|X2} = 0.35 * (0.35 + [Y \text{ to } X1 * X1 \text{ to } X2])$$
$$R^2_{Y|X2} = 0.35 * (0.35 + [0.25 * 0.55])$$
$$R^2_{Y|X2} = 0.170625 \tag{1.6}$$

Combined, the proportion of variance in *Y* explained by *X*1 ($R^2_{Y|X1}$) *plus* the proportion of variance in *Y* explained by *X*2 ($R^2_{Y|X2}$) can be calculated as follows [Equation (1.7)]:

$$R^2_Y = R^2_{Y|X1} + R^2_{Y|X2}$$
$$R^2_Y = 0.110625 + 0.1706250 = \underline{0.28125} \tag{1.7}$$

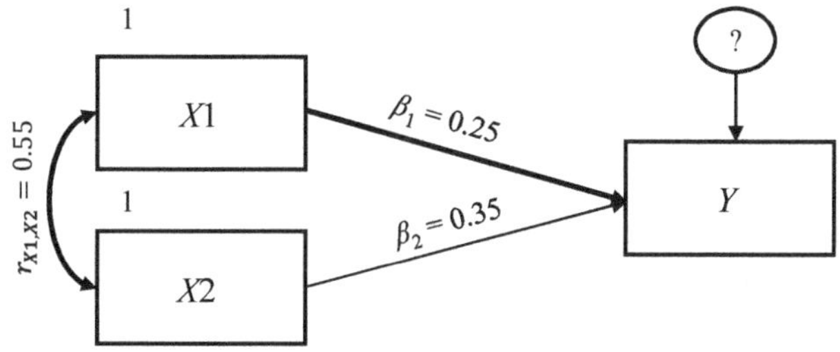

FIGURE 1.4. Indirect path from *Y* to *X*2.

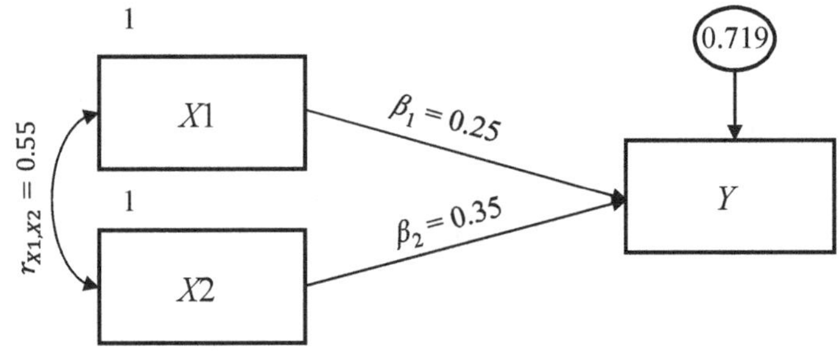

FIGURE 1.5. A fully specified regression model.

Recall that R_Y^2 is the proportion of variance in Y that is already explained by predictor variables $X1$ and $X2$. The residual variance ($\sigma^2_{\text{RESIDUAL}}$) in Y can be calculated as the difference between the total Y variance (1) and the proportion of variance in Y explained by predictor variables [R_Y^2; Equation (1.8)]:

$$\sigma^2_{\text{RESIDUAL}} = 1 - R_Y^2$$
$$\sigma^2_{\text{RESIDUAL}} = 1 - 0.28125 = \mathbf{0.71875} \tag{1.8}$$

All estimated parameters in the bivariate regression model now have specified values (Figure 1.5).

A Monte Carlo simulation power analysis can now be performed to answer the question of the minimal sample size needed to reject the null hypotheses for both β_1 and β_2 with statistical power ≥ .80. The next section shows how to conduct such a power analysis in Mplus, and thereafter in R. Sample code along with a description of coding language and interpretation will follow.

Mplus Monte Carlo Power Analysis: Bivariate Regression

To conduct a simulation in Mplus, an input model is first specified, which includes all relevant information needed to evaluate the simulation model. The full input model for the bivariate regression model is in Figure 1.5.

```
TITLE: Mplus 1.1 Bivariate Regression

MONTECARLO:
NAMES ARE Y X1 X2;
NOBSERVATIONS = 132;
NREPS = 5000;
SEED = 35170;

MODEL POPULATION:
[X1*0];
```

```
[X2*0];
X1*1;
X2*1;
X1 WITH X2*0.55;
Y ON X1*0.25;
Y ON X2*0.35;
[Y*0];
Y*0.71875;

MODEL:
Y ON X1*0.25 X2*0.35;
```

The `MONTECARLO:` command initializes the simulation algorithms in Mplus. The `NAMES ARE` specification allows researchers to provide names for the variables in the analysis model under the restriction that names must be no more than eight characters in length. `NOBSERVATIONS` allows the researcher to specify any sample size. The sample size tested here is $N = 132$ but it can be adjusted to achieve the desired level of statistical power. `NREPS`, or number of replications, allows the researcher to specify the number of sample datasets to be generated and analyzed. Here, 5,000 replications are requested and this is considered both standard and consistent with published research (Morris, White, & Crowther, 2019; Mundform et al., 2011). The `SEED` specification allows the researcher to specify a maximum eight-digit random number to facilitate data generation.

The `MODEL POPULATION:` command specifies how the simulated data should be *generated,* and all estimated parameters must have prespecified values assigned. Variable names contained within brackets [ ] refer to either the mean of a predictor variable or the intercept of a response variable. Listing a variable only by name in the syntax without brackets refers to the variance of that variable. So, the lines `[X1*0]`, `[X2*0]`, `X1*1`, and `X1*1` indicate that the two predictors both have means equal to zero and variances equal to one consistent with standardization. Further, `[Y*0]` indicates that the response variable has an intercept of zero, and the `Y*0.71875` specification is the residual variance for the response variable calculated previously with Wright's path tracing rules. The `X1 WITH X2*0.55` line indicates that $X1$ is "correlated with" $X2$ at $r = .55$. The `ON` keyword in Mplus refers to "regressed on." The proper generic format is "response variable regressed onto the predictor variable," or `Y ON X1*0.25` and `Y ON X2*0.35`. Each specific parameter to be estimated is separated from its prespecified value by an asterisk (*). This allows Mplus to introduce random variation into each estimate across all simulated replications of sample data consistent with the central limit theorem.

The `MODEL:` command specifies how the data generated by the `MODEL POPULATION:` command should be *analyzed* (*Side Note: The data generation model specified in the* `MODEL POPULATION:` *command and the data analysis model specified in the* `MODEL:` *command are not required to be identical [and will not be in subsequent chapter examples]. The models can differ to test the effects of model misspecification or analysis model assumption violations, for example.*). In this scenario, only the two regression slopes are of interest, so only the `Y ON X1*0.25 X2*0.35` line is needed. The Monte Carlo simulation power analysis results produced from the previously shown Mplus (1.1) input syntax for the bivariate regression example are shown on the next page.

```
MODEL RESULTS

                                 ESTIMATES                  S. E.     M. S. E.  95%   % Sig
                   Population    Average     Std. Dev.     Average              Cover Coeff

Y         ON
 X1                  0.250       0.2508       0.0894       0.0884     0.0080 0.948 0.802
 X2                  0.350       0.3495       0.0890       0.0885     0.0079 0.948 0.974

Intercepts
 Y                   0.000      -0.0006       0.0745       0.0734     0.0055 0.943 0.057

Residual variances
 Y                   0.719       0.7030       0.0879       0.0865     0.0080 0.927 1.000
```

The `Population` column shows the model parameter estimate values as specified by the researcher. The `Average` column shows the average for each parameter estimate, and the `Std. Dev.` shows the standard deviation for each parameter estimate, both computed across 5,000 dataset analysis replications. The `S.E. Average` column is the average of the standard error estimates for all parameters across 5,000 analysis replications. The `M. S. E.` column refers to the mean squared error for each parameter estimate, defined as the squared standard deviation for each parameter estimate plus the squared difference between the `Average` and `Population` values. For example, the M.S.E. for the residual variance for Y can be shown as [Equation (1.9)]:

$$(0.0879)^2 + (0.7030 - 0.719)^2 = 0.008 \tag{1.9}$$

The `95% Cover` column shows the proportion of instances across 5,000 analysis replications where the 95% confidence interval contained the specified `Population` value. Finally, the `% Sig Coeff` column shows the proportion of dataset replications, divided by the total number of replications requested, for which the null hypothesis for a given parameter was rejected using a two-tailed significance test at $\alpha < .05$. Said differently, this is the probability of rejecting a false null hypothesis calculated across 5,000 possible study outcomes and is the Monte Carlo estimate of statistical power. As shown in the Mplus syntax (`NOBSERVATIONS = 132;`), a researcher would need a sample size of $N = 132$ for power $\geq .80$ to reject the null hypothesis for both the β_1 and β_2 regression slope coefficients.

R Monte Carlo Power Analysis: Bivariate Regression Using lavaan and simsem

Many packages are available to conduct a simulation in R, and new packages are continually being created to address niche methodologies. Within this chapter and throughout the book, we choose to focus primarily on two commonly used packages for conducting structural equation model simulations: lavaan (Rosseel, 2012) and simsem (Pornprasertmanit, Miller, Schoenmann, & Jorgensen, 2025). Further, we use the RStudio environment to run all R code for easier accessibility and provide access to additional code and information when and where appropriate.

Unlike the Mplus approach to conducting a Monte Carlo power analysis in this book, which typically uses a single input file and results in a single output file from which results are interpreted, code in R is run in steps via a command line, and objects as well as results can be saved to the R environment for later use (for a brief introduction to using R, see Wickham & Grolemund, 2017). Although all simulation steps can be evaluated together, similar to evaluating an Mplus model input, there are checks that can be intermittently conducted to ensure that the population model is created as intended before conducting the full simulation.

To conduct a Monte Carlo power analysis, first load relevant packages and functions built and adapted for this book. The following packages will be used throughout the chapters, in combination with the GitHub project R/simsemTools.R. More details on how to use the additional functions developed and sourced in GitHub is available under the project name kayleelitson/simsemTools, which can be accessed at github.com.

```
library(simsem)
library(lavaan)
with:source("simsemTools.R")
```

Next, define the population model. Although there are many ways to define the population model using the simsem package, we focus on the method that is most similar to Mplus for greater accessibility between the two platforms. The Mplus example above is replicated using lavaan code (version .6-13; Rosseel, 2012), by first creating a Population model, and later an analysis model and other relevant objects (all saved to the R Global Environment) needed to complete the power analysis.

```
PopulationModel_Ch1 <- "
#create the population model
 X1 ~~ 1*X1          # use ~~ for (co)variances
 X2 ~~ 1*X2
 X1 ~~ 0.55*X2
 Y ~ 0.25*X1         # use ~ for regressions
   + 0.35*X2         # use + to include multiple predictors
 Y ~~ 0.71875*Y      # use ~~ also for residual variances"
```

Instead of using terms `ON`, `WITH`, `BY`, as is used in Mplus, lavaan has four simple formula types, as shown in Table 1.2, that can be used to define simple to advanced statistical models. The current model contains the regression from Y on X1 and X2 (Y ~ .25*X1 + .35*X2), three variances (X1 ~~ 1*X1, X2 ~~ 1*X2, and Y ~~ .71875*Y), and one covariance (X1 ~~ .55*X2). Since lavaan does not default to estimating means or intercepts, all means and intercepts will auto default to 0, even in the population model, unless otherwise specified. Each specific parameter to be estimated is separated from its population value by an asterisk (*). Notice that the command begins with PopulationModel_Ch1 <- . This command saves the population model to the R environment so that the object, PopulationModel_Ch1, can be called for further use.

TABLE 1.2. Primary lavaan Coding Operators

lavaan formula type	Left side	Operator	Right side	Definition	Operator Mplus equivalent
Regression	DV	~	IV	DV is regressed on IV	`ON`
Variance	var1	~~	var1	variance	`var1;`
Covariance	var1	~~	var2	Correlates/covaries with	`var1 WITH var2;`
Intercept	var1	~	1	Estimate intercept or mean	`[var1];`
Intercept	var1	~	0	Constrain intercept or mean to 0	`[var1@0];`
Define latent variable	LV	=~	var1 + var2	is measured by	`LV BY var1 var2;`

After defining the population model, an advantage in R is the ability to ensure accuracy of the covariance matrix:

```
fitted(sem(PopulationModel))$cov
```

Running this piece of code results in the covariance matrix below, which shows that the model is defined as expected and the variances are all set to 1.0 along the diagonal.

```
      Y       X1      X2
Y     1.000
X1    0.442   1.000
X2    0.488   0.550   1.000
```

An additional check that is beneficial is to determine whether the model is positive definite; if it is not, then further analysis using lavaan and simsem will be complex or impossible. To check for positive definite covariance matrix, use:

```
positive_definite(PopulationModel_Ch1)
```

which results in the following output:

```
[1] "The population model is positive definite. The determinant of the covariance matrix is
     0.501328125."
```

Once the population model has been defined and results in a positive definite covariance matrix, the next step in running an SEM simulation power analysis in R is to define the analysis model. For power analysis, this model should match the population model, but should not include the population values, unless a specific value should be fixed in the analysis model (e.g., constraining a variance to 1).

```
AnalysisModel_Ch1 <- "
X1 ~~ X1      # use ~~ for (co)variances
X2 ~~ X2
X1 ~~ X2
Y ~ X1        # use ~ for regressions
   + X2       # use + to include multiple predictors
Y ~~ Y        # use ~~ also for residual variances"
```

After specifying the population and sample models, the Monte Carlo simulation was then evaluated using the simsem package, specifically using the sim() command, which is the primary function used to complete R simulations in this book. There are many options in sim() that are not used in this book but those that are used here and throughout the book include:

nrep : the number of model replications

model : the analysis model

n : sample size

generate : the population model

rawData : a population dataset to use when generate is not possible given study constraints.

std.lv = FALSE : to estimate rather than fix factor means and variances

miss : the model of missing data, relevant for later chapters

seed : seed number to replicate exact results every time. Note that the seed does not exactly correspond to the seed number in Mplus, and results may slightly differ across the two programs.

silent = TRUE : do not print the countdown from each replication in the output.

outfun : additional lavaan output, which we will use primarily to assess missing data in future chapters

To run the sim() function, write the code as follows.

```
output_Ch1 <-  sim(nRep = 5000,
               n = 132,
               model = AnalysisModel_Ch1,
               generate = PopulationModel_Ch1,
               std.lv = FALSE,
               seed = 35170,
               silent = TRUE)
```

To evaluate output from the simulation, use the summary() command.

```
summary(output)
```

which results in two pieces of output: the overall summary of the simulation, including a section called Replications, which shows the number of replications that converged and the reasons why results did not converge.

```
================= Replications =====================
Number of replications = 5000
Number of converged replications = 5000
Number of nonconverged replications:
   1. Nonconvergent Results = 0
   2. Nonconvergent results from multiple imputation = 0
   3. At least one SE were negative or NA = 0
   4. Nonpositive-definite latent or observed (residual) covariance matrix
      (e.g., Heywood case or linear dependency) = 0
```

Also provided are 10 columns of output (Table 1.3), including the statistical power output.

Although the primary estimate of interest is the Power (not equal 0) column, other columns can be interpreted as follows.

1. **Estimate average** is the average parameter estimate computed across all replications.
2. **Estimate SD** is the average standard deviation estimates computed across all replications.
3. **Average SE** is the average of the standard error estimates computed across all replications.
4. **Power (not equal 0)** shows the proportion of instances across all analysis replications divided by the total number of replications requested, for which the null hypothesis for a given parameter was rejected using a two-tailed significance test at $\alpha < 0.05$. This is the Monte Carlo estimate of power.
5. **Std Est** is the standardized estimate average.
6. **Std Est SD** is the standardized estimate SD.
7. **Std Ave SE** is the standardized average SE.
8. **Average Param** is the population parameter value, which should theoretically be the average value of the sample parameter.
9. **Average Bias** is the difference between estimate average and average parameter.
10. **Coverage** indicates the proportion of instances across 5,000 replications where the 95% confidence interval contained the specified Population parameter value.

TABLE 1.3. Chapter 1 Regression Power Analysis Output

	Estimate average	Estimate SD	Average SE	Power (not equal 0)	Std Est	Std Est SD	Std Ave SE	Average param	Average nias	Coverage
X1~~X1	.993	.123	.122	1	1	0	0	1	−.007	.937
X2~~X2	.993	.124	.122	1	1	0	0	1	−.007	.934
X1~~X2	.547	.1	.099	1	.55	.061	.06	.55	−.003	.944
Y~X1	0251	.09	.088	.801	.25	.088	.086	.25	.001	.947
Y~X2	.349	.09	.088	.972	.348	.086	.084	.35	−.001	.951
Y~~Y	.703	.089	.087	1	.71	.065	.065	.719	−.015	.917

It is also possible to examine only power for the model parameters of interest using the getPower() command, combined with the name of the parameter of interest,

```
getPower(output_Ch1) [c("Y~X1", "Y~X2")]
```

which results in the following output:

```
Y~X1   Y~X2
0.8008 0.9720
```

As shown in the summary power estimate for the regression paths of interest, a researcher would need a sample size of $N = 132$ for power ≥ 0.80 to reject the null hypothesis for **both** the β_1 and β_2 regression slope coefficients.

A Comparison Research Question Power Analysis

Cohen's d is an effect size estimate used to describe response variable mean differences between two independent variable groups, such as a treatment group versus a control group, in standard deviation units and is calculated by [Equation (1.10)]

$$\text{Cohen's } d = \frac{\bar{X}_{\text{Treatment}} - \bar{X}_{\text{Control}}}{\sqrt{\frac{(n_{\text{Treatment}} - 1) * SD^2_{\text{Treatment}} + (n_{\text{Control}} - 1) * SD^2_{\text{Control}}}{(n_{\text{Treatment}} + s_{\text{Control}}) - 2}}} \tag{1.10}$$

Notice how the computational formulas for z-score standardization and Cohen's d both contain standard deviation (SD) in their respective denominators. The advantage of this insight can be illustrated with a hypothetical treatment group versus control group comparison of mean differences on a continuous outcome variable. Assume that sample sizes ($n_{\text{Treatment}} = ?\ n_{\text{Control}} = ?$) are unknown, and that response variable scores for both groups were standardized so that $SD_{\text{Treatment}} = SD_{\text{Control}} = 1$. Assume also that the response variable means for the two groups were known: $\bar{X}_{\text{Treatment}} = 0.55$ and $\bar{X}_{\text{Control}} = 0.20$. It can quickly be shown by substitution that the Cohen's d effect size for this scenario is $d = 0.35$ even though the sample sizes are unknown [Equation (1.11)]:

$$\begin{aligned} d &= \frac{0.55 - 0.20}{\sqrt{\frac{(n_{\text{Treatment}} - 1) * 1^2_{\text{Group\_1}} + (n_{\text{Control}} - 1) * 1^2_{\text{Group\_2}}}{(n_{\text{Treatment}} + n_{\text{Control}}) - 2}}} \\ &= \frac{0.35}{\sqrt{\frac{(n_{\text{Treatment}} + n_{\text{Control}}) - 2}{(n_{\text{Treatment}} + n_{\text{Control}}) - 2}}} = \frac{0.35}{\sqrt{1}} = 0.35 \end{aligned} \tag{1.11}$$

By assuming standardization, researchers can compute statistical power estimates for various Cohen's d effect size difference assumptions directly in the numerator because the denominator of the computational formula will always equal one (1) regardless of sample size.

In the previous example, the sample sizes for the treatment and control groups were assumed to be unknown for illustrations purposes. Keeping with the previous example, let's assume a researcher: (1) planned to test an intervention by randomly assigning participants to either a treatment or a control condition, (2) assumed standardization for the dependent variable (DV) of interest, (3) suspected based on previous research that the intervention will produce an effect size difference of $d = 0.35$ between the treatment and control groups, and (4) needed to know the minimum number of participants per condition needed for statistical power $\geq .80$. This sample size question can be answered with an independent-samples *t*-test power analysis in either Mplus or R.

Mplus Monte Carlo Power Analysis: Two-Group Comparison

As with every Monte Carlo simulation for power analysis in Mplus, an input model is first specified.

```
TITLE: Mplus 1.2 Independent Samples t-Test

MONTECARLO:
NAMES ARE DV;
NGROUPS = 2;
NOBSERVATIONS = 126 126;
NREPS = 5000;
SEED = 58459;

MODEL POPULATION:

[DV*0.55];
DV*1;

MODEL POPULATION-g2:

[DV*0.20];
DV*1;

MODEL:

[DV*0.55](a);
DV*1;

MODEL g2:

[DV*0.20](b);
DV*1;

MODEL CONSTRAINT:
NEW (MEANDIFF*0.35);
MEANDIFF = a-b;
```

The Mplus input syntax for conducting an independent samples *t*-test power analysis shown above differs from the input syntax for a bivariate regression power analysis shown previously in several important ways. The `NGROUPS = 2` specification allows a researcher to declare the number of independent variable groups to be used in both the data generation and data analysis phases of the simulation power analysis. Because `NGROUPS = 2` has been specified, the `NOBSERVATIONS` specification requires that the sample sizes for both independent variable groups be listed and separated by a space. Notice also that there are now two data generation commands, `MODEL POPULATION:` and `MODEL POPULATION-g2:` as well as two data analysis commands, `MODEL:` and `MODEL g2:`. These specifications allow separate data generation and data analysis models to be specified within both of the independent variable groups (data generation and data analysis models for a third independent variable group could be added using `MODEL POPULATION-g3:` and `MODEL g3:` specifications). Consistent with an independent samples *t*-test power analysis assuming standardization, only the response variable (DV) means (in brackets) and variances need to be specified.

Notice also that the `(a)` and `(b)` specifications have been included to the right of the mean ([]) treatment group and control group response variable values in the `MODEL:` and `MODEL g2:` commands. These specifications allow the response variable mean values for the treatment and control groups for each simulated dataset replication (recall that these mean values will deviate randomly around their specified values consistent with central limit theorem) to be assigned to the variables `(a)` and `(b)`, respectively. These specifications, together with the `MODEL CONSTRAINT:` command, allow a `NEW` variable to be calculated based on estimates obtained from the `MODEL:` command. In this case, a `NEW` mean difference (`MEANDIFF`) variable can be defined as the mean of the treatment group minus the mean of the control group, or `MEANDIFF = a – b`, for each simulated dataset replication.

The Monte Carlo simulation power analysis results produced from the above Mplus input syntax (Mplus 1.2) for the independent samples *t*-test example are shown below.

```
MODEL RESULTS

                              ESTIMATES              S. E.     M. S. E.  95%  % Sig
                 Population   Average   Std. Dev.   Average             Cover Coeff

Group G1

 Means
  DV                 0.550     0.5502     0.0901     0.0886     0.0081 0.945 1.000

 Variances
  DV                 1.000     0.9939     0.1245     0.1252     0.0155 0.941 1.000

Group G2

 Means
  DV                 0.200     0.2001     0.0880     0.0885     0.0077 0.948 0.614

 Variances
  DV                 1.000     0.9913     0.1254     0.1249     0.0158 0.938 1.000

New/Additional Parameters
  MEANDIFF           0.350     0.3501     0.1256     0.1254     0.0158 0.949 0.805
```

All definitions for all columns of output remain the same. The only difference between the outputs for the independent samples *t*-test compared to the previous bivariate regression example is that results are shown separately for the treatment (`Group G1`) and control (`Group G2`) groups, and that a statistical power estimate has been included for the mean difference variable (`MEANDIFF`) created from the `MODEL CONSTRAINT:` command. As shown in the results above, a researcher would need a sample size of $n_{\text{Treatment}} = n_{\text{Control}} = 126$, or $N = 252$ for power $\geq .80$ to detect a mean difference effect size of $d = 0.35$.

R Monte Carlo Power Analysis: Two-Group Comparison

Like the previous example in R, the first step to conducting the two-group *t*-test power analysis using lavaan style syntax is to first define the population model.

```
PopulationModel2_Ch1 <- "
DV ~ c(0.55, 0.20)*1   #c(group 1 mean, group 2 mean)
DV ~~ 1.0*DV
MEANDIFF := 0.35"
```

There are many differences between this population model and the bivariate regression example presented earlier. First, to combine two populations into a single population model, relevant parameters that differ across groups must be specified for each of the respective groups. This can be done in R using concatenation, or the command, c(), as shown in the line DV ~ c(0.55, 0.20)*1, which reflects a two-group model where the mean is 0.55 in group 1 and 0.20 in group 2. Parameters that do not differ across groups can have a single value, as shown in the line DV ~~ 1.0*DV, which shows that the variance(s) of DV are constrained to 1.0 across both groups.

Notice that there is a new piece of information called MEANDIFF := 0.35. Since this analysis is intended to compare means across groups, the mean difference must be assigned a name and population value against which it should be compared, similar to the Mplus `MODEL CONSTRAINT` command. Once the population model is specified, the analysis model should now be specified.

```
AnalysisModel2_Ch1 <- "
DV ~ c(a, b)*1 #estimating means across groups
DV ~~ 1.0*DV #constraining variances to 1 across groups
MEANDIFF := a - b"
```

Instead of specifying the population parameters, names are assigned to the sample values in the line DV ~ c(a, b)*1and MEANDIFF := a - b. Because of the multigroup nature of this dataset, a simple approach to the simulation that was shown earlier in the chapter is not possible. Instead, a two-step approach was used, where data were first generated using the simulateDatasets(), then evaluated using sim().

```
SampleDatasets2_Ch1 <- simulateDataSets(PopulationModel2_Ch1,
  nIterations = 5000,
  nObservations = c(126, 126),
  seed = 58459)
```

```
output2_Ch1 <-  sim(model = AnalysisModel2_Ch1,
     rawData =  SampleDatasets2_Ch1,
     group =    "group",
     silent =   TRUE)

getPower(output2_Ch1)["MEANDIFF"]
```

The output from the analysis showed

```
MEANDIFF
0.7766
```

indicating power of .7766 to detect the mean difference. Note that this power estimate is not above .80, unlike in Mplus, potentially due to minor differences across the two programs. An additional analysis was completed to determine what sample size was needed, using lavaan, to obtain a power estimate above .80.

```
SampleDatasets2a_Ch1 <- simulateDatasets(PopulationModel2_Ch1,
nIterations = 5000,
nObservations = c(131, 131),
seed = 58459)
output2a_Ch1 <- sim(model = AnalysisModel2_Ch1,
rawData =           SampleDatasets2a_Ch1,
     group =        "group",
     silent =       TRUE)
getPower(output2a_Ch1)["MEANDIFF"]

MEANDIFF
0.8006
```

As shown in the results above, a researcher would need a sample size of $n_{\text{Treatment}} = n_{\text{Control}} =$ 131, or $N = 262$ for power $\geq .80$ to detect a mean difference effect size of $d = 0.35$, according to this power analysis.

Conclusion

Criticisms of the two Monte Carlo simulation power analysis examples shown above could include: (1) these examples are far too simplistic; independent samples *t*-tests and bivariate regressions are unlikely to be the research designs and statistical analyses submitted either for grant funding or for publication consideration, (2) there were no control covariates included in either model; covariate inclusion is needed to control for confounding influences, explain noise variance in the response variable, and increase statistical power, and (3) there was no consideration of missing data; data collected from sample sizes between N = 132–252 will likely have missing data that will negatively impact power. An additional criticism may be that the sample sizes produced across programs can differ slightly, highlighting the importance of clearly describing, documenting, and reporting software along with the packages and versions used to obtain statistical power analysis results for future replication.

The chapters that follow consider more complex cross-sectional and longitudinal designs that answer both comparison-based and relationship-based research questions. Many of the examples will include control covariates, and a demonstration of how to specify and include a reasonable amount of missing data to a simulation power analysis will also be included. However, two important themes will be demonstrated throughout the remainder of the book: (1) standardization simplifies, and (2) assuming a correctly specified analytic model, Monte Carlo simulation statistical power estimates are no more difficult to obtain than the mathematical calculations (R syntax scripts will be provided in each chapter to assist) needed to verify an admissible correlation matrix.

SUGGESTED READINGS

- Anvari, F., & Lakens, D. (2021). Using anchor-based methods to determine the smallest effect size of interest. *Journal of Experimental Social Psychology, 96,* 1–11.
- Fernández-García, M. P., Vallejo-Seco, G., Livácic-Rojas, P., & Herrero-Díez, F. J. (2025). Proposal of an alternative way of reporting the results of comparative simulation studies. *Frontiers in Psychology, 16,* 1–21.
- Geiser, C. (2012). *Data analysis with Mplus.* Guilford Press.
- Lakens, D. (2014). Performing high-powered studies efficiently with sequential analyses. *European Journal of Social Psychology, 44*(7), 701–710.
- Maxwell, S. E. (2004). The persistence of underpowered studies in psychological research: Causes, consequences, and remedies. *Psychological Methods, 9*(2), 147–163.
- Pornprasertmanit, S., Miller, P., Schoemann, A. M., & Jorgensen, T. D. (2025). simsem: SIMulated structural equation modeling. R package version 0.5-17. Retrieved from *https://CRAN.R-project.org/package=simsem*
- Riesthuis, P. (2024). Simulation-based power analyses for the smallest effect size of interest: A confidence-interval approach for minimum-effect and equivalence testing. *Advances in Methods and Practices in Psychological Science, 7*(2), 1–14.
- Rosseel, Y. (2012). lavaan: An R Package for Structural Equation Modeling. *Journal of Statistical Software, 48*(2), 1–36.
- Wickham, H., & Grolemund, G. (2022). *R for data science* (2nd ed.). O'Reilly Media. *https://r4ds.hadley.nz*
- Witte, E. H., & Zenker, F. (2022). The statistical, theoretical, and practical aspect of an empirical effect—On the smallest effect of interest for theory construction in behavioral science. *osf.io*
- Zimmer, F., & Debelak, R. (2025). Simulation-based design optimization for statistical power: Utilizing machine learning. *Psychological Methods, 30*(3), 513–536. Advance online publication.

Appendix 1.1

Chapter Addendum

The Fundamentals

Suppose, for example, a scientific researcher wanted to conduct a simple experiment to test a treatment they believe will effectively increase scores on a response variable (Y) of interest. Ideally, a researcher would obtain a random sample of participants from the population they are interested in, and then randomly assign participants to either the treatment condition or a control condition. However, before conducting this experiment, the researcher should state the null (H_0:) and alternative (H_A:) hypotheses to be tested by their research study. The null and alternative hypotheses could be stated this way:

$$H_0\!: \bar{Y}_{\text{Treatment}} = \bar{Y}_{\text{Control}} \text{ (or } \bar{Y}_{\text{Treatment}} - \bar{Y}_{\text{Control}} = 0)$$

$$H_A\!: \bar{Y}_{\text{Treatment}} > \bar{Y}_{\text{Control}} \text{ (or } \bar{Y}_{\text{Treatment}} - \bar{Y}_{\text{Control}} > 0)$$

The null hypothesis (H_0:) states that the mean, or average, response variable score for participants receiving the treatment will equal the mean score for participants randomly assigned to the control condition. Stated another way, the null hypothesis states that the difference in response variable score means between the treatment and control groups will be zero. Either way, the null hypothesis implies an ineffective treatment. The alternative hypothesis states that the treatment being tested will result in a mean response variable score for the treatment group that is greater than the mean response variable score for the control group.

Now suppose the researcher conducts the study, collects the data, and is ready to determine whether their treatment is effective (H_A:), or not (H_0:). Stated more correctly, the researcher is ready to determine, based on data analysis results, whether the null hypothesis should be retained or rejected. Prior to conducting any statistical analysis, the researcher could examine the distribution of response variable scores in the treatment and control groups, as shown in Figure 1A.1.

As shown in the figure, response variable scores from participants randomly assigned to the control condition vary randomly around a mean of zero, as indicted by the black bell curve and solid black vertical line to the left. Response variable scores from participants randomly assigned to the treatment condition vary randomly around a mean that is greater than zero, as indicted by the gray bell curve and dashed black vertical line to the right. So, the question now becomes: Is the observed difference in response variable means between the treatment and control groups indicative of a truly effective treatment, or could the difference in means be due to random chance variation, implying a truly ineffective treatment? The nominal alpha level ($\alpha < .05$) states that, *assuming the null hypothesis is true in the population*, if the observed difference in the response variable means between the treatment and control groups shown above were to occur in less than 5% of samples of size N drawn from the population (or, has a probability [p] of occurrence of less than 5%, or $p < .05$), a researcher would reject the null hypothesis and infer a true treatment effect in the popula-

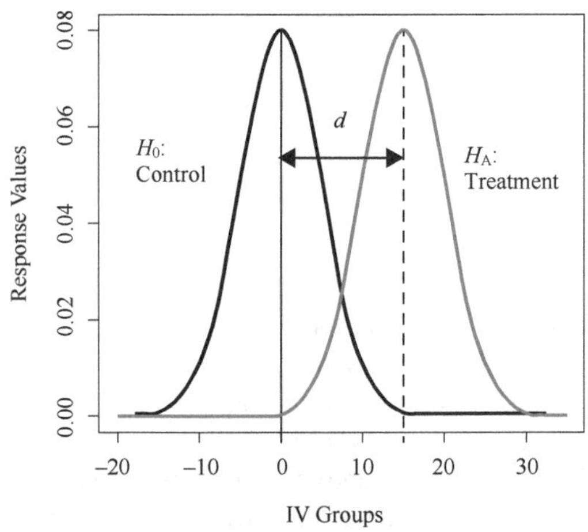

FIGURE 1A.1 A hypothetical two-group distribution example.

tion. If the observed difference in the response variable means were found in 5% or more samples of size N drawn randomly from the population, a researcher would retain the null hypothesis and conclude the treatment produces no difference in the population ($p \geq .05$). Before analyzing the data to make such a determination, it would be helpful to review the four possible inferences researchers can make, shown in Figure 1A.2, from the results of study data statistical analyses.

Shown in Figure 1A.2 are the four possible inferences that could be made as a result of conducting a research study, statistically analyzing the data, and drawing a conclusion regarding the null hypothesis. The two columns indicate the truth regarding the null hypothesis in the population: it is either true or false, but this reality is unknown to a researcher. The two rows reflect the intent of the research study: to determine the truth regarding the

H_0: Conclusion from Study Result	H_0: In the Population: TRUE	H_0: In the Population: FALSE
RETAINED	Correct Retention	Fail to Reject a False Null Hypothesis Type-2 Error (β)
REJECTED	Reject A True Null Hypothesis Type-1 Error (α)	Correct Rejection Statistical Power ($1 - \beta$)

FIGURE 1A.2 Four possible statistical inferences.

null hypothesis by analyzing a representative sample of data from the population. From the results of the study data analysis, a researcher either retains or rejects the null hypothesis. The four cells within Figure 1A.2 indicate the four possible conclusions that could be drawn regarding the null hypothesis: two of the inferences are correct, two are incorrect.

The top left cell of Figure 1A.2 shows a scenario in which a researcher analyzes their study data and obtains a probability value (p-value) greater than the nominal alpha ($p > .05$), leading the researcher to retain the null hypothesis. If the null hypothesis were, in fact, true in the population, this would indicate a correct retention of the null hypothesis. The lower left cell of Figure 1A.2 shows a scenario in which a researcher obtains a p-value less than the nominal alpha ($p < .05$), leading the researcher to infer that the null hypothesis in the population is false and should be rejected. If the null hypothesis in the population is true in reality, this would indicate an incorrect rejection of a true null hypothesis, commonly referred to as a Type 1 error. The nominal alpha ($\alpha = .05$) determines the probability of committing a Type 1 inference error. Said differently, $\alpha = .05$ means that researchers acknowledge a 5% chance of drawing a sample from a population where the null hypothesis is true that produces data analysis results ($p < .05$) that lead a researcher to falsely reject the null hypothesis (i.e., committing a Type 1 error). The top right cell of Figure 1A.2 shows a scenario in which a researcher observes a data analysis $p > .05$, which leads them to infer that the null hypothesis is true in the population. If the null hypothesis were actually false in the population, this would indicate an incorrect retention of a false null hypothesis, referred to as a Type 2 error. The probability of committing a Type 2 error is referred to as β, and the nominal probability of committing a Type 2 error is typically set at $\beta = .20$ for reasons explained next. The lower right cell shows a scenario in which a researcher obtains a p-value less than the nominal alpha ($p < .05$), which leads the researcher to infer that the null hypothesis in the population is false when it is, in fact, false in the population. The probability of a researcher rejecting a null hypothesis that is false in the population is one minus the Type II error probability ($1 - \beta$, or $1 - .20 = .80$) and is the definition of statistical power (similar to $\alpha < .05$, statistical power $[1 - \beta] = .80$ is considered a scientific research standard). Statistical power is directly impacted by four quantities: (1) sample size (N), (2) effect size (d), (3) response variable variance, and (4) the nominal alpha level (α).

For example, if a researcher lowers the nominal alpha from .05 to .01, they have decreased the probability of a Type 1 error but have also decreased their statistical power because a lower observed probability (p) value is needed to reject the null hypothesis. Raising the nominal alpha ($\alpha = .10$) would increase statistical power because a researcher could reject the null hypothesis with a higher observed probability value, but such an increase would also increase the likelihood of committing a Type 1 error. Response variable variation can also impact statistical power. Referring back to the two distributions in Figure 1A.1, the width of the black and gray bell curves for the control and treatment groups give an indication of the variability in response variable scores within the two groups. Further, there appears to be relatively little overlap in the distributions of the two groups, which might tend to suggest a rejection of the null hypothesis. However, shown in Figure 1A.3 is the distributions of scores for the control and treatment groups after the variation in both has been tripled.

Figure 1A.3 represents the same distance (d) between the means of the two groups but it now shows the effect of response variable variation on statistical power. The two distributions show far more overlap and a decrease in statistical power, which could suggest the null hypothesis be retained.

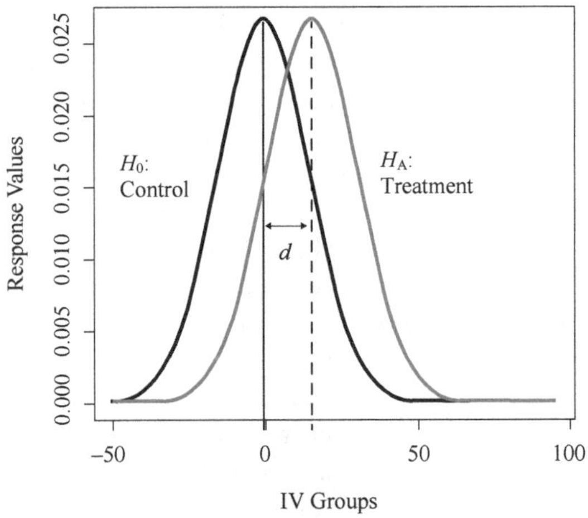

FIGURE 1A.3 A hypothetical two-group distribution, variances tripled.

As important as the influences of the nominal alpha level and response variable variation are on subsequent statistical power, the two quantities that have the greatest impact on statistical power are the *effect size* and the *sample size*. Notice how in both Figures 1A.1 and 1A.3, which show the response variable score distributions for the treatment and control groups, the difference in means between the two groups is indicated by a double-headed arrow labeled *d*. This refers to the difference, or distance, between the means of the two groups. Cohen's *d* is a standardized measure of effect size that quantifies the difference between two groups in response variable standard deviation units and is calculated by (Equation 1A.1)

$$\text{Cohen's } d = \frac{\bar{X}_{\text{Treatment}} - \bar{X}_{\text{Control}}}{\sqrt{\dfrac{(n_{\text{Treatment}} - 1) * SD^2_{\text{Treatment}} + (n_{\text{Control}} - 1) * SD^2_{\text{Control}}}{(n_{\text{Treatment}} + n_{\text{Control}}) - 2}}} \qquad \text{(A.1)}$$

For example, IQ scores are standardized at a mean of 100 and a standard deviation of 15 in the population. If two groups differed in their mean IQ scores by 7.5 points, the effect size for the mean difference on IQ scores would be $d = 0.50$, or one-half of a standard deviation. Defined broadly, effect sizes are standardized quantities that allow researchers to classify the effects of predictor or independent variables (such as random assignment to a treatment or control condition) on response or dependent variables using a common measurement scale. For example, shown in Table 1A.1 are values for three effect sizes that indicate "small," "medium," or "large" effects according to Cohen (1992). The calculation and explanation for Cohen's *d* is given above, however, calculations and explanations for R^2 and odds ratios will be considered in subsequent chapters.

Furthermore, to illustrate the impact that effect sizes, such as Cohen's *d*, have on statistical power, assume the mean difference in Figure 1A.1 indicates a $d = 0.50$, or "medium" effect size. Shown in Figure 1A.4 is the effect of increasing the effect size shown in Figure 1A.1 to $d = 0.75$, or closer to a "large" ($d = 0.80$) effect size.

TABLE 1A.1. Common Effect Size Metrics

		Magnitude	
Effect size	"Small"	"Medium"	"Large"
Cohen's *d*	0.20	0.50	0.80
R^2	0.02	0.13	0.26
Odds ratio	1.75	2.50	3.25

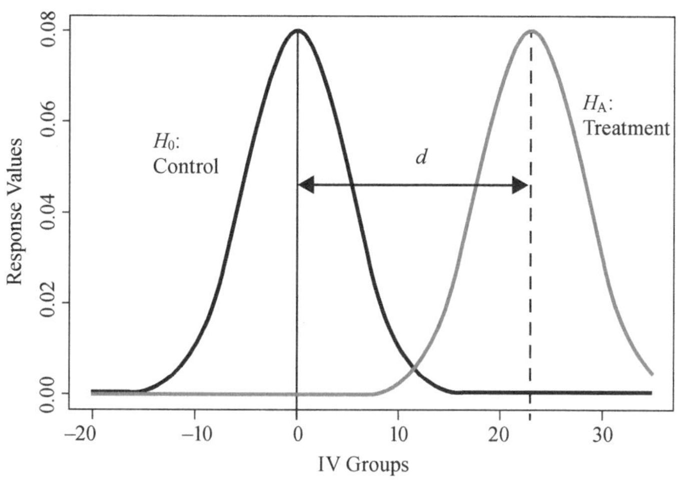

FIGURE 1A.4 Hypothetical two-group distribution; effect size increased.

Increasing the effect size from $d = 0.50$ to $d = 0.75$, as shown in Figure 1A.4, results in much less overlap between the distributions and greater statistical power to reject the null hypothesis.

All of this leads back to the original question shown in Figure 1A.1: Are the mean differences statistically significant ($p < .05$; reject H_0:), or not ($p > .05$; retain H_0:)? As stated previously, of the four influences on statistical power (nominal alpha level, response variable variation, effect size, and sample size), the two most closely tied to statistical power are effect size and sample size. Acknowledging that population effect sizes are unknown to a scientific researcher prior to conducting a study, the one influence on statistical power completely under the control of the researcher is *sample size*. Returning to Figure 1A.1, it is easy to imagine obtaining a p-value well below .05 if the data shown were obtained from a sample size of $N = 500$ ($n = 250$ for both groups). It would be somewhat more difficult to imagine obtaining a p-value well below .05 if the data shown were obtained from a sample size of $N = 40$ ($n = 20$ for both groups). Why? The answer comes from tracing the relationship between parameter estimate standard errors, test statistics, and p-values.

All p-values quantify the probability of obtaining an observed test statistic value if the null hypothesis were true. All test statistics (e.g., F, t, χ^2, Wald z, etc.) follow a similar generic computational formula [Equation (1A.2)]:

$$\text{Test statistic} = \frac{\text{Parameter estimate}}{\text{Standard error}}$$

where

$$\text{Standard error} = \frac{\sigma}{\sqrt{N}} \quad \text{(1A.2)}$$

Standard error, as shown in Equation 1A.2, is defined as the population standard deviation of a parameter estimate (σ) divided by the square root of the sample size (N). Conceptually, population standard deviation assumes that a researcher could conduct their experiment a large number of times at the same sample size N, record the parameter estimate obtained each time the experiment was conducted, and compute the standard deviation for all of the accumulated parameter estimates. Returning to our example from Figure 1A.1, assuming all other values remain the same, and assuming a sample size of $N = 500$ produced the results, the denominator of the test statistic formula shown above would contain a relatively small value, resulting in a relatively large test statistic value and a small p-value, which would increase the likelihood of a researcher rejecting the null hypothesis. By contrast, assuming a sample size of $N = 40$ produced the results, the denominator of the test statistic formula shown above would contain a relatively larger value, resulting in a relatively smaller test statistic value and a larger p-value, which would tend to decrease the likelihood of a researcher rejecting the null hypothesis. Knowing the sample size needed to reject a false null hypothesis with power $\geq .80$ requires a power analysis.

2

A Multivariate, Two-Group, Pretest–Posttest Power Analysis

Pretest–posttest research designs involving random assignment to a treatment or a control condition are both a budgetary cost-effective and statistically efficient means for testing a treatment intervention in which (1) participants are recruited and pretest data are collected on all response variables of interest, (2) participants are then randomly assigned to a treatment condition to receive the intervention to be tested, or to a control condition to receive a "treatment as usual" or another inert procedure, and (3) following an acceptable amount of exposure to the treatment or control conditions, posttest data are again collected on all response variables of interest. A pretest–posttest randomized design allows for posttest scores to be compared against "baseline" pretest scores both within the treatment and control groups, and between the treatment and control conditions at posttest. Furthermore, both the comparative-based and relationship-based power analysis examples shown in Chapter 1 dealt with a single (univariate) response variable. However, researchers are likely to be interested in changes in multiple related (multivariate) response variables operating simultaneously.

Researchers would, understandably, be tempted to analyze changes in multiple related response variables from a pretest–posttest random assignment design with a mixed-factorial (within factor: pretest vs. posttest; between factor: treatment vs. control) multivariate analysis. However, a mixed-factorial multivariate comparative design only optimizes statistical power if the correlation between pretest and posttest response variable scores is $r_{\text{Pretest,Posttest}} > .50$. Treating such a research design as purely cross-sectional by analyzing posttest mean differences between the independent variable groups after controlling for pretest scores as covariates in a multivariate *co*variance analysis is a more statistically powerful option. Compared to a mixed-factorial design, statistical power is optimized in a covariate inclusion design for *any nonzero* pretest–posttest correlation. However, a covariate design assumes homogeneity of the covariate regression slope coefficients, which means the effects of any pretest covariate on any posttest response variable must be equivalent across the independent variable groups. If the assumption of homogeneity of covariate regression slopes is not met, a covariate is essentially functioning as an additional independent variable in analysis. This means that any significant effect for the treatment of interest could be due to treatment efficacy or could be due to a violation of the homogeneity of covariate regression slopes assumption.

For a multivariate, cross-sectional comparative statistical power analysis example, let's consider a specific medical research scenario (this specific scenario will prove very helpful in explaining how to specify and incorporate missing data into Monte Carlo simulation power analyses in Chapter 6). Let's assume a researcher wishes to use a pretest/posttest data collection design with random assignment to a treatment condition or a control condition (independent variable) to test an intervention believed to improve medication adherence (`ADH`), medical disease activity (`DA`), daily functional activity (`FA`) and overall health-related quality of life (`QOL`) ratings, all of which are assumed to be correlated. Let's further assume that, to maximize statistical power, the medical researcher plans to use the four-response variable pretest scores as covariates in a multivariate data analysis design. Let's also finally assume that the medical researcher suspects, based on a review of previous publications, that the intervention will produce an effect size difference (Δ) between the treatment and control groups for all four response variables at posttest of $\Delta d = 0.45$. A model for this data analysis design is shown in Figure 2.1.

The multivariate covariance analysis model is presented separately for the treatment (upper pane) and control (lower pane) groups to indicate that the same multiple group approach in both Mplus and R used for the independent samples *t*-test power analysis from Chapter 1 will again be used for this example. The curved, double-headed arrows on the left and right sides of the analysis model indicate correlated pretest and posttest response variables. The question marks (?) both within the circles above the posttest response variables and on the single-headed regression arrows indicate unknown but related quantities that must be specified. The amount of posttest variable variance left unexplained (question marks within the circles) is contingent upon the amount of posttest variance explained by the pretest scores as predictors (question marks on the regression slopes).

Recall that Wright's (1921, 1934) path tracing rules and general form equation [Equation (1.2) from Chapter 1] for computing variance explained (R_Y^2) in any posttest response variable (Y) are given as follows:

1. A path tracing cannot involve the same variable twice.
2. A path tracing can involve only one correlation (i.e., double-headed curved arrow).
3. A path tracing can involve tracing both backward (from the arrowhead of a regression arrow back to its source) and forward (from the source of the arrow to its arrowhead), but once a forward trace is made, additional backward traces are prohibited.
4. A path tracing can involve as many backward and forward tracings as is permissible.

$$R_Y^2 = \text{Direct path} *(\text{Direct path} + [\text{Indirect path product}])$$

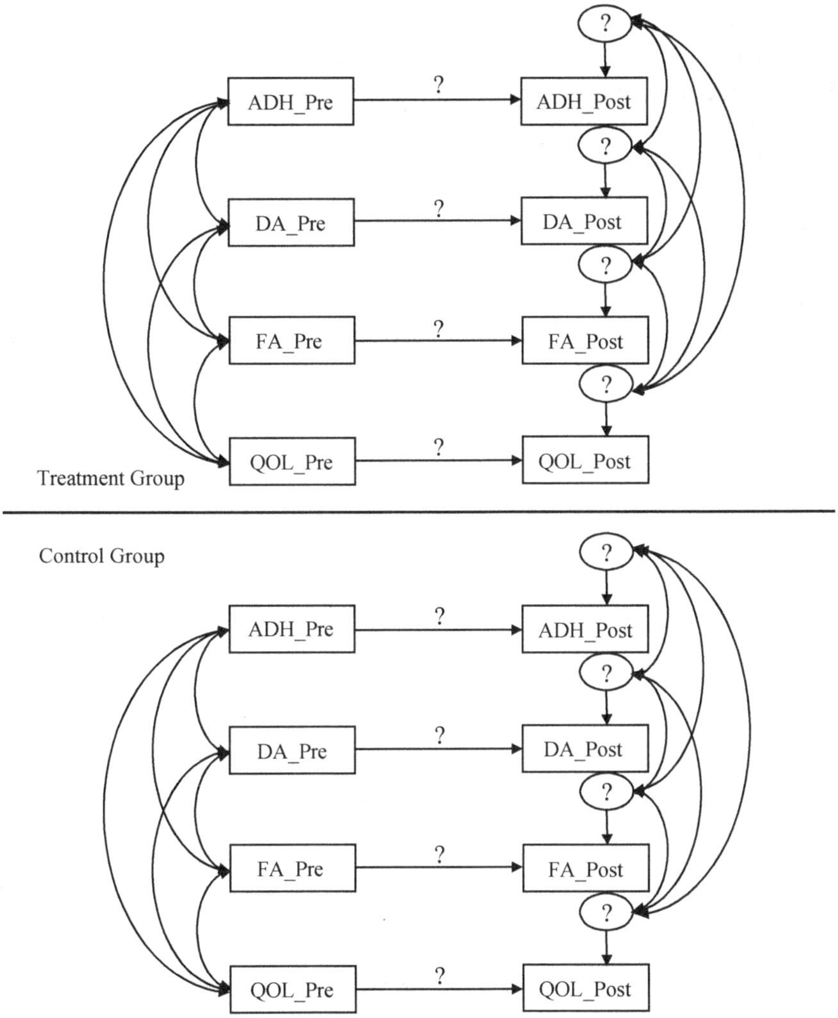

FIGURE 2.1. A multivariate two-group model.

Furthermore, assuming standardization, residual variance ($\sigma^2_{\text{RESIDUAL}}$) for each posttest response variable is calculated as ($\sigma^2_{\text{RESIDUAL}} = 1 - R^2_Y$). Equation 1.2 from Chapter 1 for calculating variance explained can be simplified further because, for the MANCOVA example, the direct path for each posttest response variable is the regression slope for its respective pretest as a predictor. Note, there are no admissible indirect paths because any indirect path tracing for the relationship between any pretest variable and its respective posttest variable would involve more than one correlation (curved, double-headed arrow) path, which is inadmissible. To illustrate, assume an indirect path tracing for pretest adherence predicting posttest adherence (`ADH_Pre` → `ADH_Post`) is needed. Starting at pretest adherence, a researcher could use any curved, double-headed arrow as a path to any other pretest variable, and then follow the regression arrow forward to the pretest variable's respective posttest variable. But getting from any posttest variable back to posttest adherence would require taking a second curved, double-headed arrow path, which is inadmissible under path tracing rule #2. The residual variance calculation for any posttest response variable then reduces to exclude the indirect path ($\sigma^2_{\text{RESIDUAL}} = 1 - [\text{Direct path}^2]$). Suppose that after a literature search, the medical researcher is willing to assume that a standardized regression slope of $\beta = 0.40$ best quantifies the prediction of all posttest variables by their respective pretest scores. This implies that ($R^2_{\text{Post-test}} = [0.40]^2 = 0.16$) 16% of posttest variance is explained by pretest scores across both groups and ($\sigma^2_{\text{RESIDUAL}} = 1 - [0.40^2] = 0.84$) 84% of posttest variance remains unexplained. Using these now known values, it is possible to conduct a Monte Carlo simulation power analysis in either Mplus or R (see Figure 2.2).

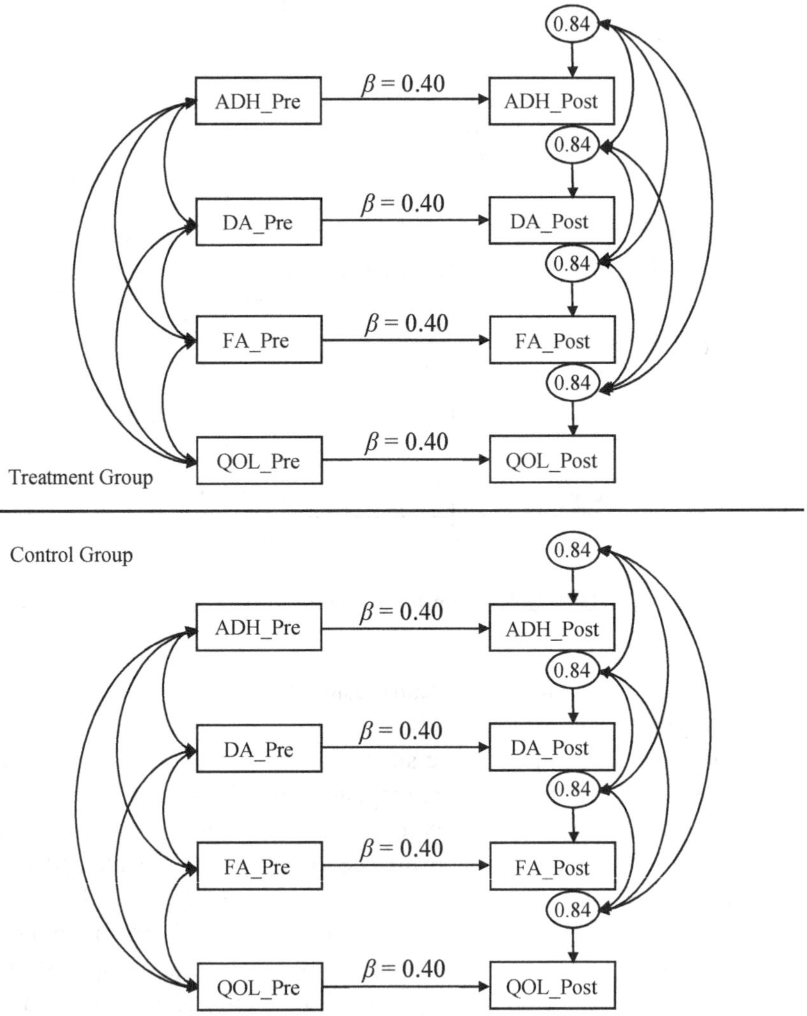

FIGURE 2.2. A fully specified multivariate two-group model.

Mplus Monte Carlo Power Analysis: Multivariate Two-Group Comparison

The complete multivariate two-group comparison Monte Carlo simulation power analysis Mplus input syntax is shown next.

```
TITLE: Mplus 2.1 Multivariate Two-Group Comparison

MONTECARLO:
NAMES ARE
ADH_pre  DA_pre  FA_pre  HRQ_pre
ADH_post DA_post FA_post HRQ_post;
NOBSERVATIONS = 66 66;
NGROUPS = 2;
NREPS = 5000;
SEED = 10127;

! IV: Control Group;
MODEL POPULATION:

[ADH_pre*0];
[DA_pre*0];
[FA_pre*0];
[HRQ_pre*0];
ADH_pre*1;
DA_pre*1;
FA_pre*1;
HRQ_pre*1;

[ADH_post*0.16];
[DA_post*0.16];
[FA_post*0.16];
[HRQ_post*0.16];

ADH_post*.84;
DA_post*.84;
FA_post*.84;
HRQ_post*.84;

ADH_post DA_post FA_post WITH DA_post*0.3 FA_post*0.3 HRQ_post*0.3;
ADH_pre DA_pre FA_pre WITH DA_pre*0.3 FA_pre*0.3 HRQ_pre*0.3;

ADH_post ON ADH_pre*.4(1);
DA_post ON DA_pre*.4(2);
FA_post ON FA_pre*.4(3);
HRQ_post ON HRQ_pre*.4(4);

! IV: Treatment Group;
MODEL POPULATION-g2:

[ADH_pre*0];
[DA_pre*0];
[FA_pre*0];
[HRQ_pre*0];
```

```
ADH_pre*1;
DA_pre*1;
FA_pre*1;
HRQ_pre*1;

[ADH_post*0.61];
[DA_post*0.61];
[FA_post*0.61];
[HRQ_post*0.61];

ADH_post*.84;
DA_post*.84;
FA_post*.84;
HRQ_post*.84;

ADH_post DA_post FA_post WITH DA_post*0.3 FA_post*0.3 HRQ_post*0.3;
ADH_pre DA_pre FA_pre WITH DA_pre*0.3 FA_pre*0.3 HRQ_pre*0.3;

ADH_post ON ADH_pre*.4(1);
DA_post ON DA_pre*.4(2);
FA_post ON FA_pre*.4(3);
HRQ_post ON HRQ_pre*.4(4);

MODEL: !IV: Control Group;
ADH_post DA_post FA_post WITH DA_post*0.3 FA_post*0.3 HRQ_post*0.3;

ADH_post ON ADH_pre*.4(1);
DA_post ON DA_pre*.4(2);
FA_post ON FA_pre*.4(3);
HRQ_post ON HRQ_pre*.4(4);

[ADH_post*0.16](E);
[DA_post*0.16](F);
[FA_post*0.16](G);
[HRQ_post*0.16](H);

ADH_post*.84;
DA_post*.84;
FA_post*.84;
HRQ_post*.84;

MODEL g2: ! IV: Treatment Group;
ADH_post DA_post FA_post WITH DA_post*0.3 FA_post*0.3 HRQ_post*0.3;

ADH_post ON ADH_pre*.4(1);
DA_post ON DA_pre*.4(2);
FA_post ON FA_pre*.4(3);
HRQ_post ON HRQ_pre*.4(4);

[ADH_post*0.61](A);
[DA_post*0.61](B);
[FA_post*0.61](C);
[HRQ_post*0.61](D);

ADH_post*.84;
DA_post*.84;
```

```
FA_post*.84;
HRQ_post*.84;

MODEL CONSTRAINT:
NEW (ADH_DIFF*.45 DA_DIFF*.45 FA_DIFF*.45 HRQ_DIFF*.45);
ADH_DIFF = A-E;
DA_DIFF = B-F;
FA_DIFF = C-G;
HRQ_DIFF = D-H;
```

To facilitate ease of learning, the Mplus syntax above is presented in later sections.

```
MONTECARLO:
NAMES ARE
ADH_pre   DA_pre   FA_pre   HRQ_pre
ADH_post  DA_post  FA_post  HRQ_post;
NGROUPS = 2;
NOBSERVATIONS = 66 66;
NREPS = 5000;
SEED = 10127;
```

Rather than list a single response variable for a univariate independent samples t-test power analysis, as was done in Chapter 1, the names of the four pretest covariate variables and their respective posttest variables are all listed after `NAMES ARE`. The `NGROUPS = 2` indicates a two-group (treatment vs. control) comparison, the `NOBSERVATIONS = 66 66` specification indicates that the medical researcher is testing an $N = 132$ ($n = 66$ per independent variable group; group-specific sample sizes are entered separately on the '`NOBSERVATIONS =`' line separated by a space and can be adjusted as needed) sample size for power ≥ .80 to detect a posttest difference between the treatment and control groups of $\Delta d = 0.45$.

```
! IV: Control Group;
MODEL POPULATION:
[ADH_pre*0];
[DA_pre*0];
[FA_pre*0];
[HRQ_pre*0];

ADH_pre*1;
DA_pre*1;
FA_pre*1;
HRQ_pre*1;

[ADH_post*0.16];
[DA_post*0.16];
[FA_post*0.16];
[HRQ_post*0.16];

ADH_post*.84;
DA_post*.84;
FA_post*.84;
HRQ_post*.84;
```

As shown near the top of the `MODEL POPULATION:` data generation statement, all pretest response variables are assumed to be standardized with means equal to zero and variances equal to one. In the lower portion of the `MODEL POPULATION:` statement, the means of the posttest response variables in the control condition are specified to be `0.16` based on meta-analysis research that shows control condition participants experience a response variable improvement of $d = 0.16$, on average (Kahana, Drotar, & Frazier, 2008). Finally, as shown, posttest response variable variances are specified as `0.84` based on the above residual variance calculations.

```
ADH_post DA_post FA_post WITH DA_post*0.3 FA_post*0.3 HRQ_post*0.3;
ADH_pre DA_pre FA_pre WITH DA_pre*0.3 FA_pre*0.3 HRQ_pre*0.3;
```

The next two statements are a shortcut method for specifying all pretest and posttest response variable correlations at $r = .30$. These values can be adjusted based on previous research or length of time between pretest and posttest assessments. Shorter time intervals between assessments tend to dictate higher correlations among response variables.

```
ADH_post ON ADH_pre*.4(1);
DA_post ON DA_pre*.4(2);
FA_post ON FA_pre*.4(3);
HRQ_post ON HRQ_pre*.4(4);
```

The syntax lines shown above indicate a standardized regression slope coefficient of $\beta = 0.40$ for each pretest response variable predicting its respective posttest counterpart. Notice also that integer values between 1 and 4 are listed in parentheses after each `ON` statement. Integer values listed in parentheses indicate *equality constraints*. Recall that for any univariate or multivariate covariance analysis, the assumption of homogeneity of covariate regression slope coefficients must be met. Recall also that the asterisk (*) indicates that the covariate regression slope values will differ randomly around the `0.40` specified slope value consistent with central limit theorem. The integer values listed in parentheses, together with asterisks, indicate that the standardized regression slope values can vary separately for each response variable, but such variation must be constrained to equality between the treatment and control conditions for each response variable to meet the homogeneity of covariate regression slopes assumption. For example, within the treatment group for a given replication of simulated data, the slope for the effect of adherence pretest scores (`ADH_Pre`) as a predictor of adherence posttest (`ADH_Post`) scores could be $\beta = 0.43$, while the effect of disease activity pretest scores (`DA_Pre`) as a predictor of disease activity posttest scores could be $\beta = 0.37$ (`DA_Post`). The integer values in parentheses specify that, within the same dataset replication, the effects of adherence pretest scores (`ADH_Pre`) as a predictor of adherence posttest (`ADH_Post`) scores and disease activity pretest scores (`DA_Pre`) as a predictor of disease activity posttest scores must also be $\beta = 0.43$ and $\beta = 0.37$, respectively, in the control condition for that specific dataset replication. The data-generating syntax for the treatment condition is exactly the same as the syntax specified above for the control condition, with one exception.

```
! IV: Treatment Group;
MODEL POPULATION-g2:
```

```
[ADH_post*0.61];
[DA_post*0.61];
[FA_post*0.61];
[HRQ_post*0.61];
```

The posttest means for the four response variables in the treatment condition are specified as $d = 0.61$. Recall that the medical researcher expected a treatment ($d = 0.61$) versus control ($d = 0.16$) response variable effect size difference at posttest of ($0.61 - 0.16 =$) $\Delta d = 0.45$.

The data analysis statements for the control group (`MODEL:`) and the treatment group (`MODEL g2:`) are the same as the data-generating `MODEL POPULATION:` and `MODEL POPULATION-g2:` statements with one exception.

```
! IV: Control Group;
MODEL:

[ADH_post*0.16](E);
[DA_post*0.16](F);
[FA_post*0.16](G);
[HRQ_post*0.16](H);

! IV: Treatment Group;
MODEL g2:

[ADH_post*0.61](A);
[DA_post*0.61](B);
[FA_post*0.61](C);
[HRQ_post*0.61](D);
```

As shown in the `MODEL g2:` statement above, the treatment group response variable intercept values (0.61; not means, because posttest scores are predicted by their respective pretest counterparts) for adherence (`ADH_post`), disease activity (`DA_post`), functional activity (`FA_post`), and health-related quality of life (`HRQ_post`) are assigned to variables `A-D`, respectively. Similarly, in the `MODEL:` statement, the control group response variable intercept values (0.16) for adherence (`ADH_post`), disease activity (`DA_post`), functional activity (`FA_post`), and health-related quality of life (`HRQ_post`) are assigned to variables `E-H`, respectively.

```
MODEL CONSTRAINT:
NEW
(ADH_DIFF*.45 DA_DIFF*.45 FA_DIFF*.45 HRQ_DIFF*.45);
ADH_DIFF = A-E;
DA_DIFF = B-F;
FA_DIFF = C-G;
HRQ_DIFF = D-H;
```

As shown above, the MODEL CONSTRAINT: command together with the NEW specification allows treatment group minus control group intercept difference (‘ `_DIFF'`) variables to be created from the group-specific intercept values assigned to variables `A-H`. Each of the four difference variables are assigned the value (`.45`) to indicate the medical researcher's hypothesized (0.61 – 0.16 =) $\Delta d = 0.45$ posttest treatment effect difference. The abbreviated results produced from the above syntax (Mplus 2.1) are shown below.

```
MODEL RESULTS

                              ESTIMATES                  S. E.      M. S. E.  95%   % Sig
                Population    Average    Std. Dev.     Average               Cover  Coeff

New/Additional Parameters
  ADH_DIFF            0.450     0.4476      0.1576      0.1582      0.0248 0.949 0.808
  DA_DIFF             0.450     0.4509      0.1600      0.1581      0.0256 0.943 0.809
  FA_DIFF             0.450     0.4482      0.1594      0.1580      0.0254 0.947 0.804
  HRQ_DIFF            0.450     0.4474      0.1584      0.1580      0.0251 0.946 0.808
```

As shown in the results above, a sample size of ($n_{\text{Treatment}} = n_{\text{Control}} = 66$; $N = 132$) is needed for power ≥ .80 to detect any treatment group minus control group intercept difference of $\Delta d = 0.45$ at posttest. Also, the Monte Carlo simulation power analysis was conducted assuming that both response variable pretest scores and posttest scores were correlated at $r = .30$. Response variable pretest and posttest correlations represent information a researcher may not have. However, additional sensitivity simulation power analyses showed that assuming response variable correlations as low as $r = .10$ or as high as $r = .50$ produced no appreciable change in the sample size needed for power ≥ .80.

With quick, simple adjustments to the above syntax, a quick admissibility verification check can be conducted in two steps. The previous Monte Carlo simulation power analysis was conducted in a single step, sometimes referred to as an *internal* power analysis. An admissibility verification involves a two-step, or *external* power analysis. In the first step, the following two lines (**bolded**) are added to the previous '`NAMES ARE:`' syntax as follows:

```
TITLE: Mplus 2.2 Admissibility Check, Part 1

MONTECARLO:
NAMES ARE
ADH_pre  DA_pre  FA_pre  HRQ_pre
ADH_post DA_post FA_post HRQ_post;
NOBSERVATIONS = 66 66;
NGROUPS = 2;
NREPS = 5000;
SEED = 10127;
REPSAVE = ALL;
SAVE = NAME_*.dat;
```

The '`REPSAVE = ALL;`' syntax results in Mplus writing out all 5,000 Monte Carlo simulation data files. The '`SAVE = NAME_*.dat;`' syntax allows the researcher to assign any name to the replication datasets, and the '_*' specification automatically assigns a value from 1 to 5,000 for all datasets. For example, if a researcher specified

```
REPSAVE = ALL;
SAVE = MANCOVA_*.dat;
```

Mplus would write out 5,000 datasets named MANCOVA_1.dat, MANCOVA_2.dat,. . . MANCOVA_5000.dat. and also, by default, Mplus will write out an additional file named 'MANCOVA_list.dat'. The 'MANCOVA_list.dat' file contains the names of all 5,000 datasets in a single column.

```
MANCOVA_1.dat
MANCOVA_2.dat
...
MANCOVA_5000.dat
```

As will be shown, the ' `_list.dat`' file is used by Mplus to automate the process of reading in and analyzing the 5,000 datasets. In addition, at the bottom of the output file in the '`SAVEDATA INFORMATION`' section, Mplus will print the '`Order of variables`' for the 5000 datasets as shown.

```
SAVEDATA INFORMATION

  Order of variables

    ADH_POST
    DA_POST
    FA_POST
    HRQ_POST
    ADH_PRE
    DA_PRE
    FA_PRE
    HRQ_PRE
    GROUP
```

In the second step, and using the '`Order of variables`' and the '*`NAME`*`_list.dat`' file, Mplus can automate the reading-in and analysis of all data files with the following syntax commands:

```
TITLE: Mplus 2.3 Admissibility Check, Part 2
DATA:
File = MANCOVA_list.dat;
Type = MONTECARLO;
```

Notice how the '`MANCOVA_list.dat;`' file is given as the input file in the first line. This specification, followed on the next line by the '`Type = MONTECARLO;`' specification automates the reading-in and analyzing of all 5,000 datasets.

```
VARIABLE:

NAMES =

ADH_POST
DA_POST
FA_POST
```

```
HRQ_POST
ADH_PRE
DA_PRE
FA_PRE
HRQ_PRE
GROUP;
```

The order of the variable names given in the 'NAMES =' specification *must* be in the same order given in the output file that generated the 5,000 datasets.

```
GROUPING IS GROUP (1=Control 2 = Treat);
```

The 5,000 datasets were generated using the multiple-group format, so the last variable generated, as shown above, is 'GROUP'. Based on the syntax that generated the datasets, the first group specified ('MODEL POPULATION') was the control condition, the second ('MODEL POPULATION-g2') group was the treatment condition. To analyze the 5,000 datasets in a multiple-group model, the values in the 'GROUP' variable are assigned the labels '(1=Control 2 = Treat);' so that the 'MODEL:' statement refers to the control group, and 'MODEL TREAT:' refers to the treatment group as follows:

```
MODEL: !IV: Control Group;

ADH_post WITH DA_post*0.3 FA_post*0.3 HRQ_post*0.3;
DA_post WITH FA_post*0.3 HRQ_post*0.3;
FA_post WITH HRQ_post*0.3;

ADH_post ON ADH_pre*.4(1);
DA_post ON DA_pre*.4(2);
FA_post ON FA_pre*.4(3);
HRQ_post ON HRQ_pre*.4(4);

[ADH_post*0.16](E);
[DA_post*0.16](F);
[FA_post*0.16](G);
[HRQ_post*0.16](H);

ADH_post*.84;
DA_post*.84;
FA_post*.84;
HRQ_post*.84;

MODEL Treat: !IV: Treatment Group;

ADH_post WITH DA_post*0.3 FA_post*0.3 HRQ_post*0.3;
DA_post WITH FA_post*0.3 HRQ_post*0.3;
FA_post WITH HRQ_post*0.3;

ADH_post ON ADH_pre*.4(1);
DA_post ON DA_pre*.4(2);
FA_post ON FA_pre*.4(3);
HRQ_post ON HRQ_pre*.4(4);
```

```
[ADH_post*0.61](A);
[DA_post*0.61](B);
[FA_post*0.61](C);
[HRQ_post*0.61](D);

ADH_post*.84;
DA_post*.84;
FA_post*.84;
HRQ_post*.84;

MODEL CONSTRAINT:
NEW (ADH_DIFF*.45 DA_DIFF*.45 FA_DIFF*.45 HRQ_DIFF*.45);

ADH_DIFF = A-E;
DA_DIFF = B-F;
FA_DIFF = C-G;
HRQ_DIFF = D-H;
```

After running the above syntax (Mplus 2.2 and 2.3), and also by default, Mplus will print to the output file model-reproduced correlation matrices for both the treatment and control groups averaged across the 5,000 datasets, as shown:

```
SAMPLE STATISTICS

NOTE: These are average results over 5000 data sets.

     SAMPLE STATISTICS FOR CONTROL
          ADH_POST DA_POST  FA_POST HRQ_POST ADH_PRE  DA_PRE   FA_PRE  HRQ_PRE
          ________ ________ ________ ________ ________ ________ ________ ________
 ADH_POST    1
  DA_POST  0.350      1
  FA_POST  0.348    0.350      1
 HRQ_POST  0.349    0.347    0.349      1
  ADH_PRE  0.403    0.124    0.124    0.123      1
   DA_PRE  0.123    0.401    0.122    0.120    0.301      1
   FA_PRE  0.119    0.123    0.403    0.123    0.300    0.302      1
  HRQ_PRE  0.122    0.121    0.122    0.402    0.302    0.302    0.302      1

      SAMPLE STATISTICS FOR TREAT
          ADH_POST DA_POST  FA_POST HRQ_POST ADH_PRE  DA_PRE   FA_PRE  HRQ_PRE
          ________ ________ ________ ________ ________ ________ ________ ________
 ADH_POST    1
  DA_POST  0.351      1
  FA_POST  0.348    0.348      1
 HRQ_POST  0.349    0.348    0.346      1
  ADH_PRE  0.398    0.120    0.119    0.116      1
   DA_PRE  0.121    0.401    0.117    0.119    0.299      1
   FA_PRE  0.118    0.119    0.399    0.118    0.298    0.298      1
  HRQ_PRE  0.120    0.120    0.120    0.400    0.297    0.300    0.298      1
```

As shown above, the model-reproduced correlation matrices are *admissible*, which is defined as both matrices showing values of exactly one on the main diagonal elements, and correlations between zero and one on the off-diagonal elements. However, this was a post hoc model admissibility check, performed in a two-step external process after having obtained Monte Carlo statistical power estimates. In all subsequent chapters, model admissibility checks will be performed *prior to* Monte Carlo simulation power estimation to ensure model admissibility. Rather than performing the somewhat cumbersome external or two-step admissibility check using Mplus, a priori model admissibility checks will be performed using matrix syntax in base R and show how to compute even simpler admissibility checks using lavaan syntax.

R Monte Carlo Power Analysis: Multivariate Two-Group Comparison

The first step in evaluating the multivariate two-group comparison Monte Carlo simulation power analysis in R, specifically by using the combination of lavaan and simsem packages, is to specify and save the population model.

```
PopulationModel_Ch2 <- "
 ADH_pre ~ 0                               # means are set to 0 for documentation
 DA_pre ~ 0
 FA_pre ~ 0
 HRQ_pre ~ 0
 ADH_pre ~~ 1*ADH_pre                      # variances are constrained to 1
 DA_pre ~~ 1*DA_pre
 FA_pre ~~ 1*FA_pre
 HRQ_pre ~~ 1*HRQ_pre

 ADH_post ~ c(0.16, 0.61)*1                # mean values differ across populations
 DA_post ~ c(0.16, 0.61)*1
 FA_post ~ c(0.16, 0.61)*1
 HRQ_post ~ c(0.16, 0.61)*1
 ADH_post ~~ 0.84*ADH_post                 # residual variances are constrained to .84
 DA_post ~~ 0.84*DA_post
 FA_post ~~ 0.84*FA_post
 HRQ_post ~~ 0.84*HRQ_post

 ADH_post ~~ 0.3*DA_post + 0.3*FA_post + 0.3*HRQ_post
 DA_post ~~ 0.3*FA_post + 0.3*HRQ_post
 FA_post ~~ 0.3*HRQ_post
 ADH_pre ~~ 0.3*DA_pre + 0.3*FA_pre + 0.3*HRQ_pre
 DA_pre ~~ 0.3*FA_pre + 0.3*HRQ_pre
 FA_pre ~~ 0.3*HRQ_pre

 ADH_post ~ 0.4*ADH_pre + a1*ADH_pre       # constrain parameters equal across groups
 DA_post ~ 0.4*DA_pre + a2*DA_pre
 FA_post ~ 0.4*FA_pre + a3*FA_pre
 HRQ_post ~ 0.4*HRQ_pre + a4*HRQ_pre

 ADH_DIFF := .45                           # set population value mean difference
 DA_DIFF := .45
 FA_DIFF := .45
 HRQ_DIFF := .45 "
```

Within this set of code that is used to define the population model, multiple sections are explained. The first section:

```
ADH_pre ~ 0                  # means are set to 0 for documentation
DA_pre ~ 0
FA_pre ~ 0
HRQ_pre ~ 0
ADH_pre ~~ 1*ADH_pre         # variances are constrained to 1
DA_pre ~~ 1*DA_pre
FA_pre ~~ 1*FA_pre
HRQ_pre ~~ 1*HRQ_pre
```

constrains all pretest means and variances to 0 and 1, respectively. The second section:

```
ADH_post ~ c(0.16, 0.61)*1     # mean values differ across groups
DA_post ~ c(0.16, 0.61)*1
FA_post ~ c(0.16, 0.61)*1
HRQ_post ~ c(0.16, 0.61)*1
ADH_post ~~ 0.84*ADH_post      # residual variances are set to .84
DA_post ~~ 0.84*DA_post
FA_post ~~ 0.84*FA_post
HRQ_post ~~ 0.84*HRQ_post
```

establishes the posttest means and variances across the two groups. The first group is assigned posttest mean values of 0.16 while the second group is assigned posttest mean values of 0.61. Both groups are assigned posttest residual variances of 0.84. The third section of code:

```
ADH_post ~~ 0.3*DA_post + 0.3*FA_post + 0.3*HRQ_post
DA_post ~~ 0.3*FA_post + 0.3*HRQ_post
FA_post ~~ 0.3*HRQ_post
ADH_pre ~~ 0.3*DA_pre + 0.3*FA_pre + 0.3*HRQ_pre
DA_pre ~~ 0.3*FA_pre + 0.3*HRQ_pre
FA_pre ~~ 0.3*HRQ_pre
```

designates correlation values among the posttest scores and the pretest scores, separately, while the fourth section of code:

```
ADH_post ~ 0.4*ADH_pre    # regression estimates are set to 0.4 across groups
DA_post ~ 0.4*DA_pre
FA_post ~ 0.4*FA_pre
HRQ_post ~ 0.4*HRQ_pre
```

sets the regression between each pre- and posttest score at 0.4. Finally, the last section of the population model code:

```
ADH_DIFF := .45 # set population value mean difference
DA_DIFF := .45
FA_DIFF := .45
HRQ_DIFF := .45
```

provides the expected difference value between pre- and posttest scores to indicate the medical researcher's hypothesized (0.61 – 0.16 =) $\Delta d = 0.45$ posttest treatment effect difference.

Once the population model is defined, the analysis model can now be written.

```
AnalysisModel_Ch2 <- "
  ADH_pre ~~ ADH_pre
  DA_pre ~~ DA_pre
  FA_pre ~~ FA_pre
  HRQ_pre ~~ HRQ_pre

  ADH_post ~ c(E, A)*1          # mean label across groups
  DA_post ~ c(F, B)*1
  FA_post ~ c(G, C)*1
  HRQ_post ~ c(H, D)*1
  ADH_post ~~ ADH_post
  DA_post ~~ DA_post
  FA_post ~~ FA_post
  HRQ_post ~~ HRQ_post

  ADH_post ~~ DA_post + FA_post + HRQ_post
  DA_post ~~ FA_post + HRQ_post
  FA_post ~~ HRQ_post
  ADH_pre ~~ DA_pre + FA_pre + HRQ_pre
  DA_pre ~~ FA_pre + HRQ_pre
  FA_pre ~~ HRQ_pre

  ADH_post ~ a1*ADH_pre          # label parameter and constrain equal across groups
  DA_post ~ a2*DA_pre
  FA_post ~ a3*FA_pre
  HRQ_post ~ a4*HRQ_pre

  #Creating mean difference values
  ADH_DIFF := A-E
  DA_DIFF := B-F
  FA_DIFF := C-G
  HRQ_DIFF := D-H "
```

There are three primary differences between the analysis model and the population model. First, parameter values are not specified in the analysis model since doing so sets the parameter equal to that exact value in all sample analyses (equivalent to the Mplus `@` specification). Second, parameter *labels* are included in two sections of the analysis model code:

```
ADH_post ~ c(E, A)*1 # mean labels across groups
DA_post ~ c(F, B)*1
FA_post ~ c(G, C)*1
HRQ_post ~ c(H, D)*1
```

and

```
ADH_post ~ a1*ADH_pre # label a parameter and constrain it equal across groups
DA_post ~ a2*DA_pre
```

```
FA_post ~ a3*FA_pre
HRQ_post ~ a4*HRQ_pre
```

The first set of parameter labels, denoted c(E, A) through c(H, D), name each posttest mean value according to its group, where, for example, the mean value of ADH_post in group 1 will be named E and the mean value of ADH_post in group 2 will be named A. The second set of parameter labels, denoted a1 through a4, label the pre–post regression estimates, constraining them equal across groups in the analysis phase of the simulation. The last difference between the population and analysis model is shown as follows:

```
ADH_DIFF := A-E
DA_DIFF := B-F
FA_DIFF := C-G
HRQ_DIFF := D-H
```

Unlike the population model, which provided exact difference values for the difference variables, the analysis model uses parameter labels to estimate the difference found within each sample model. In the power analysis simulation, these sample difference estimates will be compared to the previously specified population difference parameters.

Because of the multigroup nature of this dataset, a two-step approach was used to conduct the simulation analysis, where sample datasets were first generated using the simulateDatasets(),

```
SampleDatasets_Ch2 <- simulateDataSets(PopulationModel_Ch2,
                                        nIterations = 5000,
                                        nObservations = c(66, 66),
                                        seed = 10127)
```

then output was evaluated using sim().

```
output_Ch2 <- sim(model = AnalysisModel_Ch2,
                  rawData = SampleDatasets_Ch2,
                  group = "group",
                  silent = TRUE)
```

Initial examination of the output summary showed that all replications converged, and provided the following power estimates:

```
ADH_DIFF  DA_DIFF   FA_DIFF   HRQ_DIFF
0.82      0.82      0.86      0.83
```

Statistical power is above .80, so a sample size of ($n_{\text{Treatment}} = n_{\text{Control}} = 66$; $N = 132$) is adequate for power ≥ .80 to detect any treatment group minus control group intercept difference of $\Delta d = 0.45$ at posttest. Additional smaller sample sizes could be estimated, if desired, yet those will not be shown here for brevity.

To evaluate the model-reproduced correlation matrices and determine admissibility, a much simpler approach in R is available than that shown in Mplus. In single group models, only one additional line of code (shown below) will be necessary to determine admissibility. However, in the multigroup approach, minimal additional coding is necessary to first specify each population group model separately before examining admissibility within each group. Instead of writing the multigroup model as a single object, specify each group as its own object. For the control group,

```
Population1_Ch2 <- "
 ADH_pre ~ 0
 DA_pre ~ 0
 FA_pre ~ 0
 HRQ_pre ~ 0
 ADH_pre ~~ 1*ADH_pre
 DA_pre ~~ 1*DA_pre
 FA_pre ~~ 1*FA_pre
 HRQ_pre ~~ 1*HRQ_pre

 ADH_post ~ 0.16*1
 DA_post ~ 0.16*1
 FA_post ~ 0.16*1
 HRQ_post ~ 0.16*1
 ADH_post ~~ 0.84*ADH_post
 DA_post ~~ 0.84*DA_post
 FA_post ~~ 0.84*FA_post
 HRQ_post ~~ 0.84*HRQ_post

 ADH_post ~~ 0.3*DA_post + 0.3*FA_post + 0.3*HRQ_post
 DA_post ~~ 0.3*FA_post + 0.3*HRQ_post
 FA_post ~~ 0.3*HRQ_post
 ADH_pre ~~ 0.3*DA_pre + 0.3*FA_pre + 0.3*HRQ_pre
 DA_pre ~~ 0.3*FA_pre + 0.3*HRQ_pre
 FA_pre ~~ 0.3*HRQ_pre

 ADH_post ~ 0.4*ADH_pre
 DA_post ~ 0.4*DA_pre
 FA_post ~ 0.4*FA_pre
 HRQ_post ~ 0.4*HRQ_pre "
```

and for the treatment group,

```
Population2_Ch2 <- "
#Treatment Group
 ADH_pre ~ 0
 DA_pre ~ 0
 FA_pre ~ 0
 HRQ_pre ~ 0
 ADH_pre ~~ 1*ADH_pre
 DA_pre ~~ 1*DA_pre
 FA_pre ~~ 1*FA_pre
 HRQ_pre ~~ 1*HRQ_pre

 ADH_post ~ 0.61*1
 DA_post ~ 0.61*1
 FA_post ~ 0.61*1
 HRQ_post ~ 0.61*1
```

```
ADH_post ~~ 0.84*ADH_post
DA_post ~~ 0.84*DA_post
FA_post ~~ 0.84*FA_post
HRQ_post ~~ 0.84*HRQ_post

ADH_post ~~ 0.3*DA_post + 0.3*FA_post + 0.3*HRQ_post
DA_post ~~ 0.3*FA_post + 0.3*HRQ_post
FA_post ~~ 0.3*HRQ_post
ADH_pre ~~ 0.3*DA_pre + 0.3*FA_pre + 0.3*HRQ_pre
DA_pre ~~ 0.3*FA_pre + 0.3*HRQ_pre
FA_pre ~~ 0.3*HRQ_pre

ADH_post ~ 0.4*ADH_pre
DA_post ~ 0.4*DA_pre
FA_post ~ 0.4*FA_pre
HRQ_post ~ 0.4*HRQ_pre "
```

The accuracy of the model-implied covariance matrices and mean vectors can then be evaluated by calling the function combination fitted(sem()), as follows:

```
fitted(sem(Population1_Ch2))
fitted(sem(Population2_Ch2))
```

which produces covariance matrices and mean vectors for each group.

```
$cov
          ADH_ps   DA_pst   FA_pst   HRQ_ps   ADH_pr   DA_pre   FA_pre   HRQ_pr
ADH_post      1
DA_post   0.348        1
FA_post   0.348    0.348        1
HRQ_post  0.348    0.348    0.348        1
ADH_pre     0.4     0.12     0.12     0.12        1
DA_pre     0.12      0.4     0.12     0.12      0.3        1
FA_pre     0.12     0.12      0.4     0.12      0.3      0.3        1
HRQ_pre    0.12     0.12     0.12      0.4      0.3      0.3      0.3        1

$mean
        ADH_post  DA_post  FA_post HRQ_post  ADH_pre   DA_pre   FA_pre  HRQ_pre
            0.16     0.16     0.16     0.16        0        0        0        0

$cov
          ADH_ps   DA_pst   FA_pst   HRQ_ps   ADH_pr   DA_pre   FA_pre   HRQ_pr
ADH_post      1
DA_post   0.348        1
FA_post   0.348    0.348        1
HRQ_post  0.348    0.348    0.348        1
```

```
ADH_pre       0.4      0.12      0.12      0.12        1
DA_pre       0.12       0.4      0.12      0.12      0.3        1
FA_pre       0.12      0.12       0.4      0.12      0.3      0.3        1
HRQ_pre      0.12      0.12      0.12       0.4      0.3      0.3      0.3        1

$mean
         ADH_post  DA_post  FA_post  HRQ_post  ADH_pre   DA_pre   FA_pre  HRQ_pre
             0.61     0.61     0.61      0.61        0        0        0        0
```

As shown above, the model-reproduced correlation matrices are *admissible*, defined as both matrices showing values of exactly one on the main diagonal elements, and correlations between zero and one on the off-diagonal elements. Although this admissibility check was conducted post hoc, admissibility checks can be conducted before completing the power analysis.

Simulation Power Analysis Write-Up: Multivariate Two-Group Comparison

Finally, an example of a Monte Carlo simulation power analysis write-up is shown below and consists of four sections: (1) a statement of the power analysis question; (2) a description of how power was calculated, including the data analysis model assumed, and the statistical software package and version used; (3) a clear statement of all power analysis assumptions, including specific parameter estimate values; and (4) a clear answer to the power analysis question that includes the number of simulated dataset replications requested, the effect size assumed, and the sample size needed to achieve power ≥.80. Here, the write-up is shown using the Mplus results.

> "The power analysis question involves the smallest sample size needed to achieve power ≥.80 to detect a posttest mean effect size difference (Δd) between the treatment and control conditions of $\Delta d = 0.45$ after controlling for pretest scores as covariates. A Monte Carlo simulation power analysis was conducted using Mplus (version 8.6) assuming: (1) a multivariate covariance data analysis model where pretest response variables are included as covariates for each of their respective posttest variables (adherence, disease activity, functional activity and health-related quality of life); (2) standardization of all pretest and posttest response variables; (3) random assignment results in equivalent groups across the four response variables at the pretest assessment; (4) the control condition will experience a minimal pretest to posttest difference ($\Delta d = 0.16$; Kahana et al., 2008); (5) the treatment condition will experience a pretest to posttest difference of ($\Delta d = 0.61$), resulting in a treatment versus control group difference of ($\Delta d = 0.61 - 0.16 = 0.45$) at posttest; (6) the assumption of homogeneity of covariate regression slopes (i.e., the effect of each posttest response variable regressed onto their respective pretest counterparts is equal across the treatment and control groups) will be ensured via parameter estimate equality constraints; (7) the use of pretest scores as

covariates will explain ($R^2 = 0.16$) 16% of response variable error variance; and (8) all four response variables will be correlated at a medium effect size (i.e., $r_{\text{Pearson}} = 0.30$) at both the pretest and posttest assessments. Monte Carlo simulation power analysis results aggregated over 5,000 replications showed power ≥.80 for the anticipated treatment versus control posttest difference ($\Delta d = 0.45$) if $N = 132$ ($n_{\text{Treatment}} = n_{\text{Control}} = 66$) is available for analysis."

SUGGESTED READINGS

- Cao, C. (2020). Review of univariate and multivariate general linear models: Theory and applications with SAS. *Structural Equation Modeling: A Multidisciplinary Journal, 27,* 825–827.
- D'Amico, E. J., Neilands, T. B., & Zambarano, R. (2001). Power analysis for multivariate and repeated measures designs: A flexible approach using the SPSS MANOVA procedure. *Behavior Research Methods, Instruments, & Computers, 33,* 479–484.
- Denis, D. J. (2021). *Applied univariate, bivariate, and multivariate statistics: Understanding statistics for social and natural scientists, with applications in SPSS and R* (2nd ed.). Wiley.
- Enders, C. K. (2003). Performing multivariate group comparisons following a statistically significant MANOVA. *Measurement and Evaluation in Counseling and Development, 36,* 40–56.
- Enders, L. R., Boykin, G. L., & Rice, V. J. (2020). Effects of neurocognitive temporal training on weapon firing performance. *Perceptual and Motor Skills, 127,* 939–959.
- Huberty, C. J., & Olejnik, S. (2006). *Applied MANOVA and discriminant analysis* (Vol. 498). Wiley.
- Lüdtke, O., & Robitzsch, A. (2025). ANCOVA versus change score for the analysis of two-wave data. *The Journal of Experimental Education, 93*(2), 363–395.
- Nelson, S., Cunningham, N., Peugh, J., Jagpal, A., Arnold, L. M., Lynch-Jordan, A., & Kashikar-Zuck, S. (2017). Clinical profiles of young adults with juvenile-onset fibromyalgia with and without a history of trauma. *Arthritis Care & Research, 69,* 1636–1643.
- Perugini, M., Gallucci, M., & Costantini, G. (2018). A practical primer to power analysis for simple experimental designs. *International Review of Social Psychology, 31*(1).
- Raudenbush, S. W. (1993). Hierarchical linear models and experimental design. In L. K. Edwards (Ed.), *Applied analysis of variance in behavioral science* (pp. 459–496). Marcel Dekker.

3

Path Analysis

A path analysis model is considered to be the simplest structural equation model because it involves predictions among observed variables similar to a regression model. However, unlike the bivariate regression model example in Chapter 1 that showed a clear delineation between the predictor variables (*X*1 and *X*2) and the response variable (*Y*), a path analysis extends a regression model using *exogenous* and *endogenous* variables. The distinction between exogenous and endogenous variables can be illustrated using the path analysis model shown (Figure 3.1), adapted from McDonald and Clelland's (1984) "union sentiment" model (as shown in Bollen, 1989, p. 83).

Exogenous variables are, by definition, variables that are not predicted by any variable, but rather predict other variables. The variables *X*1 and *X*2 in the model above fit the definition of exogenous variables: neither are predicted by any other variable, and both are involved in the prediction of variables *Y*1–*Y*3. *Endogenous variables* are, by definition, variables that are predicted either by exogenous variables *or other endogenous variables.* The variables *Y*1–*Y*3 fit the definition of endogenous variables: *Y*1 and *Y*2 are both being predicted by the exogenous variable *X*2, and *Y*3 is being predicted by both the exogenous variable *X*1 and both endogenous *Y*1 and *Y*2 variables. The distinction between a regression model and a path analysis model is clearly shown by variables *Y*1 and *Y*2: both variables are being predicted by *X*2, and both are also simultaneously predicting *Y*3.

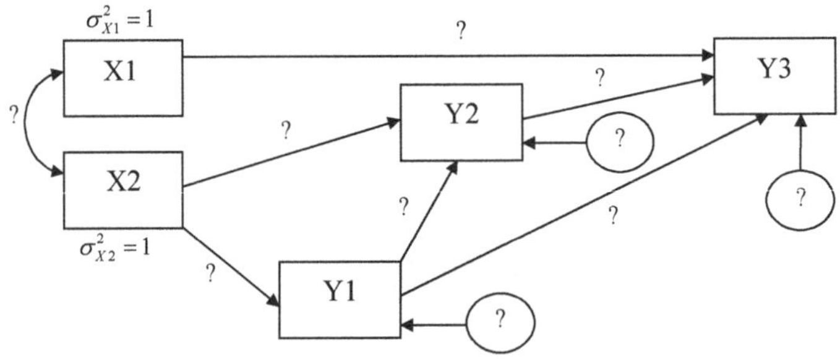

FIGURE 3.1. An example path analysis model.

Furthermore, assuming standardization, only two quantities in the path analysis model are known at this point: the variances of the two exogenous variables equal one ($\sigma^2_{X1} = \sigma^2_{X2} = 1$) by definition. The 10 question marks (?) shown in the path analysis model in Figure 3.1 indicate unknown values that must be specified prior to conducting a Monte Carlo simulation power analysis, including: (1) the correlation between $X1$ and $X2$, indicated by the curved, double-headed arrow, (2) the six regression coefficients shown by the single-headed arrows, and (3) the three residual variances for $Y1$–$Y3$, indicated by the question marks within the circles. Let's assume that following an extensive search of the published literature, or based on reasonable assumptions, a researcher specified the following (Figure 3.2). The only values that remain to be specified are the residual variances for the endogenous ($Y1$–$Y3$) variables.

Recall from previous chapters that, assuming standardization, the residual variance ($\sigma^2_{\text{RESIDUAL}}$) for a response variable can be computed by one minus the variance explained (R^2_{Yn}; $\sigma^2_{\text{RESIDUAL}} = 1 - R^2_{Yn}$), and the variance explained in each response variable (R^2_{Yn}) can be calculated by Equation (3.1)

$$R^2_{Yn} = (\text{Direct effect} * (\text{Direct effect} + [\text{Sum of indirect effects products}])) \quad (3.1)$$

Recall also that the sum of indirect effects products can be obtained by using the four path tracing rules developed by Sewall Wright (1921, 1934):

1. A path cannot involve tracing through the same variable twice.
2. A path can involve only one correlation tracing (i.e., double-headed curved arrow).
3. A path can involve tracing both backward (from the arrowhead of a regression arrow back to its source) and forward (from the source of the arrow to its arrowhead), but once a forward tracing is made, additional backward tracings are prohibited.
4. A path can involve as many backward and forward tracings as is permissible.

For example, as shown in the path analysis model, the endogenous variable $Y1$ is predicted by only one exogenous variable, $X2$. The variance explained in Equation (3.1) and substitution can be used to compute the variance in $Y1$ explained by $X2$ [$R^2_{Y1|X2}$; Equation (3.2)]:

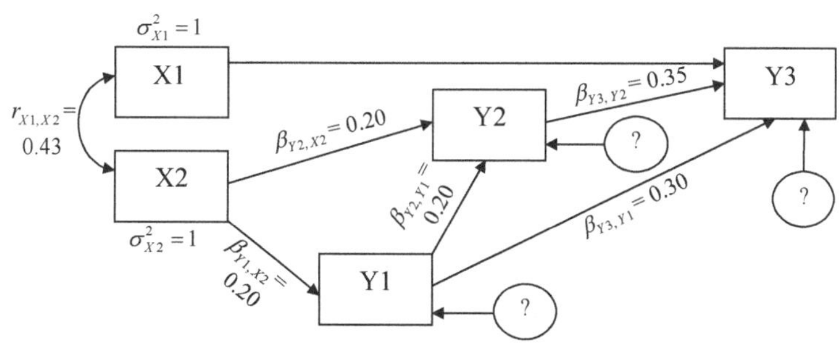

FIGURE 3.2. Path analysis model with standardized slope estimates.

$$R^2_{Y1|X2} = (\text{Direct effect} * (\text{Direct effect} + [\text{Sum of indirect effects products}]))$$

$$R^2_{Y1|X2} = (\beta_{Y1,X2} * (\beta_{Y1,X2} + [\text{Sum of indirect effects products}]))$$

$$R^2_{Y1|X2} = (0.20 * (0.20 + [\text{Sum of indirect effects products}])) \quad (3.2)$$

At this point, it is important to notice that, under Wright's path tracing rules, there are no permissible indirect effects, because any indirect path tracing would have to involve tracing forward, then backward, which is inadmissible under path tracing rule #3, so [Equation (3.3)]

$$R^2_{Y1|X2} = (0.20 * (0.20 + [0]))$$

$$R^2_{Y1|X2} = (0.20^2) = \underline{0.04}$$

so $$\sigma^2_{\text{RESIDUAL}\_Y1} = 1 - R^2_{Y1|X2} = 1 - 0.04 = \mathbf{0.96} \quad (3.3)$$

The endogenous variable *Y*2 is predicted by an exogenous variable (*X*2) and an endogenous variable (*Y*1), so the total variance explained in *Y*2 can be shown as the sum of variance in *Y*2 explained by *X*2 ($R^2_{Y2|X2}$) plus the variance in *Y*2 explained by *Y*1 [$R^2_{Y2|Y1}$; Equation (3.4)]

$$R^2_{Y2} = R^2_{Y2|X2} + R^2_{Y2|Y1}$$

or $$R^2_{Y2} = (\beta_{Y2,Y1} * (\beta_{Y2,Y1} + [\text{Indirect effects products}]))$$

$$+ (\beta_{Y2,X2} * (\beta_{Y2,X2} + [\text{Indirect effects products}])) \quad (3.4)$$

To better illustrate the use of Wright's path tracing rules to determine indirect effects, the two equations above are solved separately as Equation (3.5)

$$R^2_{Y2|Y1} = (\beta_{Y2,Y1} * (\beta_{Y2,Y1} + [\text{Indirect effects products}]))$$

$$= (0.20 * (0.20 + [\text{Indirect effects products}])) \quad (3.5)$$

According to Wright's rules, there is only one permissible indirect path from *Y*1 to *Y*2 (all other possible paths involve tracing forward, then backward, which is impermissible): the path from *Y*1 to *X*2 (backward), then the path from *X*2 to *Y*2 (forward), or [Figure 3.3 and Equation (3.6)]

$$(0.20 * (0.20 + [Y1 \text{ to } X2 * X2 \text{ to } Y2]))$$

$$(0.20 * (0.20 + [0.20 * 0.20]))$$

$$= R^2_{Y2|Y1} = \underline{0.048} \quad (3.6)$$

$$R^2_{Y2|X2} = (\beta_{Y2,X2} * (\beta_{Y2,X2} + [\text{Indirect effects products}]))$$

$$= (0.20 * (0.20 + [\text{Indirect effects products}])) \quad (3.7)$$

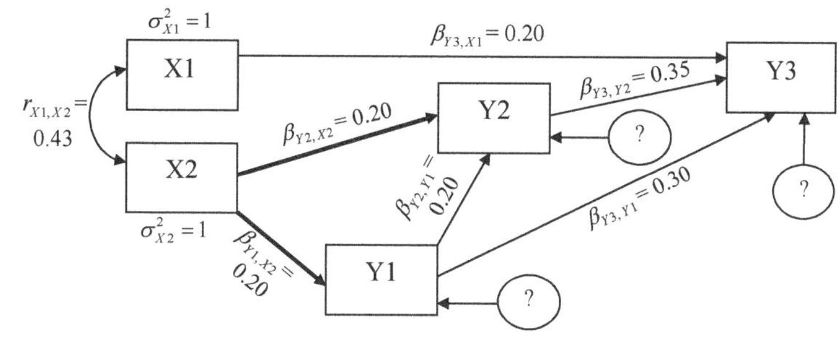

FIGURE 3.3. Indirect path from *Y*1 to *Y*2.

There is also only one permissible indirect path, based on Wright's rules, from *X*2 to *Y*2 (all other possibilities would again involve tracing forward, then backward, which is impermissible): the path from *X*2 to *Y*1, and then the path from *Y*1 to *Y*2, or [Equations 3.7–3.8 and Figure 3.4)

$$= (0.20 * (0.20 + [X2 \text{ to } Y1 * Y1 \text{ to } Y2]))$$

$$= (0.20 * (0.20 + [0.20 * 0.20]))$$

$$= R^2_{Y2|Y1} = \underline{0.048}$$

so

$$R^2_{Y2} = R^2_{Y2|X2} + R^2_{Y2|Y1}$$

or

$$R^2_{Y2} = \underline{0.048} + \underline{0.048} = \underline{0.096}$$

and

$$\sigma^2_{\text{RESIDUAL\_}Y2} = 1 - R^2_{Y2} = 1 - 0.096 = \mathbf{0.904} \tag{3.8}$$

The last endogenous variable, *Y*3, is predicted by one exogenous variable (*X*1) and two endogenous variables (*Y1* and *Y*2). The total variance explained in *Y*3 (R^2_{Y3}) is again shown as the sum of the variance in *Y*3 explained by *X*1 ($R^2_{Y3|X1}$) plus the variance in *Y*3 explained by *Y*1 ($R^2_{Y3|Y1}$) plus the variance in *Y*3 explained by *Y*2 ($R^2_{Y3|Y2}$), or Equation (3.9)

$$R^2_{Y3} = R^2_{Y3|X1} + R^2_{Y3|Y1} + R^2_{Y3|Y2}$$

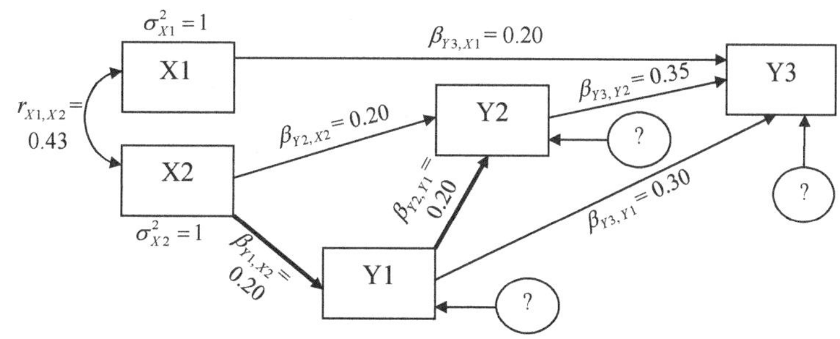

FIGURE 3.4. Indirect path from *X2* to *Y*2.

and by substitution

$$R^2_{Y3} = (\beta_{Y3,X1} * (\beta_{Y3,X1} + [\text{Indirect effects products}]))$$
$$+ (\beta_{Y3,Y2} * (\beta_{Y3,Y2} + [\text{Indirect effects products}]))$$
$$+ (\beta_{Y3,Y1} * (\beta_{Y3,Y1} + [\text{Indirect effects products}])) \quad (3.9)$$

Again, to better illustrate the use of Wright's path tracing rules to obtain the Indirect effects products, the three equations for computing variance explained in $Y3$ will be solved separately [Equation (3.10)]

$$R^2_{Y3|X1} = (\beta_{Y3,X1} * (\beta_{Y3,X1} + [\text{Indirect effects products}]))$$
$$= (0.20 * (0.20 + [\text{Indirect effects products}])) \quad (3.10)$$

According to Wright's rules, there are three permissible indirect paths for $Y3$ to $X1$. The first is the path from $X1$ to $X2$, then the path from $X2$ to $Y2$, then the path from $Y2$ to $Y3$, as shown in Figure 3.5. The second indirect path is from $X1$ to $X2$, then the path from $X2$ to $Y1$, then the path from $Y1$ to $Y2$, then the path from $Y2$ to $Y3$, as shown in Figure 3.6. The third indirect path is from $X1$ to $X2$, then the path from $X2$ to $Y1$, then the path from $Y1$ to $Y3$, as shown in Figure 3.7. So in Equations (3.11) and (3.12),

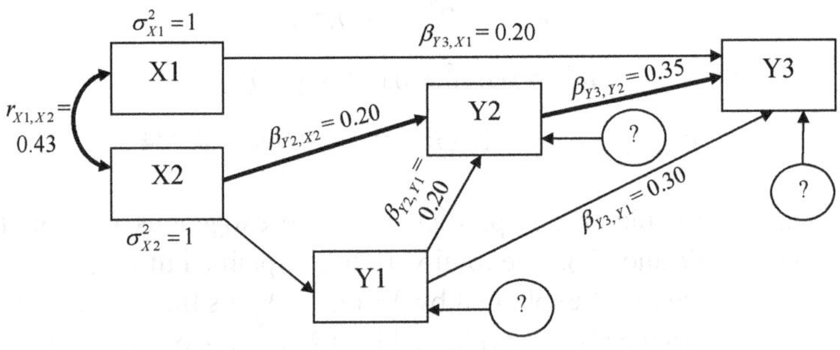

FIGURE 3.5. Indirect path from $X1$ to $Y3$.

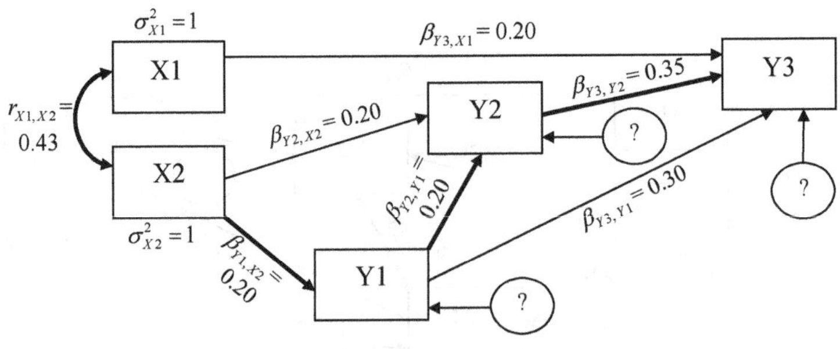

FIGURE 3.6. A second indirect path from $X1$ to $Y3$.

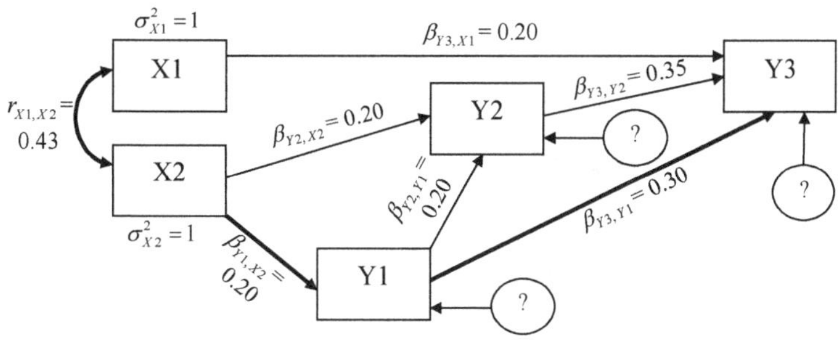

FIGURE 3.7. A third indirect path from $X1$ to $Y3$.

$$R^2_{Y3|X1} = (0.20 * (0.20 + [\text{Indirect effects products}]))$$

$$= (0.20 * (0.20 + [X1 \text{ to } X2 * X2 \text{ to } Y2 * Y2 \text{ to } Y3] + [X1 \text{ to } X2 * X2 \text{ to } Y1 * Y1 \text{ to } Y2 * Y2 \text{ to } Y3] + [X1 \text{ to } X2 * X2 \text{ to } Y1 * Y1 \text{ to } Y3]))$$

$$= (0.20 * (0.20 + [0.43 * 0.20 * 0.35] + [0.43 * 0.20 * 0.20 * 0.35] + [0.43 * 0.20 * 0.30])$$

$$= (0.20 * (0.20 + [0.0301] + [0.00602] + [0.0258]) = \underline{0.052384} \quad (3.11)$$

$$R^2_{Y3|Y2} = (\beta_{Y3,Y2} * (\beta_{Y3,Y2} + [\text{Indirect effects products}]))$$

$$= (0.35 * (0.35 + [\text{Indirect effects products}])) \quad (3.12)$$

There are four permissible indirect paths [Equation (3.12)] for $Y3$ to $Y2$. The first is the path from $Y2$ to $Y1$, then the path from $Y1$ to $Y3$, as shown in Figure 3.8. The second is the path from $Y2$ to $X2$, then the path from $X2$ to $Y1$, then the path from $Y1$ to $Y3$, as shown in Figure 3.9. The third is the path from $Y2$ to $X2$, then the path from $X2$ to $X1$, then the path from $X1$ to $Y3$, as shown in Figure 3.10. The fourth and final indirect path for $Y3$ to $Y2$ is the path from $Y2$ to $Y1$, then the path from $Y1$ to $X2$, then the path from $X2$ to $X1$, then the path from $X1$ to $Y3$, as shown in Figure 3.11. So [Equation (3.13)],

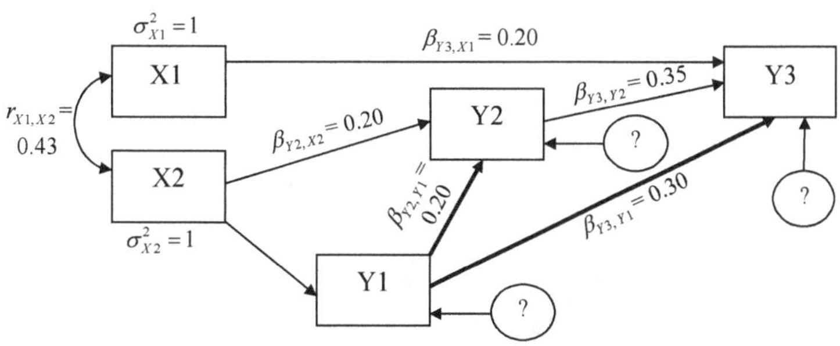

FIGURE 3.8. First indirect path from $Y2$ to $Y3$.

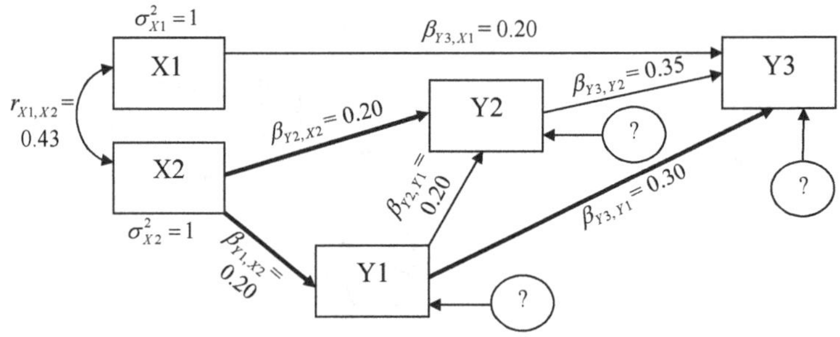

FIGURE 3.9. Second indirect path from *Y*2 to *Y*3.

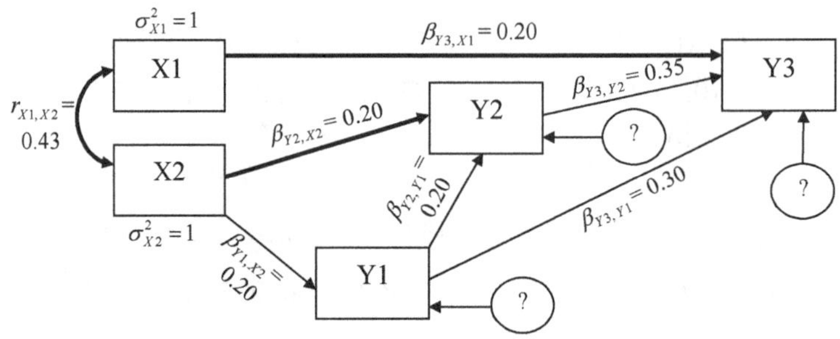

FIGURE 3.10. Third indirect path from *Y*2 to *Y*3.

$$R^2_{Y3|Y2} = (0.35 * (0.35 + [\text{Indirect effects products}]))$$

$$= (0.35 * (0.35 + [Y2 \text{ to } Y1 * Y1 \text{ to } Y3\}] + [Y2 \text{ to } X2 * X2 \text{ to } Y1 * Y1 \text{ to } Y3] + [Y2 \text{ to } X2 * X2 \text{ to } X1 * X1 \text{ to } Y3] + [Y2 \text{ to } Y1 * Y1 \text{ to } X2 * X2 \text{ to } X1 * X1 \text{ to } Y3])$$

$$= (0.35 * (0.35 + [0.20 * 0.30] + [0.20 * 0.20 * 0.30] + [0.20 * 0.43 * 0.20] + [0.20 * 0.20 * 0.43 * 0.20])$$

$$= (0.35 * (0.35 + [0.06] + [0.012] + [0.0172] + [0.00344]) = \underline{0.154924} \quad (3.13)$$

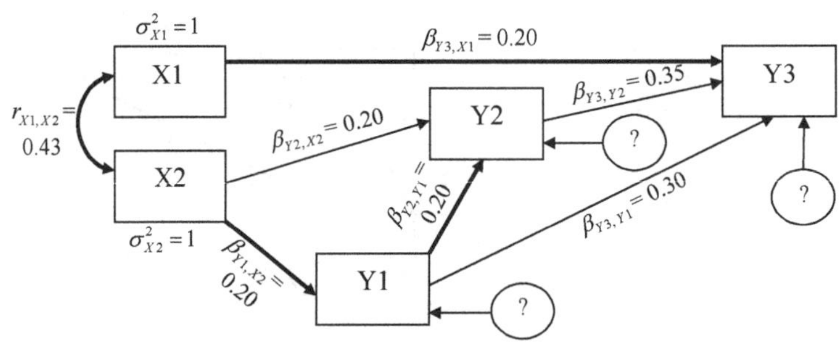

FIGURE 3.11. Fourth indirect path from *Y*2 to *Y*3.

$$R^2_{Y3|Y1} = (\beta_{Y3,Y1} * (\beta_{Y3,Y1} + [\text{Indirect effects products}]))$$
$$= (0.30 * (0.30 + [\text{Indirect effects products}])) \quad (3.14)$$

There are three permissible indirect effects [Equation (3.14)] for *Y*3 to *Y*1. The first is the path from *Y*1 to *Y*2, then the path from *Y*2 to *Y*3, as shown in Figure 3.12. The second is the path from *Y*1 to *X*2, then the path from *X*2 to *Y*2, then the path from *Y*2 to *Y*3, as shown in Figure 3.13. The third is the path from *Y*1 to *X*2, then the path from *X*2 to *X*1, then the path from *X*1 to *Y*3, as shown in Figure 3.14. So [Equation (3.15)],

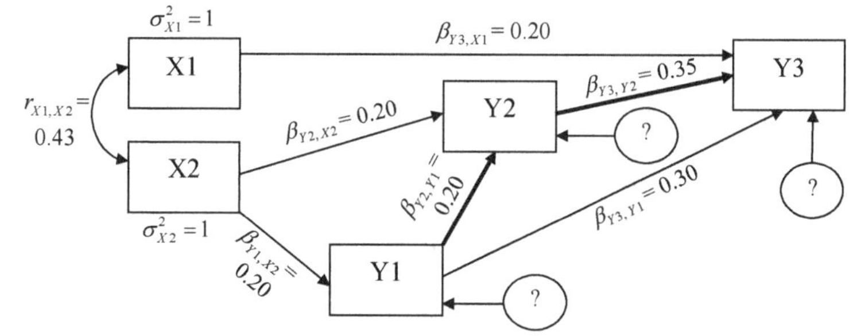

FIGURE 3.12. First indirect path from *Y*1 to *Y*3.

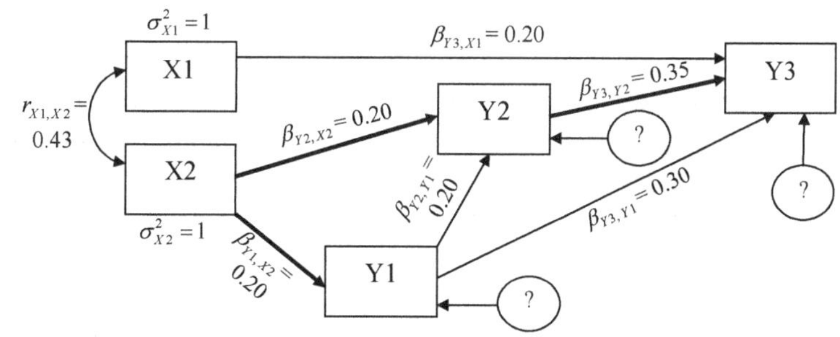

FIGURE 3.13. Second indirect path from *Y*1 to *Y*3.

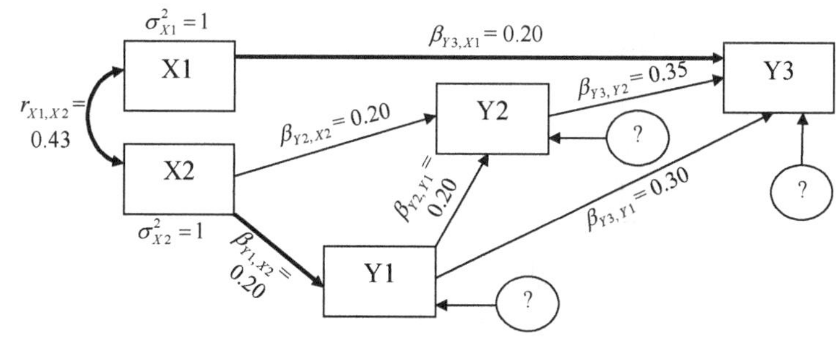

FIGURE 3.14. Third indirect path from *Y*1 to *Y*3.

$$R^2_{Y3|Y1} = (0.30 * (0.30 + [\text{Indirect effects products}]))$$

$$= (0.30 * (0.30 + [Y1 \text{ to } Y2 * Y2 \text{ to } Y3] + [Y1 \text{ to } X2 * X2 \text{ to } Y2 * Y2 \text{ to } Y3] + [Y1 \text{ to } X2 * X2 \text{ to } X1 * X1 \text{ to } Y3]))$$

$$= (0.30 * (0.30 + [0.20 * 0.035] + [0.20 * 0.20 * 0.35] + [0.20 * 0.43 * 0.20]))$$

$$= (0.30 * (0.30 + [0.07] + [0.014] + [0.0172])) = \underline{0.12036} \quad (3.15)$$

So in Equation (3.16),

$$R^2_{Y3} = R^2_{Y3|X1} + R^2_{Y3|Y1} + R^2_{Y3|Y2}$$

or

$$R^2_{Y3} = \underline{0.052384} + \underline{0.12036} + \underline{0.154924} = 0.327668$$

and

$$\sigma^2_{\text{Residual\_}Y3} = 1 - R^2_{Y3} = 1 - 0.327444 = \mathbf{0.672332} \quad (3.16)$$

Now all required values for the path analysis model have been specified and the computed residual variances can be added (Figure 3.15).

At this point, two practical concerns need to be addressed. First, a considerable amount of path tracing and calculations were needed to obtain the three residual variances for *Y*1–*Y*3, leaving open the possibility for errors in both the path tracing and in the subsequent computations. Second, although the values specified in the path analysis model above appear to be both face-valid and plausible, a Monte Carlo simulation power analysis cannot be performed on an inadmissible analysis model that results in an estimation error. Common estimation errors include analysis models that produce negative variance estimates or correlations that exceed ± 1. The admissibility and accuracy of the path analysis model specified above can be checked by computing a *model-reproduced correlation matrix*.

For example, if a researcher had a sample of data, computing the correlations among two or more analysis variables in any statistical analysis software package would be a simple procedure. A correlation matrix computed based on observed data is commonly referred to by the notation (**Σ**). In similar fashion, but somewhat less well-known, is the fact that a correlation matrix for a set of analysis variables can also be computed based on parameter values from any structural equation model, and this is commonly referred to as a *model-reproduced correlation matrix*, by the notation (**Σθ**), indicating a correlation matrix (**Σ**) based on structural equation model parameter estimate values (**θ**) instead of observed data.

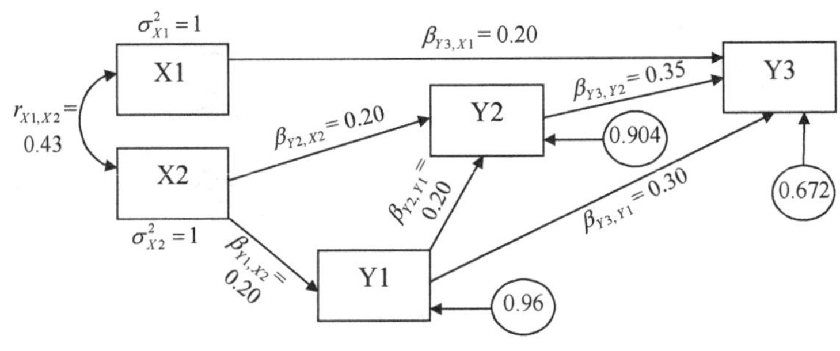

FIGURE 3.15. Path analysis model with residual variances added.

As an additional example, consider that the issue of structural equation model "fit" bears directly on the extent to which the data analysis variable relationships quantified by structural equation model parameter estimates ($\boldsymbol{\Sigma\theta}$) match the data analysis variable relationships computed from a sample of data ($\boldsymbol{\Sigma}$). Obviously, no sample data are available at this point, but a model-reproduced correlation matrix ($\boldsymbol{\Sigma\theta}$) can still be calculated based on the specified parameter values to check both the accuracy and admissibility of the above path analysis model.

As shown in Bollen (1989, p. 86) and assuming standardization, the equations for computing a path analysis model-reproduced correlation matrix [$\boldsymbol{\Sigma\theta}$; Equation (3.17)] are

$$\boldsymbol{\Sigma\Theta} = \begin{bmatrix} (\mathbf{I}-\mathbf{B})^{-1}(\boldsymbol{\Gamma\Phi\Gamma}^{T}+\boldsymbol{\Psi})(\mathbf{I}-\mathbf{B})^{-1T} & (\mathbf{I}-\mathbf{B})^{-1}\boldsymbol{\Gamma\Phi} \\ \boldsymbol{\Phi\Gamma}^{T}(\mathbf{I}-\mathbf{B})^{-1T} & \boldsymbol{\Phi} \end{bmatrix} \tag{3.17}$$

As shown, five matrices are needed: phi ($\boldsymbol{\Phi}$), gamma ($\boldsymbol{\Gamma}$), beta ($\mathbf{B}$), psi ($\boldsymbol{\Psi}$), and identity ($\mathbf{I}$). All of the information needed for the five matrices has already been specified in the above path analysis model. It is now only a matter of placing the values from the path analysis model above correctly into the five matrices.

First, the dimensions of the phi ($\boldsymbol{\Phi}$) matrix are defined as the number of rows and the number of columns both equal to the number of exogenous variables (2; $X1$ and $X2$) in the path analysis model. The phi ($\boldsymbol{\Phi}$) matrix here is a two-row by two-column matrix of exogenous variable variances (as main diagonal elements) and correlations (as off-diagonal elements). Assuming standardization, the variances of $X1$ and $X2$ are both one, and the correlation between $X1$ and $X2$ has been specified as $r_{X1,X2} = 0.43$, so [Equation (3.18)]

$$\boldsymbol{\Phi} = \begin{array}{c|cc|} & X1 & X2 \\ X1 & 1 & 0.43 \\ X2 & 0.43 & 1 \end{array} \tag{3.18}$$

The dimensions of the gamma ($\boldsymbol{\Gamma}$) matrix will have a number of rows equal to the number of endogenous variables, and the number of columns will equal the number of exogenous variables. So, here the gamma ($\boldsymbol{\Gamma}$) matrix is a three-row (three endogenous variables, $Y1$–$Y3$) by two-column (two exogenous variables, $X1$ and $X2$) matrix that contains regression coefficient values for exogenous variables predicting endogenous variables, or Equation (3.19)

$$\boldsymbol{\Gamma} = \begin{array}{c|cc|} & X1 & X2 \\ Y1 & 0 & 0.20 \\ Y2 & 0 & 0.20 \\ Y3 & 0.20 & 0 \end{array} \tag{3.19}$$

In the left column of the gamma ($\boldsymbol{\Gamma}$) matrix, the first two entered values are zeros because $X1$ does not predict either $Y1$ or $Y2$. The last value in the left column of the gamma ($\boldsymbol{\Gamma}$) matrix (0.20) indicates $X1$ does predict $Y3$, and the value specified is $\beta_{Y3,X1} = 0.20$. Similarly, in the right column of the gamma ($\boldsymbol{\Gamma}$) matrix, the first two entered values are the specified values for $X2$ as a predictor of both $Y1$ ($\beta_{Y1,X2} = 0.20$) and $Y2$ ($\beta_{Y2,X2} = 0.20$), but the last value is zero, indicating that $X2$ is not specified as a predictor of $Y3$.

The dimensions of the beta (**B**) matrix are defined as the number of rows and the number of columns both equal to the number of endogenous variables ($Y1$–$Y3$). The beta (**B**) matrix here is a three-row by three-column matrix that contains regression coefficient values for endogenous variables predicting other endogenous variables, or Equation (3.20)

$$\mathbf{B} = \begin{array}{c|ccc|} & Y1 & Y2 & Y3 \\ Y1 & 0 & 0 & 0 \\ Y2 & 0.20 & 0 & 0 \\ Y3 & 0.30 & 0.35 & 0 \end{array} \tag{3.20}$$

In the first column of the beta (**B**) matrix, the values 0.20 and 0.30 are the specified regression coefficients for $Y1$ as a predictor of both $Y2$ ($\beta_{Y2,Y1} = 0.20$) and $Y3$ ($\beta_{Y3,Y1} = 0.30$). In the second column of the beta (**B**) matrix, the last value (0.35) is the specified regression coefficient for $Y2$ as a predictor of $Y3$ ($\beta_{Y3,Y2} = 0.35$). No other endogenous predictions are specified, so all other values in the beta (**B**) matrix are zeros.

The dimensions of the psi (**Ψ**) matrix are also defined as the number of rows and the number of columns both equal to the number of endogenous variables ($Y1$–$Y3$). The psi (**Ψ**) matrix here is a three-row by three-column matrix that contains residual variances as main diagonal elements, and residual variance correlations (if applicable) as off-diagonal elements, or Equation (3.21)

$$\mathbf{\Psi} = \begin{array}{c|ccc|} & Y1 & Y2 & Y3 \\ Y1 & 0.96 & 0 & 0 \\ Y2 & 0 & 0.904 & 0 \\ Y3 & 0 & 0 & 0.672332 \end{array} \tag{3.21}$$

The main diagonal elements of the psi (**Ψ**) matrix are the residual variances for the endogenous $Y1$–$Y3$ variables calculated using Wright's path tracing rules. All off-diagonal elements are zeros because there are no residual variance correlations (i.e., there are no curved, double-headed arrows connecting any residual variance circles in the above path analysis model) specified.

Finally, the identity (**I**) matrix shown in Equation (3.22) is also defined as the number of rows and the number of columns both equal to the number of endogenous variables ($Y1$–$Y3$). The main diagonal elements will always be values of one. The off-diagonal elements will always be zeros. This remains true regardless of the structural equation model under consideration.

$$\mathbf{I} = \begin{array}{c|ccc|} & Y1 & Y2 & Y3 \\ Y1 & 1 & 0 & 0 \\ Y2 & 0 & 1 & 0 \\ Y3 & 0 & 0 & 1 \end{array} \tag{3.22}$$

Now that all five matrices have been defined and the correct values specified for each, the five matrices can be used to solve the model-reproduced correlation matrix ($\boldsymbol{\Sigma\theta}$) equations. This can be done in three steps using base R statistical analysis syntax specified as follows. The first step involves creating five matrix variables, each containing the correct data.

```
Gamma <- matrix(c(0, .2, 0, .2, .2, 0), ncol = 2, byrow = TRUE)
Beta <- matrix(c(0, 0, 0, .2, 0, 0, .3, .35, 0), ncol = 3, byrow = TRUE)
Phi <- matrix(c(1, .43, .43, 1), nrow = 2, byrow = TRUE)
I <- matrix(c(1, 0, 0, 0, 1, 0, 0, 0, 1), nrow = 3, byrow = TRUE)
Psi <- matrix(c(.96, 0, 0, 0, .904, 0, 0, 0, .672332), nrow = 3, byrow = TRUE)
```

To the left of each <- are the names of the variables that will contain matrix data. The values for each of the five matrices are entered into the parenthetical expression following the matrix(c(specification, starting with the top left value within each matrix and moving across each row, separating each value with a comma. The ncol = or nrow = statements, together with the command byrow = TRUE ensures that the comma-separated data contained within each parenthetical expression is parsed into the correct number of rows and columns for each matrix.

The second step involves combining matrices to calculate quadrants of the model-reproduced covariance matrix. Notice how the model-reproduced correlation matrix ($\boldsymbol{\Sigma\theta}$) equation is a combination of four separate equations: an "upper left" equation ($(\mathbf{I} - \mathbf{B})^{-1}(\boldsymbol{\Gamma\Phi\Gamma}^T + \boldsymbol{\Psi})(\mathbf{I} - \mathbf{B})^{-1T}$), an "upper right" equation ($(\mathbf{I} - \mathbf{B})^{-1}\boldsymbol{\Gamma\Phi}$), a "lower left" equation ($\boldsymbol{\Phi\Gamma}^T(\mathbf{I} - \mathbf{B})^{-1T}$), and a "lower right" equation ($\boldsymbol{\Phi}$). Each of the four separate equations can be solved with the following base R syntax:

```
upper_left <- solve(I-Beta) %*% (Gamma %*% Phi %*% t(Gamma) + Psi) %*% t(solve(I-Beta))

upper_right <- solve(I-Beta) %*% (Gamma %*% Phi)

lower_left <- (Phi) %*% t(Gamma) %*% t(solve(I-Beta))
lower_right <- (Phi),
```

where the expression %*% specifies matrix multiplication, the solve() expression specifies computing the inverse ($^{-1}$) of a matrix, and the t() expression specifies transposing (^{T}) a matrix.

The final step to computing the model-implied correlation matrix requires merging the "upper left," "upper right," "lower left," and "lower right" results into a single correlation matrix using base R code,

```
upper <- cbind(upper_left, upper_right)
lower <- cbind(lower_left, lower_right)

corr_matrix <- rbind(upper, lower),
```

where the cbind() specification unites both the "upper left" and "upper right" results, as well as the "lower left" and "lower right" results, by merging, or binding, the columns of each by matching their respective rows. The rbind() specification merges the "upper" and "lower" results by binding their respective rows by matching their columns.

The complete and integrated R syntax for computing the path analysis model-implied correlation matrix is shown below.

```
Gamma <- matrix(c(0, .2, 0, .2, .2, 0), ncol = 2, byrow = TRUE)
Beta <- matrix(c(0, 0, 0, .2, 0, 0, .3, .35, 0), ncol = 3, byrow = TRUE)
Phi <- matrix(c(1, .43, .43, 1), nrow = 2, byrow = TRUE)
I <- matrix(c(1, 0, 0, 0, 1, 0, 0, 0, 1), nrow = 3, byrow = TRUE)
Psi <- matrix(c(.96, 0, 0, 0, .904, 0, 0, 0, .672332), nrow = 3, byrow = TRUE)

upper_left <-
solve(I-Beta) %*% (Gamma %*% Phi %*% t(Gamma) + Psi) %*% t(solve(I-Beta))
upper_right <- solve(I-Beta) %*% (Gamma %*% Phi)
lower_left <- (Phi) %*% t(Gamma) %*% t(solve(I-Beta))
lower_right <- (Phi)

upper <- cbind(upper_left, upper_right)
lower <- cbind(lower_left, lower_right)
corr_matrix <- rbind(upper, lower)

corr_matrix
```

The final statement, corr_matrix, results in the correlation matrix output. This correlation matrix is saved in the Global environment as the object corr_matrix and can be called into further functions for additional analysis, if desired.

	Y1	*Y2*	*Y3*	*X1*	*X2*
Y1	1	0.240	0.401	0.086	0.200
Y2	0.240	1	0.443	0.103	0.240
Y3	0.401	0.443	1	0.262	0.230
X1	0.086	0.103	0.262	1	0.430
X2	0.200	0.240	0.230	0.430	1

Here again is an example of how standardization simplifies the results. Notice how the resulting correlation matrix is *admissible*, which is defined as having values of exactly one on the main diagonal and correlations between ± 1 as off-diagonal elements. This means the path analysis model specifications are admissible and a Monte Carlo simulation power analysis can be conducted. If the result of solving the model-reproduced correlation matrix ($\boldsymbol{\Sigma\theta}$) equations produced negative values on the main diagonal, or values exceeding ± 1 on the off-diagonal, such a model is inadmissible and would produce an estimation error. Furthermore, if solving the model-reproduced correlation matrix ($\boldsymbol{\Sigma\theta}$) equations produced values other than one on the main diagonal, this could indicate one or more path tracings that were missed, incorrect computations, or both.

Now that an admissible path analysis model has been verified, a Monte Carlo simulation power analysis can be performed. However, let's assume that the power analysis question specifically involves the minimal sample size needed to detect the effect of *Y*2 as a *mediator* of the relationship between *Y*1 and *Y*3 after controlling for the influence of variables *X*1 and *X*2. The power analysis can be conducted in either Mplus or R, as shown below.

Mplus Monte Carlo Power Analysis: Mediated Path Analysis

In Mplus, the mediated path analysis model input consists of information about the Monte Carlo simulation, a population model, an analysis model, and model constraints.

```
TITLE: MPLUS 3.1 MEDIATED PATH ANALYSIS

MONTECARLO:
NAMES ARE X1 X2 Y1 Y2 Y3;
NOBSERVATIONS = 207;
NREPS = 5000;
SEED = 47586;
```

The `MONTECARLO:` specifications are similar to previous simulation examples, except that the `NAMES ARE` specification has changed to include the names of the variables in the path analysis model, and a new random number is provided for the `SEED` = specification. Specifying the data generation model in the `MODEL POPULATION:` command involves converting the information contained in the four (phi, gamma, beta, and psi; identity excluded) matrices into Mplus syntax as follows

```
MODEL POPULATION:

!Phi Matrix;
X1*1;
X2*1;
X1 WITH X2*0.43;

!Gamma Matrix;
Y1 ON X2*0.20;
Y2 ON X2*0.20;
Y3 ON X1*0.20;

!Beta Matrix;
Y2 ON Y1*0.20;
Y3 ON Y2*0.35;
Y3 ON Y1*0.30;

!Psi Matrix;
Y1*0.96;
Y2*0.904;
Y3*0.672332;
```

Recall that `WITH` specifies "correlated with," `ON` specifies "response variable regressed on predictor variable," and referring to the name of a variable only refers to an exogenous variable's variance or an endogenous variable's residual variance. The data analysis model specified in the `MODEL:` command is the same as the data-generating model specified in the `MODEL POPULATION:` command with two exceptions: (1) the phi matrix information can be excluded and (2) testing the statistical power for a mediated pathway involves specifying two additional variables.

```
MODEL:

!Psi Matrix;
Y1*0.96;
Y2*0.904;
Y3*0.672332;

!Gamma Matrix;
Y1 ON X2*0.20;
Y2 ON X2*0.20;
Y3 ON X1*0.20;

!Beta Matrix;
Y2 ON Y1*0.20(A);
Y3 ON Y2*0.35(B);
Y3 ON Y1*0.30;
```

Testing the statistical power of a mediated pathway involves testing the product of two regression coefficients: the regression coefficient for the independent variable that predicts the mediator (in this case, $\beta_{Y2,Y1} = 0.20$) and the regression coefficient for the mediator as a predictor of the response variable (in this case, $\beta_{Y3,Y2} = 0.35$), or ($\beta_{Y2,Y1} * \beta_{Y3,Y2} = 0.20 * 0.35$). In the `MODEL:` statement, the regression coefficient for the independent variable predicting the mediator (`Y2 ON Y1*0.20`) is assigned to the variable`(A)`, and the regression coefficient for the mediator predicting the response variable (`Y3 ON Y2*0.35`) is assigned to the variable`(B)`.

```
MODEL CONSTRAINT:
New(Med*0.07);
Med = A*B;
```

By assigning the specific components of the mediated pathway to the variables `(A)` and `(B)`, the `MODEL CONSTRAINT:` command can be used to create a `New` "mediation" (`Med`) variable that is the joint product of the two regression coefficients that define the mediated, or indirect, path. The "mediation" (`Med`) variable is given the specified value of (0.20 * 0.35 =) 0.07.

The annotated results from the Monte Carlo simulation power analysis (Mplus 3.1) are shown below.

```
MODEL RESULTS

                                ESTIMATES                S. E.      M. S. E.  95%   % Sig
                    Population   Average    Std. Dev.   Average              Cover  Coeff
New/Additional Parameters
  MED                    0.070    0.0695      0.0267     0.0266      0.0007  0.944  0.802
```

Results of the Monte Carlo simulation power analysis show that a minimal sample size of $N = 207$ is needed for power $\geq .80$ to detect a standardized mediated pathway coefficient of (`A * B` =) 0.07.

R Monte Carlo Power Analysis: Mediated Path Analysis

Similarly, a power analysis can be conducted using R packages simsem and lavaan. First, use lavaan specification to create the population model shown in this chapter:

```
library(simsem)
library(lavaan)

PopulationModel_Ch3 <- "
  !Phi Matrix
  X1 ~~ 1*X1                  #Variance of X1
  X2 ~~ 1*X2                  #Variance of X2
  X1 ~~ 0.43*X2               #Covariance of X1 with X2

  !Gamma Matrix
  Y1 ~ 0.20*X2                #Regression of Y1 on X2
  Y2 ~ 0.20*X2                #Regression of Y2 on X2
  Y3 ~ 0.20*X1                #Regression of Y3 on X1

  !Beta Matrix
  Y2 ~ 0.20*Y1                #Regression of Y2 on Y1
  Y3 ~ 0.35*Y2                #Regression of Y3 on Y2
  Y3 ~ 0.30*Y1                #Regression of Y3 on Y1

  !Psi Matrix
  Y1 ~~ 0.96*Y1               #Residual variance of Y1
  Y2 ~~ 0.904*Y2              #Residual variance of Y2
  Y3 ~~ 0.672332*Y3           #Residual variance of Y3

  !New Variable, Med = 0.07
  Med := 0.07     "           # Med, is the product Y2~Y1 * Y3~Y2 = .20 * .35 = .07
```

Before moving forward, check the accuracy of the model-implied covariance matrix.

```
fitted(sem(PopulationModel))
```

The results from this model-implied covariance matrix contains 1's along the diagonal and values between 0 and 1 on the off-diagonal, indicating that it is a correlation matrix and is admissible.

```
     Y1      Y2      Y3      X2      X1
Y1   1.000
Y2   0.240   1.000
Y3   0.401   0.443   1.000
X2   0.200   0.240   0.230   1.000
X1   0.086   0.103   0.262   0.430   1.000
```

Note that this population model-implied correlation matrix matches the corr_matrix solved earlier in the chapter. The population model accurately reflects the intended population model.

Next, use the lavaan specification to write the analysis model.

```
AnalysisModel_Ch3 <- "
 !Gamma Matrix
 Y1 ~ X2
 Y2 ~ X2
 Y3 ~ X1

 !Beta Matrix
 Y2 ~ A*Y1
 Y3 ~ B*Y2
 Y3 ~ Y1

 !Psi Matrix
 Y1 ~~ Y1
 Y2 ~~ Y2
 Y3 ~~ Y3

 !New Variable, Med = 0.07, as defined in the Population Model command
 Med := A*B     "    #Med is the product Y2~Y1 * Y3~Y = A * B, which should equal .07
```

As in prior chapters, the sample model introduces parameter labels to compute a new variable; in the present case, that variable is Med, which is the joint product of the pathway A and B. After specifying the population and sample models, evaluate the Monte Carlo simulation using the simsem package. Since this model is a single group model, a single-step analysis using the single function sim() can be used to run the full simulation. Although it was not a concern with less complicated models, note that once you begin running the simulation code in R, the process can be stopped, but all progress will be lost in stopping the process. For this reason, it is a good idea to run a "test" model with fewer replications (e.g., $n = 20$) before conducting the full power analysis. The full power analysis is shown below.

```
output_Ch3 <-  sim(nRep = 5000,
               n = 207,
               model = AnalysisModel_Ch3,
               generate = PopulationModel_Ch3,
               std.lv = FALSE,
               seed = 47586,
               silent = TRUE)
```

An overall summary of the Monte Carlo simulation can then be examined by running the code summary(output_Ch3). This overall summary contains two elements: A summary of the model fit and convergence, and a dataframe that contains the Monte Carlo simulation model estimate(s). First, it's important to assess convergence to ensure that no major errors happened during computation.

```
================= Replications =====================
Number of replications = 5000
Number of converged replications = 5000
```

All replications converged. Next, check the statistical power for the parameters of interest. Although this power estimate can be obtained by examining summary output, it is only necessary to evaluate the statistical power estimate for the parameter(s) of interest, which can be obtained by using the getPower() function in combination with the name of the output file and the parameter name; this function is very useful when many parameters are included in the model.

```
getPower(output)["Med"]
0.804
```

Power results are almost the exact same as they were in Mplus, although minor variations (due to seed, program, etc.) may result in slightly different findings across programs.

Simulation Power Analysis Write-Up: Mediated Path Analysis

Finally, an example mediated path analysis Monte Carlo simulation power analysis write-up is shown below and consists of four sections: (1) a statement of the power analysis question; (2) a description of how power was calculated, including the data analysis model assumed, and the statistical software package and version used; (3) a clear statement of all power analysis assumptions, including specific parameter estimate values; and (4) a clear answer to the power analysis question that includes the number of simulated dataset replications requested, the effect size assumed, and the sample size needed to achieve power ≥ .80:

> "The power analysis question involves the smallest sample size needed to achieve power ≥ 0.80 to detect a standardized effect for *Y*2 as a mediator of the relationship between *Y*1 and *Y*3. A Monte Carlo simulation power analysis was conducted using Mplus (version 8.5) [or R, using simsem v. 0.5-16 (Pornprasertmanit et al., 2025) and lavaan v. 0.6-12 (Rosseel et al., 2012)] assuming: (1) standardization of all variables included in the path analysis model, (2) the exogenous variables (*X*1 and *X*2) are correlated at $r_{X1,X2} = 0.43$, (3) the standardized effects of the exogenous (*X*1 and *X*2) variables as predictors of endogenous response variables were all specified to be $\beta = 0.20$, (4) the standardized effects of endogenous variables predicting other endogenous variables ranged between β = 0.20 – 0.35, (5) residual variances for the three endogenous variables ranged between (0.672 – 0.96), and (6) the admissibility of the path analysis model specifications was verified by computing a model-reproduced correlation matrix. Monte Carlo simulation power analysis results aggregated over 5,000 replications showed power ≥.80 for any standardized joint indirect pathway, indicating *Y*2 as a mediator of the relationship between *Y*1 and *Y*3 (A = 0.20 * B = 0.35) of A * B ≥ 0.07 if *N* = <u>207</u> is available for analysis."

SUGGESTED READINGS

- Agler, R., & De Boeck, P. (2017). On the interpretation and use of mediation: multiple perspectives on mediation analysis. *Frontiers in Psychology, 8*, 1–11.
- Cole, D. A., & Preacher, K. J. (2014). Manifest variable path analysis: Potentially serious and misleading consequences due to uncorrected measurement error. *Psychological Methods, 19*, 300–315.

- Fritz, M. S., Cox, M. G., & MacKinnon, D. P. (2015). Increasing statistical power in mediation models without increasing sample size. *Evaluation & The Health Professions, 38,* 343–366.
- Götz, M., O'Boyle, E. H., Gonzalez-Mulé, E., Banks, G. C., & Bollmann, S. S. (2021). The "Goldilocks Zone": (Too) many confidence intervals in tests of mediation just exclude zero. *Psychological Bulletin, 147,* 95–114.
- Goldstein, B. L., Finsaas, M. C., Olino, T. M., Kotov, R., Grasso, D. J., & Klein, D. N. (2021). Three-variable systems: An integrative moderation and mediation framework for developmental psychopathology. *Development and Psychopathology, 35*(1), 1–12.
- Lachowicz, M. J., Preacher, K. J., & Kelley, K. (2018). A novel measure of effect size for mediation analysis. *Psychological Methods, 23,* 244–261.
- Liu, X., & Wang, L. (2019). Sample size planning for detecting mediation effects: A power analysis procedure considering uncertainty in effect size estimates. *Multivariate Behavioral Research, 54,* 822–839.
- MacKinnon, D. P., Lockwood, C. M., & Williams, J. (2004). Confidence limits for the indirect effect: Distribution of the product and resampling methods. *Multivariate Behavioral Research, 39,* 99–128.
- MacKinnon, D. P., Valente, M. J., & Gonzalez, O. (2020). The correspondence between causal and traditional mediation analysis: The link is the mediator by treatment interaction. *Prevention Science, 21,* 147–157.
- McDonald, J. A., & Clelland, D. A. (1984). Textile workers and union sentiment. *Social Forces, 63,* 502–521.
- Miočević, M., MacKinnon, D. P., & Levy, R. (2017). Power in Bayesian mediation analysis for small sample research. *Structural Equation Modeling: A Multidisciplinary Journal, 24*(5), 666–683.
- Qin, X. (2024). Sample size and power calculations for causal mediation analysis: A Tutorial and Shiny App. *Behavior Research Methods, 56*(3), 1738–1769.
- Reif, L. L., Schulman, M. D., & Belyea, M. J. (1988). The social bases of union support: An analysis of Southern textile workers. *Journal of Political & Military Sociology, 16*(1), 57–75.
- Schoemann, A. M., Boulton, A. J., & Short, S. D. (2017). Determining power and sample size for simple and complex mediation models. *Social Psychological & Personality Science, 8,* 379–386.
- Streiner, D. L. (2005). Finding our way: An introduction to path analysis. *The Canadian Journal of Psychiatry, 50,* 115–122.
- Thoemmes, F., MacKinnon, D. P., & Reiser, M. R. (2010). Power analysis for complex mediational designs using Monte Carlo methods. *Structural Equation Modeling, 17,* 510–534.
- VanderWeele, T. (2015). *Explanation in causal inference: Methods for mediation and interaction.* Oxford University Press.
- Wolfle, L. M. (2003). The introduction of path analysis to the social sciences, and some emergent themes: An annotated bibliography. *Structural Equation Modeling, 10,* 1–34.
- Zhang, Z. (2014). Monte Carlo based statistical power analysis for mediation models: Methods and software. *Behavior Research Methods, 46,* 1184–1198.

4

Structural Equation Model

Various medical health variables, such as the amount of more than a dozen component chemicals in blood, hormone levels, and cholesterol levels, can be measured and quantified to a very exact level of specificity and precision with the aid of sophisticated analytic equipment. In contrast to these medical absolutes, many of the variables of interest to educational and social and psychological researchers, such as cognitive ability, marital satisfaction, state or trait anxiety, and mild to moderate depression, are far more difficult to measure and quantify accurately because they are *theoretical constructs* rather than medical absolutes. The sophisticated analytic approaches needed to measure and quantify exact levels of these constructs do not exist; these constructs cannot be measured using methods that are free of uncertainty or error. Researchers can only pose questions in the form of stimulus items that imperfectly and incompletely capture various aspects of the construct under consideration. Furthermore, the response options available to participants for each stimulus item, to varying degrees, limit the expression and quantification of the true level of the construct that is present. *Structural equation modeling* (SEM) has been described as a combination of a measurement model plus a prediction (or structural) model, or the combination of a confirmatory factor analysis (CFA) model and a path analysis model (shown in Chapter 3). It is this combination that affords SEM a distinct advantage over other data analytic techniques: the ability to simultaneously estimate complex predictive relationships among several interrelated and co-occurring constructs in a manner that excludes measurement error.

Measurement Model: CFA

With regard to the measurement of constructs, a fundamental psychometric theory states that the variability in a participant's observed construct score (O) is a combination of their true (T) value or level for that construct plus the influence of measurement error (E), or $O = T + E$. By theoretical extension, a participant's true (T) value or level for a construct could be obtained from an observed construct score (O), assuming measurement error (E) could be removed: T = O – E. The goal of a CFA model is to quantify participants' true scores on a construct based on observed indicators by removing measurement error. An example CFA model for the constructs of depression and anxiety is shown in Figure 4.1.

In the CFA model, the rectangles to the left represent observed scores for the Beck Depression Inventory-2 (BDI-II), Hamilton Rating Scale for Depression (Hamilton), and a depression assessment used by the World Health Organization (WHO). These observed scores are referred to as *indicators of depression.* The rectangles to the right represent State-Trait Anxiety Inventory (STAI), Beck Anxiety Inventory (BAI), and Hospital Anxiety and Depression Scale–Anxiety (HADS-A). These observed scores are referred to as *indicators of anxiety.* The large ovals indicate unobserved, or latent, factors that represent true depression and anxiety scores. The smaller ovals indicate measurement errors (or residual variances) for the three depression (ε_1, ε_2, and ε_3) and three anxiety (ε_4, ε_5, and ε_6) observed scores. Finally, the curved, double-headed arrow represents the anticipated correlation between depression and anxiety. The previous conceptual CFA equation (T = O – E) can be rewritten in terms of the CFA model presented in Figure 4.1 as (DEPRESSION = [BDI-II, HAMILTON, WHO] – [ε_1, ε_2, and ε_3]) and (ANXIETY = [STAI, BAI, HADS-A] – [ε_4, ε_5, and ε_6]).

Notice how the regression prediction arrows, or factor loadings, point from the latent depression factor to the BDI-II, HAMILTON, and WHO observed indicators, as well as from the latent anxiety factor to the STAI, BAI, and HADS-A observed indicators. This is also consistent with psychometric theory: an individual's latent and unobserved true level of depression influences, predicts, or drives their observed BDI-II, HAMILTON, and WHO depression scores. Likewise, an individual's latent and unobserved true level of anxiety influences, predicts, or drives their observed STAI, BAI, and HADS-A anxiety scores. Two additional observations can be gleaned from this CFA model. First, notice how the observed depression scores are predicted by the latent depression factor only. Likewise, the observed anxiety scores are predicted only by the anxiety latent factor. Stated differently, each of the three depression indicators, as well as the three anxiety indicators, is predicted by (or load onto) their respective latent factors only. Second, notice also that there are no curved arrows either among the measurement errors (ε_1–ε_6), or between the measurement errors of the latent depression and anxiety factors. The measurement errors are neither intercorrelated

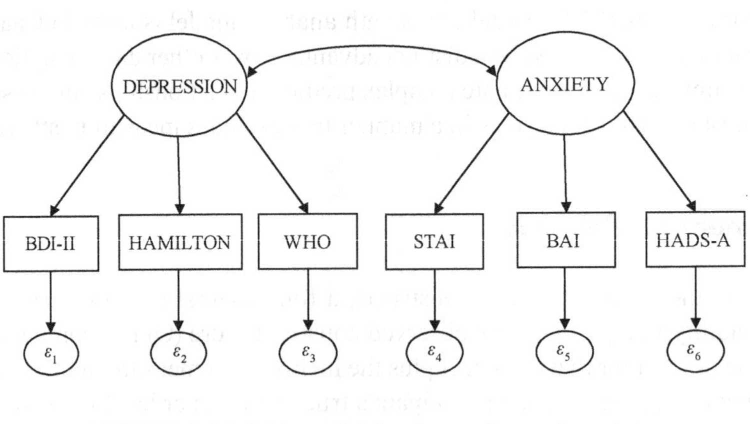

FIGURE 4.1. CFA model for depression and anxiety.

nor correlated with either latent factor. Taken together, these two observations constitute a *simple structure*.

Furthermore, two additional and related methodological considerations warrant discussion: (1) establishing a measurement scale for the latent depression and anxiety factors and (2) confirming that the CFA model is identified. As shown in the model, the latent factor depression is measured by observed BDI-II, Hamilton, and WHO scores; the latent factor anxiety is measured by STAI, BAI, and HADS-A scores. Assuming that each of the observed variables is measured on different metrics, this begs the question of how the measurement scale of the latent variables is to be determined. The two most common methods for establishing the measurement scales for latent factor scores are the unit measurement loading constraint or the unit factor variance constraint. An example of the unit measurement loading constraint is shown in Figure 4.2.

Constraining, or fixing, the loadings of the BDI-II onto the depression latent factor and the STAI onto the latent anxiety factor (which is the default in many SEM statistical analysis software packages) places latent depression scores on the BDI-II measurement scale and latent anxiety scores on the STAI measurement scale. An example of the unit factor variance constraint is shown in Figure 4.3.

In contrast to the unit loading constraint, constraining or fixing the depression and anxiety latent factor variances to unity places both latent depression and latent anxiety scores on a standardized or *z*-score measurement metric.

Staying with the unit latent factor variance example CFA model shown in Figure 4.3, the second methodological question to answer is that of model identification. Model identification is the answer to the question of whether there are more unique pieces of information contained in a sample of data than there are parameters estimated in an analysis model. As a simple example, the equation $X + 5 = 12$, from a model identification perspective, is an identified model. It has only one solution because there are more unique pieces of information contained in the sample data (5 and 12) than there are unknowns (or parameters) that need to be estimated (X). If the equation changes to $X + Y = 12$, the solutions for X and Y are not unique but numerous because the number of unique pieces of sample data (12) is less than the number of unknowns (X and Y). To obtain a single, unique set of estimates for a SEM, there must be more unique pieces of information contained in the sample data than

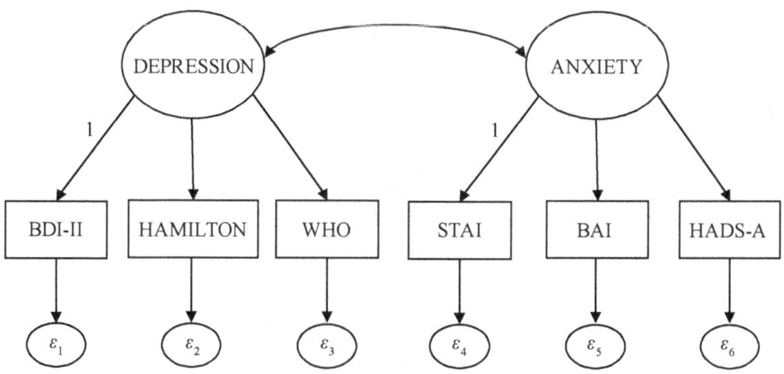

FIGURE 4.2. CFA model for depression and anxiety with fixed factor loadings.

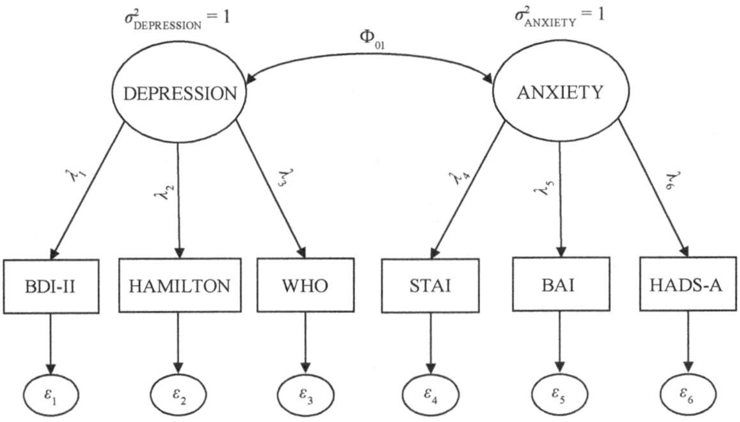

FIGURE 4.3. CFA model for depression and anxiety with fixed latent factor variances.

there are parameters to be estimated in the analysis model; the model must be identified. If P represents the number of variables included in an analysis, the number of unique pieces of information contained in P analysis variables can be determined by solving (P [P + 1] / 2). Furthermore, if Q represents the number of parameters estimated in an analysis model, the analysis model is identified if the result of ($df = P\,[P + 1] / 2) - Q$ is greater than or equal to zero. Using the unit latent factor constrained CFA model, three observed depression and anxiety variables each means there are (6[7] / 2) or 21 unique pieces of information. If latent depression and anxiety variances are constrained to unity, there are 13 (six factor loadings [$\lambda_1 - \lambda_6$], six [$\varepsilon_1 - \varepsilon_6$] measurement errors, and one factor correlation [Φ_{01}]) parameters to be estimated. The model is identified because there are eight (21 – 13) more unique pieces of sample data information than needed parameter estimates. Equivalently, the model has eight degrees of freedom ($df = 8$).

Furthermore, let's assume a researcher wanted to conduct a power analysis using the unit constrained latent variance CFA model shown, and let's further assume a researcher, based on a literature search or a reasonable suspicion, is willing to assume the correlation between depression and anxiety is $\Phi_{01} = r = .50$. As shown in Figure 4.4, and as indicated by the question marks ('?'), 12 additional estimates (six factor loadings and six residual variances) are needed before a Monte Carlo simulation power analysis could be performed.

Again, here is where the assumption of standardization simplifies. An additional literature search could easily produce the following (internal consistency) reliability estimates (R_{xx}) for the six indicator variable total scores: BDI-II: $R_{xx} = 0.91$, Hamilton: $R_{xx} = 0.79$, WHO: $R_{xx} = 0.90$; STAI: $R_{xx} = 0.93$, BAI: $R_{xx} = 0.94$, HADS-A: $R_{xx} = 0.89$. Assuming simple structure and standardization, it can be further shown that: (1) standardized loading estimates (λ_β) can be obtained from reliability estimates by: $\lambda_\beta = \sqrt{R_{xx}}$, and (2) measurement errors (ε) can be estimated by $\varepsilon = 1 - R_{xx}$, or equivalently, $1 - (\lambda_\beta)^2$ (see Cole & Preacher, 2014; Hayduk, 1987; McDonald, 1999; Muthén & Muthén, 2002). Substituting the reliability estimates for the six indicator variables into both equations results in the 12 needed estimates (see Figure 4.5).

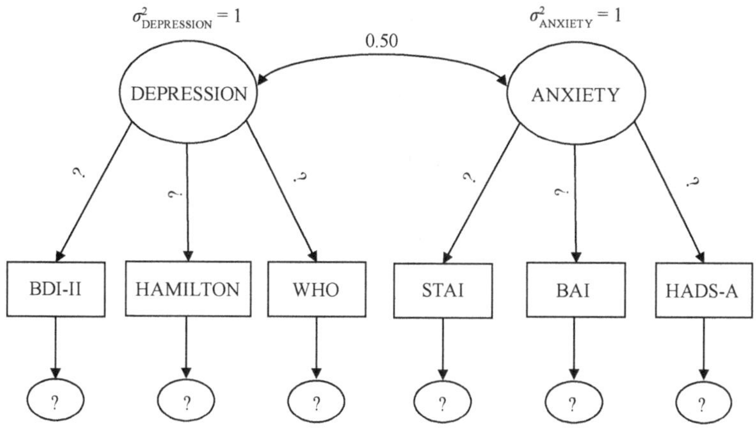

FIGURE 4.4. CFA for depression and anxiety with missing factor loadings and residual variances.

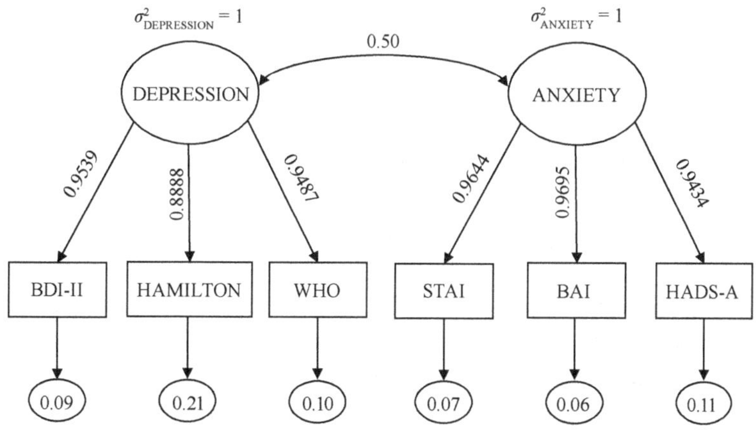

FIGURE 4.5. Fully specified CFA for depression and anxiety.

$$\lambda_{\beta \text{BDI-II}} = \sqrt{0.91} = 0.9539 \qquad \varepsilon_{\text{BDI-II}} = 1 - .91 = 0.09$$
$$\lambda_{\beta \text{HAMILTON}} = \sqrt{0.79} = 0.8888 \qquad \varepsilon_{\text{HAMILTON}} = 1 - .79 = 0.21$$
$$\lambda_{\beta \text{WHO}} = \sqrt{0.90} = 0.9487 \qquad \varepsilon_{\text{WHO}} = 1 - .90 = 0.10$$
$$\lambda_{\beta \text{STAI}} = \sqrt{0.93} = 0.9644 \qquad \varepsilon_{\text{STAI}} = 1 - .93 = 0.07$$
$$\lambda_{\beta \text{BAI}} = \sqrt{0.94} = 0.9695 \qquad \varepsilon_{\text{BAI}} = 1 - .94 = 0.06$$
$$\lambda_{\beta \text{HADS-A}} = \sqrt{0.89} = 0.9434 \qquad \varepsilon_{\text{HADS-A}} = 1 - .89 = 0.11$$

All the estimates specified above can be verified by performing a CFA model admissibility check.

Equation (4.1) for a CFA model-reproduced correlation matrix ($\boldsymbol{\Sigma\theta}$) is

$$\boldsymbol{\Sigma\theta} = \boldsymbol{\Lambda\Phi\Lambda}^T + \boldsymbol{\Psi} \tag{4.1}$$

where the three ($\boldsymbol{\Lambda}$, $\boldsymbol{\Phi}$, $\boldsymbol{\Psi}$) matrices are defined as follows. The dimensions of the lambda ($\boldsymbol{\Lambda}$) matrix are defined as the number of rows equal to the number of observed analysis variables (6: BDI-II, HAMILTON, WHO, STAI, BAI, HADS-A), the number of columns equals the number of latent factors (2: Depression and Anxiety), and the cells contain the factor loading values, as in Equation (4.2).

$\boldsymbol{\Lambda}$ =	Depression	Anxiety
BDI-II	0.9539	0
HAMILTON	0.8888	0
WHO	0.9487	0
STAI	0	0.9644
BAI	0	0.9695
HADS-A	0	0.9434

(4.2)

The dimensions of the phi ($\boldsymbol{\Phi}$) matrix are defined as the number of rows and columns both equal to the number of latent factors and the cells of the matrix that contain the latent factor variances and correlation, as in Equation (4.3).

$\boldsymbol{\Phi}$ =	Depression	Anxiety
Depression	1	0.50
Anxiety	0.50	1

(4.3)

Finally, the dimensions of the psi ($\boldsymbol{\Psi}$) matrix shown in Equation (4.4) are defined as the number of rows and columns both equal to the number of observed analysis variables, the cells on the main diagonal contain the measurement errors ($\varepsilon_1 - \varepsilon_6$), and the off-diagonal elements would contain any measurement error correlations if present.

$\boldsymbol{\Psi}$ =	BDI-II	HAMILTON	WHO	STAI	BAI	HADS-A
BDI-II	0.09	0	0	0	0	0
HAMILTON	0	0.21	0	0	0	0
WHO	0	0	0.10	0	0	0
STAI	0	0	0	0.07	0	0
BAI	0	0	0	0	0.06	0
HADS-A	0	0	0	0	0	0.11

(4.4)

The model-reproduced correlation matrix equation can be solved using the information contained in the three matrices using the following R syntax.

```
Lambda <- matrix(c(.9539, 0, .8888, 0, .9487, 0, 0, .9644, 0, .9695, 0, .9434),
ncol = 2, byrow = TRUE)
Phi <- matrix(c(1, .5, .5, 1), nrow = 2, byrow = TRUE)
```

```
Psi <- matrix(c(0.09, 0, 0, 0, 0, 0, 0, 0.21, 0, 0, 0, 0, 0, 0, 0.10, 0, 0, 0, 0, 0, 0, 0.07, 0, 0,
0, 0, 0, 0, 0.06, 0, 0, 0, 0, 0, 0, 0.11), nrow = 6, byrow = TRUE)
corr_matrix <- (Lambda %*% Phi %*% t(Lambda)) + Psi
corr_matrix
```

	BDI-II	HAMILTON	WHO	STAI	BAI	HADS-A
BDI-II	1.000	0.848	0.905	0.460	0.462	0.450
HAMILTON	0.848	1.000	0.843	0.429	0.431	0.419
WHO	0.905	0.843	1.000	0.457	0.460	0.448
STAI	0.460	0.429	0.457	1.000	0.933	0.910
BAI	0.462	0.431	0.460	0.933	1.000	0.915
HADS-A	0.450	0.419	0.448	0.910	0.915	1.000

Now that an admissible CFA model has been verified, a Monte Carlo simulation power analysis can now be performed, but that power analysis will not be performed here. CFA models in isolation rarely answer substantive research questions. However, the relationships between standardized factor loadings, reliability estimates, and measurement errors established with the CFA example will be useful when considering a more likely scenario needing a power analysis: a research question requiring a structural equation model (SEM).

SEM: Predictive Relationships among CFA Models

A SEM extends CFA modeling by proposing and testing predictive relationships among two or more CFA models. A hypothetical SEM is shown in Figure 4.6.

The SEM example shown assumes the following: (1) the exogenous latent variables X_1 and X_2 are identified using the unit latent factor variance constraint, (2) the latent variables X_1 and X_2 are correlated at a medium effect size ($r_{X1,X2} = 0.30$), and (3) all four latent variables

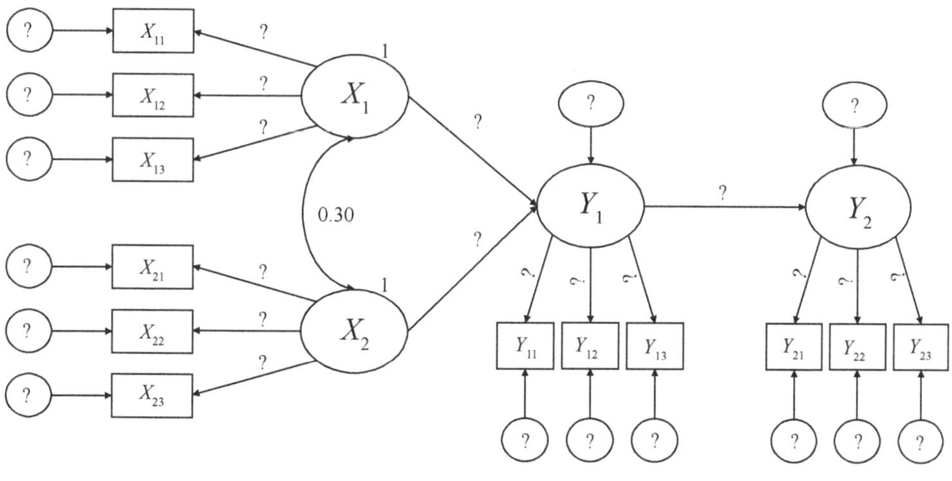

FIGURE 4.6. A hypothetical and incomplete SEM.

(X_1, X_2, Y_1, and Y_2) show simple structure. Let's further assume: (1) the observed variables (X_{11}, X_{12}, and X_{13}) measuring X_1 all show reliability estimates of $r_{xx} = 0.70$ ($\lambda_\beta = \sqrt{.70} = .8367$), (2) the observed variables (X_{21}, X_{22}, and X_{23}) measuring X_2 all show reliability estimates of $r_{xx} = 0.75$ ($\lambda_\beta = \sqrt{.75} = .866$), (3) the observed variables (Y_{11}, Y_{12}, and Y_{13}) measuring Y_1 all show reliability estimates of $r_{xx} = .80$ ($\lambda_\beta = \sqrt{.80} = .8944$), (4) the observed variables (Y_{21}, Y_{22}, and Y_{23}) measuring Y_2 all show reliability estimates of $r_{xx} = .85$ ($\lambda_\beta = \sqrt{.85} = .922$), and (5) measurement errors for all 12 observed variables ($\varepsilon_1 - \varepsilon_{12}$) were computed based, converting reliability estimates to measurement errors ($\varepsilon_1 - \varepsilon_{12} = 1 - R_{xx}$), as shown in Figure 4.7.

Let's further assume, based on a search of the empirical literature, a researcher is willing to test the following standardized regression coefficient values for X_1 and X_2 predicting Y_1 and predicting Y_2 (see Figure 4.8).

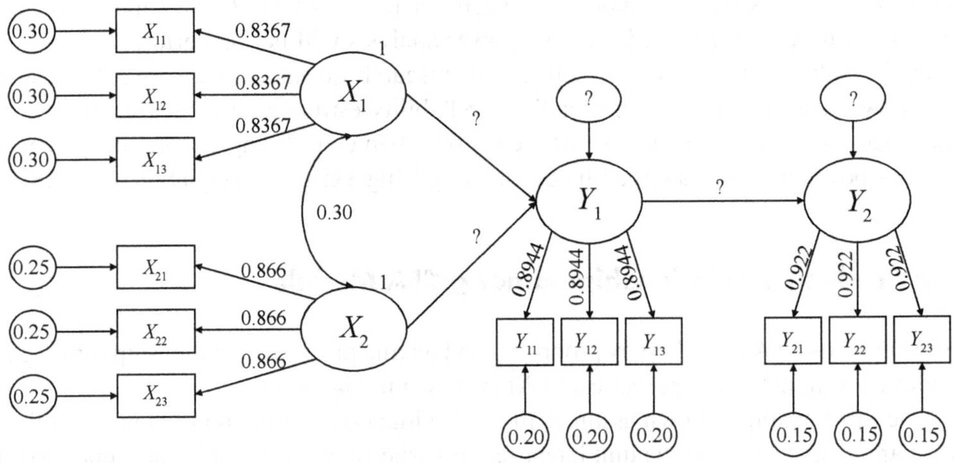

FIGURE 4.7. A hypothetical SEM with factor loadings and residual variances.

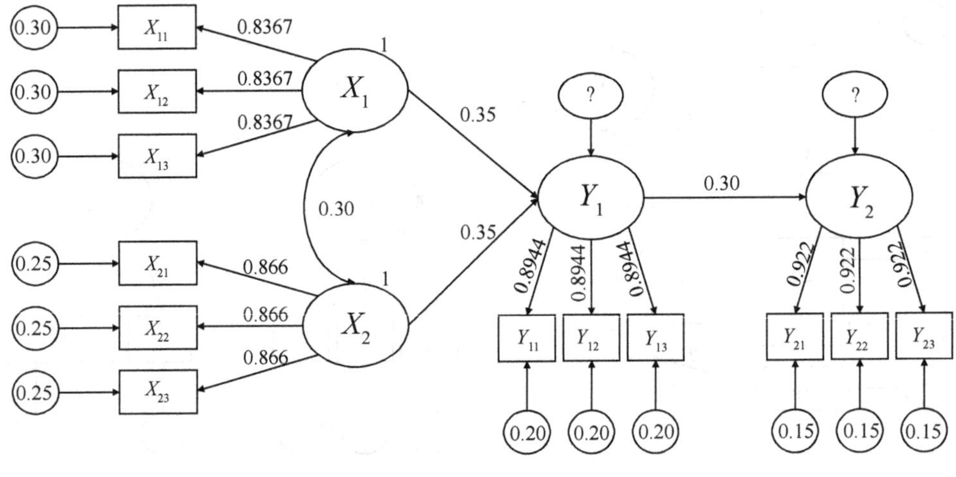

FIGURE 4.8. A hypothetical SEM with structural prediction values.

All that remains to be specified are the values for the ovals containing question marks above the Y_1 and Y_2 latent variables that refer to residual variances in Y_1 (i.e., variance unexplained by X_1 and X_2) and Y_2 (i.e., variance unexplained by Y_1). Residual variances for latent factors are commonly referred to as *disturbances*. It can quickly be seen in the example SEM that there are no indirect effects for the relationship between Y_1 and Y_2 that would not involve tracing through Y_1 more than once, which is not allowed under Wright's Rule #1. The disturbance for Y_2 can be computed by Equation (4.5):

$$R^2_{Y2|Y1} = (\beta_{Y2,Y1} * (\beta_{Y2,Y1} + [\text{Sum of indirect effects products}]))$$

$$= R^2_{Y1|Y1} = (0.30 * (0.30 + [\text{Sum of indirect effects products}]))$$

$$R^2_{Y1|X2} = (0.30 * (0.30 + [0]))$$

$$= R^2_{Y1|X2} = (0.30^2) = \underline{0.09}$$

so $$\sigma^2_{\text{DISTURBANCE}\_Y2} = 1 - R^2_{Y2|Y1} = 1 - 0.09 = \mathbf{0.91} \quad (4.5)$$

At this point, readers may notice, looking only at the structural relationships between X_1, X_2, and Y_1, this portion of the model looks very similar to the bivariate regression model example shown in Chapter 1. The $Y1$ disturbance can be computed the same way as for the residual for the bivariate regression response variable Y in Chapter 1 [Equations (4.6) and (4.7)].

For X_1:

$$R^2_{Y1|X1} = (\beta_{Y1|X1} * (\beta_{Y1|X1} + [\text{Indirect effects product}]))$$

$$R^2_{Y1|X1} = 0.35 * (0.35 + [Y_1 \text{ to } X_2, X_2 \text{ to } X_1])$$

$$R^2_{Y1|X1} = 0.35 * (0.35 + [0.35 * 0.30])$$

$$R^2_{Y1|X1} = 0.15925 \quad (4.6)$$

For X_2:

$$R^2_{Y1|X2} = \beta_{Y1|X2} * (\beta_{Y1|Xx} + [\text{Indirect effects product}])$$

$$R^2_{Y1|X2} = 0.35 * (0.35 + [Y_1 \text{ to } X_1, X_1 \text{ to } X_2])$$

$$R^2_{Y1|X2} = 0.35 * (0.35 + [0.35 * 0.30])$$

$$R^2_{Y1|X2} = 0.15925 \quad (4.7)$$

So

$$R^2_{Y1} = R^2_{Y1|X1} + R^2_{Y1|X2}$$

$$R^2_{Y1} = 0.15925 + 0.15925 = \underline{0.3185}$$

and $$\sigma^2_{\text{DISTURBANCE}\_Y1} = 1 - R^2_{Y1} == 1 - 0.3185 = \mathbf{0.6815} \quad (4.8)$$

Also see Figure 4.9.

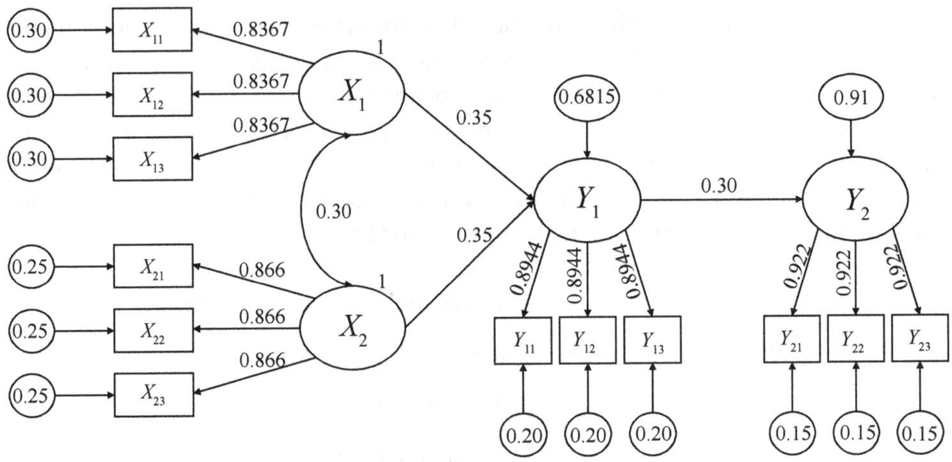

FIGURE 4.9. A complete hypothetical SEM.

With all SEM parameter estimates given specified values, the next step involves a SEM admissibility check. As shown in Bollen (1989, p. 325), the equations for computing a SEM model-reproduced correlation matrix (**Σθ**) are

$$\Sigma\theta = \begin{bmatrix} \Lambda_Y(\mathbf{I}-\mathbf{B})^{-1}(\Gamma\Phi\Gamma+\Psi)(\mathbf{I}-\mathbf{B}^T)^{-1}\Lambda_Y^T+\theta_\mu & \Lambda_Y(\mathbf{I}-\mathbf{B})^{-1}\Gamma\Phi\Lambda_X^T \\ \Lambda_X\Phi\Gamma^T(\mathbf{I}-\mathbf{B}^T)^{-1}\Lambda_Y^T & \Lambda_X\Phi\Lambda_X^T+\theta_\delta \end{bmatrix} \quad (4.9)$$

As shown in Equation (4.9), there are nine matrices ($\mathbf{\Lambda_X}$, $\mathbf{\Gamma}$, $\mathbf{\Phi}$, θ_δ, $\mathbf{\Lambda_Y}$, $\mathbf{B}$, $\mathbf{\Psi}$, $\theta\varepsilon$, and $\mathbf{I}$) used to compute a model-reproduced SEM correlation matrix. Each of the nine matrices is defined as follows.

$\mathbf{\Lambda_X}$ (Lambda_X) is a matrix with the number of rows equal to the number of observed exogenous variables (6; X_{11}–X_{23}), with the number of columns equal to the number of exogenous latent factors (2; X_1 and X_2), and the cells of the matrix contain the factor loadings, as in Equation (4.10).

$$\mathbf{\Lambda_X} = \begin{array}{c|cc|} & X_1 & X_2 \\ X_{11} & 0.8367 & 0 \\ X_{12} & 0.8367 & 0 \\ X_{13} & 0.8367 & 0 \\ X_{21} & 0 & 0.866 \\ X_{22} & 0 & 0.866 \\ X_{23} & 0 & 0.866 \end{array} \quad (4.10)$$

$\mathbf{\Gamma}$ (Gamma) is a matrix with the number of rows equal to the number of endogenous latent factors (2; Y_1 and Y_2), the number of columns equal to the number of exogenous latent factors (2; X_1 and X_2), and the cells of the matrix contain the regression coefficients for exogenous latent factors predicting endogenous latent factors, as in Equation (4.11).

$$\mathbf{\Gamma} = \begin{array}{c|cc|} & X_1 & X_2 \\ Y_1 & 0.35 & 0.35 \\ Y_2 & 0 & 0 \end{array} \tag{4.11}$$

$\mathbf{\Phi}$ (Phi) is a matrix with the number of rows and columns equal to the number of exogenous latent factors (2; X_1 and X_2) and the cells of the matrix contain the exogenous latent factor variances and correlation, as in Equation (4.12).

$$\mathbf{\Phi} = \begin{array}{c|cc|} & X_1 & X_2 \\ X_1 & 1 & 0.30 \\ X_2 & 0.30 & 1 \end{array} \tag{4.12}$$

$\mathbf{\theta_\delta}$ (Theta_delta) is a matrix with the number of rows and columns equal to the number of exogenous observed variables (6; $X_{11} - X_{23}$)) and the cells of the matrix contain the exogenous variable measurement errors ($\varepsilon_{X_{11}} - \varepsilon_{X_{23}}$), as in Equation (4.13)

$$\mathbf{\theta_\delta} = \begin{array}{c|cccccc|} & \varepsilon_{X11} & \varepsilon_{X12} & \varepsilon_{X13} & \varepsilon_{X21} & \varepsilon_{X22} & \varepsilon_{X23} \\ \varepsilon_{X11} & 0.30 & 0 & 0 & 0 & 0 & 0 \\ \varepsilon_{X12} & 0 & 0.30 & 0 & 0 & 0 & 0 \\ \varepsilon_{X13} & 0 & 0 & 0.30 & 0 & 0 & 0 \\ \varepsilon_{X21} & 0 & 0 & 0 & 0.30 & 0 & 0 \\ \varepsilon_{X22} & 0 & 0 & 0 & 0 & 0.30 & 0 \\ \varepsilon_{X23} & 0 & 0 & 0 & 0 & 0 & 0.30 \end{array} \tag{4.13}$$

$\mathbf{\Lambda_Y}$ (Lambda_Y) is a matrix with the number of rows equal to the number of observed endogenous variables (6; Y_{11}–Y_{23}), with the number of columns equal to the number of endogenous latent factors (2; Y_1 and Y_2), and the cells of the matrix contain the factor loadings, as in Equation (4.14).

$$\mathbf{\Lambda_Y} = \begin{array}{c|cc|} & Y_1 & Y_2 \\ Y_{11} & 0.8944 & 0 \\ Y_{12} & 0.8944 & 0 \\ Y_{13} & 0.8944 & 0 \\ Y_{21} & 0 & 0.922 \\ Y_{22} & 0 & 0.922 \\ Y_{23} & 0 & 0.922 \end{array} \tag{4.14}$$

B (Beta) is a matrix with the number of rows and columns equal to the number of endogenous latent factors (2; Y_1 and Y_2) and the cells of the matrix contain the regression coefficients for endogenous latent factors predicting other endogenous latent factors, as in Equation (4.15).

$$\mathbf{B} = \begin{array}{c|cc|} & Y_1 & Y_2 \\ Y_1 & 0 & 0 \\ Y_2 & 0.30 & 0 \end{array} \tag{4.15}$$

Ψ (Psi) is a matrix with the number of rows and columns equal to the number of endogenous latent factors (2; Y_1 and Y_2) and the cells of the matrix contain the endogenous latent factor disturbances, as in Equation (4.16).

$$\boldsymbol{\Psi} = \begin{array}{c|cc|} & Y_1 & Y_2 \\ Y_1 & 0.6815 & 0 \\ Y_2 & 0 & 0.91 \end{array} \tag{4.16}$$

θε (Theta_epsilon) is a matrix with the number of rows and columns equal to the number of endogenous observed variables (6; Y_{11}–Y_{23})) and the cells of the matrix contain the endogenous variable measurement errors ($\varepsilon_{X_{11}} - \varepsilon_{X_{23}}$), as in Equation (4.17).

$$\boldsymbol{\theta}_{\varepsilon} = \begin{array}{c|cccccc|} & \varepsilon_{Y11} & \varepsilon_{Y12} & \varepsilon_{Y13} & \varepsilon_{Y21} & \varepsilon_{Y22} & \varepsilon_{Y23} \\ \varepsilon_{Y11} & 0.20 & 0 & 0 & 0 & 0 & 0 \\ \varepsilon_{Y12} & 0 & 0.20 & 0 & 0 & 0 & 0 \\ \varepsilon_{Y13} & 0 & 0 & 0.20 & 0 & 0 & 0 \\ \varepsilon_{Y21} & 0 & 0 & 0 & 0.15 & 0 & 0 \\ \varepsilon_{Y22} & 0 & 0 & 0 & 0 & 0.15 & 0 \\ \varepsilon_{Y23} & 0 & 0 & 0 & 0 & 0 & 0.15 \end{array} \tag{4.17}$$

I is an identity matrix with the number of rows and columns equal to the number of endogenous latent factors (2; Y_1 and Y_2) and the cells on the diagonal of the matrix contain values of 1 and off-diagonal cells contain values of zero, as in Equation (4.18).

$$\mathbf{I} = \begin{array}{c|cc|} & Y_1 & Y_2 \\ Y_1 & 1 & 0 \\ Y_2 & 0 & 1 \end{array} \tag{4.18}$$

Finally, a SEM model-reproduced correlation matrix can be computed using the R syntax in the next section.

R Code for SEM Model-Reproduced Correlation Matrix

```
Lambda_X <- matrix(c(.8367, 0, .8367, 0, .8367, 0, 0, .866, 0, .866, 0, .866), ncol = 2, byrow =
    TRUE)
Gamma <- matrix(c(.35, .35, 0, 0), ncol = 2, byrow = TRUE)
Phi <- matrix(c(1, .3, .3, 1), nrow = 2, byrow = TRUE)
Theta_Delta <- matrix(c(.30, 0, 0, 0, 0, 0, 0, .30, 0, 0, 0, 0, 0, 0, .30, 0, 0, 0, 0, 0, 0, .25, 0, 0, 0,
    0, 0, 0, .25, 0, 0, 0, 0, 0, 0, .25), nrow = 6, byrow = TRUE)
Theta_Epsilon <- matrix(c(.20, 0, 0, 0, 0, 0, 0, .20, 0, 0, 0, 0, 0, 0, .20, 0, 0, 0, 0, 0, 0, .15, 0, 0,
    0, 0, 0, 0, .15, 0, 0, 0, 0, 0, 0, .15), nrow = 6, byrow = TRUE)
Lambda_Y <- matrix(c(.8944, 0, .8944, 0, .8944, 0, 0, .922, 0, .922, 0, .922), ncol = 2, byrow =
    TRUE)
Beta <- matrix(c(0, 0, .3, 0), ncol = 2, byrow = TRUE)
Psi <- matrix(c(.6815, 0, 0, .91), ncol = 2, byrow = TRUE)
I <- matrix(c(1, 0, 0, 1), ncol = 2, byrow = TRUE)
upper_left <- Lambda_Y %*% (solve(I-Beta)) %*% (Gamma %*% Phi %*% t(Gamma) + Psi)
    %*% t(solve(I-Beta)) %*% t(Lambda_Y) + Theta_Epsilon
upper_right <- Lambda_Y %*% (solve(I-Beta)) %*% Gamma %*% Phi %*% t(Lambda_X)
upper <- cbind(upper_left, upper_right)
lower_left <- Lambda_X %*% Phi %*% t(Gamma) %*% t(solve(I-Beta)) %*% t(Lambda_Y)
lower_right <- Lambda_X %*% Phi %*% t(Lambda_X) + Theta_Delta
lower <- cbind(lower_left, lower_right)
cov_matrix <- rbind(upper, lower)
cov_matrix
```

The admissible model-reproduced covariance matrix shows all expected relationships among variables.

	Y_{11}	Y_{12}	Y_{13}	Y_{21}	Y_{22}	Y_{23}	X_{11}	X_{12}	X_{13}	X_{21}	X_{22}	X_{23}
Y_{11}	1.000	0.800	0.800	0.247	0.247	0.247	0.340	0.340	0.340	0.357	0.357	0.357
Y_{12}	0.800	1.000	0.800	0.247	0.247	0.247	0.340	0.340	0.340	0.357	0.357	0.357
Y_{13}	0.800	0.800	1.000	0.247	0.247	0.247	0.340	0.340	0.340	0.357	0.357	0.357
Y_{21}	0.247	0.247	0.247	1.000	0.850	0.850	0.105	0.105	0.105	0.109	0.109	0.109
Y_{22}	0.247	0.247	0.247	0.850	1.000	0.850	0.105	0.105	0.105	0.109	0.109	0.109
Y_{23}	0.247	0.247	0.247	0.850	0.850	1.000	0.105	0.105	0.105	0.109	0.109	0.109
X_{11}	0.340	0.340	0.340	0.105	0.105	0.105	1.000	0.700	0.700	0.217	0.217	0.217
X_{12}	0.340	0.340	0.340	0.105	0.105	0.105	0.700	1.000	0.700	0.217	0.217	0.217
X_{13}	0.340	0.340	0.340	0.105	0.105	0.105	0.700	0.700	1.000	0.217	0.217	0.217
X_{21}	0.357	0.357	0.357	0.109	0.109	0.109	0.217	0.217	0.217	1.000	0.750	0.750
X_{22}	0.357	0.357	0.357	0.109	0.109	0.109	0.217	0.217	0.217	0.750	1.000	0.750
X_{23}	0.357	0.357	0.357	0.109	0.109	0.109	0.217	0.217	0.217	0.750	0.750	1.000

Now that the SEM example model has been verified using an admissible model-reproduced correlation matrix, a power analysis can now be performed, assuming the power analysis question of interest is the smallest sample size needed to reject the null hypotheses for all structural predictions (i.e., the three regression coefficients contained in $\mathbf{\Gamma}$ and $\mathbf{B}$) with power $\geq .80$.

Both Mplus and R can be used to complete the power analysis for this model.

Mplus Monte Carlo Power Analysis: SEM

The Mplus syntax needed to perform the power analysis is shown as follows:

```
TITLE: MPLUS 4.1 SEM

MONTECARLO:
NAMES ARE
X11 X12 X13 X21 X22 X23
Y11 Y12 Y13 Y21 Y22 Y23;

NOBSERVATIONS = 99;

NREPS = 5000;

MODEL POPULATION:
X1 BY X11*.8367 X12*.8367 X13*.8367;
X2 BY X21*.866 X22*.866 X23*.866;
Y1 BY Y11*.8944 Y12*.8944 Y13*.8944;
Y2 BY Y21*.922 Y22*.922 Y23*.922;

X1@1;
X2@1;
Y1@.6815;
Y2@.91;

X1 WITH X2*.3;

Y1 ON X1*.35 X2*.35;
Y2 ON Y1*.3;

X11-X13*.30;
X21-X23*.25;
Y11-Y13*.20;
Y21-Y23*.15;

Analysis:
estimator = ml;

MODEL:
X1 BY X11*.8367 X12*.8367 X13*.8367;
X2 BY X21*.866 X22*.866 X23*.866;
Y1 BY Y11*.8944 Y12*.8944 Y13*.8944;
Y2 BY Y21*.922 Y22*.922 Y23*.922;

X1@1;
X2@1;
Y1@.6815;
Y2@.91;
```

```
X1 WITH X2*.3;

Y1 ON X1*.35 X2*.35;
Y2 ON Y1*.3;

X11-X13*.30;
X21-X23*.25;
Y11-Y13*.20;
Y21-Y23*.15;

OUTPUT: res;
```

All the Mplus syntax interpretations remain consistent with previous examples, but with two exceptions for this example. First, notice how the `BY` keyword (meaning "measured by") is used to initialize and specify the four latent factors by relating each to their respective observed indicator variables. Second, in previous analysis examples, the asterisk (*) was used to allow random variation in all parameter estimates across simulated datasets. The asterisk is again used here for most parameters except for the specification of the exogenous latent factor variances and endogenous latent disturbances, `X1@1; X2@1; Y1@.6815; Y2@.91;`. Recall from the CFA example that the unit latent factor variance constraint was needed to establish a scale for the latent factor scores. However, because all four latent variables are measured by three observed indicators and all four latent factors show simple structure, the CFA model is not identified unless the unit latent variances are constrained to a specific value. In the present example, each latent variable is measured by three observed indicators, which means that there are (3 * [3 + 1]) / 2 = 6 unique pieces of information for each construct. Assuming the unit latent factor variance constraint is used to set the latent factor measurement scale, there are 6 parameters (3 factor loadings and 3 measurement errors) to be estimated, which means that the model has (6 – 6) or 0 degrees of freedom, so the model is *just-identified*: there is an equal amount of unique information and needed parameter estimates. Constraining the latent factor variances is accomplished by using the "at" (@) symbol (meaning "fixed at"), which does not allow random variation to be introduced into constraints needed to identify the four CFA models contained within the SEM example.

Recall that in Mplus the '`MODEL POPULATION:`' command specifies how the Monte Carlo simulation data are to be generated. Adding a '`MODEL:`' command specifies how the generated data are to be analyzed. Often, but not always (as shown in Chapter 5), researchers have two options when specifying a '`MODEL:`' command. The simplest option involves including only those statements needed to specify a SEM: the four '`BY`', two '`ON`', and one '`WITH`' statement. A second option would involve simply copying all the '`MODEL POPULATION:`' specifications and pasting them into the '`MODEL:`' command. The advantage of the latter option is that it would allow a researcher to gauge how well values specified for the 5,000 generated data replications are being reproduced in analyses. Combined syntax using the latter '`MODEL:`' command option, as well as results from running the combined Mplus syntax (Mplus 4.1), are both shown below.

```
MONTECARLO:
NAMES ARE
```

```
X11 X12 X13 X21 X22 X23
Y11 Y12 Y13 Y21 Y22 Y23;

NOBSERVATIONS = 99;

NREPS = 5000;

MODEL POPULATION:
X1 BY X11*.8367 X12*.8367 X13*.8367;
X2 BY X21*.866 X22*.866 X23*.866;
Y1 BY Y11*.8944 Y12*.8944 Y13*.8944;
Y2 BY Y21*.922 Y22*.922 Y23*.922;

X1@1;
X2@1;
Y1@.6815;
Y2@.91;

X1 WITH X2*.3;

Y1 ON X1*.35 X2*.35;
Y2 ON Y1*.3;

X11-X13*.30;
X21-X23*.25;
Y11-Y13*.20;
Y21-Y23*.15;

Analysis:
estimator = ml;

MODEL:
X1 BY X11*.8367 X12*.8367 X13*.8367;
X2 BY X21*.866 X22*.866 X23*.866;
Y1 BY Y11*.8944 Y12*.8944 Y13*.8944;
Y2 BY Y21*.922 Y22*.922 Y23*.922;

X1@1;
X2@1;
Y1@.6815;
Y2@.91;

X1 WITH X2*.3;

Y1 ON X1*.35 X2*.35;
Y2 ON Y1*.3;

X11-X13*.30;
X21-X23*.25;
Y11-Y13*.20;
Y21-Y23*.15;
```

```
MODEL RESULTS

                           ESTIMATES                S. E.     M. S. E.   95%   % Sig
              Population   Average    Std. Dev.   Average              Cover  Coeff
Y1        ON
 X1              0.350      0.3592      0.1153     0.1120     0.0134  0.950  0.916
 X2              0.350      0.3556      0.1138     0.1101     0.0130  0.946  0.917

 Y2        ON
 Y1              0.300      0.2992      0.1115     0.1084     0.0124  0.951  0.807
```

As shown in these results, a sample size of $N = 99$ is needed for power $\geq .80$ to reject the null hypothesis for all three structural predictions.

R Monte Carlo Power Analysis: SEM

Using R to accomplish the same SEM power analysis is as straightforward as it was in Mplus. Using the packages lavaan and simsem, the population model is specified as follows:

```
library(simsem)
library(lavaan)

PopulationModel_Ch4 <- "
 X1 =~ 0.8367*X11 + 0.8367*X12 + 0.8367*X13
 X2 =~ 0.866*X21 + 0.866*X22 + 0.866*X23
 Y1 =~ 0.8944*Y11 + 0.8944*Y12 + 0.8944*Y13
 Y2 =~ 0.922*Y21 + 0.922*Y22 + 0.922*Y23

 X1 ~~ 1*X1
 X2 ~~ 1*X2
 Y1 ~~ 0.6815*Y1
 Y2 ~~ 0.91*Y2

 X1 ~~ 0.30*X2

 Y1 ~ 0.35*X1 + 0.35*X2
 Y2 ~ 0.30*Y1

 X11 ~~ 0.30*X11
 X12 ~~ 0.30*X12
 X13 ~~ 0.30*X13
 X21 ~~ 0.25*X21
 X22 ~~ 0.25*X22
 X23 ~~ 0.25*X23
 Y11 ~~ 0.20*Y11
 Y12 ~~ 0.20*Y12
 Y13 ~~ 0.20*Y13
 Y21 ~~ 0.15*Y21
 Y22 ~~ 0.15*Y22
 Y23 ~~ 0.15*Y23"
```

One advantage of using simsem is the ability to automatically assess the accuracy of the covariance matrix before proceeding with the full simulation. To do this, the following code:

```
fitted(sem(PopulationModel_Ch4))
```

results in the lower half of the model-implied covariance matrix.

```
$cov
     X11   X12   X13   X21   X22   X23   Y11   Y12   Y13   Y21   Y22   Y23
X11  1.00
X12  0.70  1.00
X13  0.70  0.70  1.00
X21  0.22  0.22  0.22  1.00
X22  0.22  0.22  0.22  0.75  1.00
X23  0.22  0.22  0.22  0.75  0.75  1.00
Y11  0.34  0.34  0.34  0.35  0.35  0.35  1.00
Y12  0.34  0.34  0.34  0.35  0.35  0.35  0.80  1.00
Y13  0.34  0.34  0.34  0.35  0.35  0.35  0.80  0.80  1.00
Y21  0.11  0.11  0.11  0.11  0.11  0.11  0.25  0.25  0.25  1.00
Y22  0.11  0.11  0.11  0.11  0.11  0.11  0.25  0.25  0.25  0.85  1.00
Y23  0.11  0.11  0.11  0.11  0.11  0.11  0.25  0.25  0.25  0.85  0.85  1.00
```

The analysis model is then written:

```
AnalysisModel_Ch4 <- "
  X1 =~ X11 + X12 + X13
  X2 =~ X21 + X22 + X23
  Y1 =~ Y11 + Y12 + Y13
  Y2 =~ Y21 + Y22 + Y23

  X1 ~~ 1*X1 #constrain all factor variances to freely estimate the factor loadings
  X2 ~~ 1*X2
  Y1 ~~ 0.6815*Y1
  Y2 ~~ 0.91*Y2

  X1 ~~ X2

  Y1 ~ X1 + X2
  Y2 ~ Y1

  X11 ~~ X11
  X12 ~~ X12
  X13 ~~ X13
  X21 ~~ X21
  X22 ~~ X22
  X23 ~~ X23
  Y11 ~~ Y11
```

```
Y12 ~~ Y12
Y13 ~~ Y13
Y21 ~~ Y21
Y22 ~~ Y22
Y23 ~~ Y23"
```

Similar to the Mplus @ syntax, R can constrain loadings to a specific value using the * syntax in the analysis model. Here, the latent X variances are constrained to 1 while the endogenous latent Y variances are constrained to 0.6815 and 0.91, respectively. After specifying both the population and analysis models, the power analysis can now be completed using the sim() command in the simsem package.

```
output_Ch4 <- sim( nRep = 5000,
             n = 99,
             model = AnalysisModel_Ch4
             generate = PopulationModel_Ch4
             std.lv = FALSE,
             seed = 35170,
             silent = TRUE)
```

An overall summary of results can be obtained using summary(output_Ch4). The simulation output summary contains two elements that can be examined: (1) a summary of the model fit and convergence and (2) a dataframe that contains the Monte Carlo simulation model estimates. Examining model convergence shows that all but one replication converged; one model randomly contained a non-positive-definite sample covariance matrix. Note that one model not converging is not problematic and results can still be interpreted, given the large number of replications that did converge.

```
================== Replications =====================
Number of replications = 5000
Number of converged replications = 4999
Number of nonconverged replications:
  1. Nonconvergent Results = 0
  2. Nonconvergent results from multiple imputation = 0
  3. At least one SE were negative or NA = 0
  4. Nonpositive-definite latent or observed (residual) covariance matrix
     (e.g., Heywood case or linear dependency) = 1
```

Statistical power can be obtained by examining summary output, but it is only necessary to evaluate the statistical power estimate for the parameter(s) of interest, which can be obtained by using the getPower() function in combination with the name of the output file and the parameter name.

```
getPower(output_Ch4)[c("Y1~X1", "Y1~X2", "Y2~Y1")]
Y1~X1       Y1~X2       Y2~Y1
0.9122      0.9286      0.8046
```

The obtained power for the effects of interest are .91, .93, and .80, so a sample size of $N = 99$ is sufficient to detect the expected effects.

Impacts of Unreliability on SEM Power Estimates

In the SEM approach just shown, the statistical power was estimated assuming relatively reliable measures. One topic to consider when conducting power analyses using SEM is that indicators may *not* always be reliable, or may have varying degrees of reliability, and this should be considered when conducting the power analysis assessment. Although reliability will not inherently impact the strength of the relationships among constructs, they can impact the statistical power to find a specified strength of relationships among constructs. SEMs that contain more measurement error and lower indicator reliabilities will require higher sample sizes while SEMs that contain less measurement error and greater indicator reliabilities will require lower sample sizes. Illustrating the effect of reliability on statistical power estimates warrants an additional example. In the example SEM above, all indicator variables were specified to have reliability estimates between $R_{xx} = 0.70$ and 0.85 which reflect values generally considered acceptable. Let's assume indicator variables with questionably lower reliability estimates were used and now range between $R_{xx} = 0.50$ and 0.65 and all other specifications remain the same.

Using Mplus, the model input changes minimally and only in the population model.

Mplus Syntax for Lower Reliability SEM Power Analysis

```
TITLE: MPLUS 4.2 SEM LOWER RELIABILITY

MONTECARLO:
NAMES ARE
X11 X12 X13 X21 X22 X23
Y11 Y12 Y13 Y21 Y22 Y23;

NOBSERVATIONS = 126;

NREPS = 5000;

MODEL POPULATION:
X1 BY X11*.7071 X12*.7071 X13*.7071;
X2 BY X21*.7416 X22*.7416 X23*.7416;
Y1 BY Y11*.7746 Y12*.7746 Y13*.7746;
Y2 BY Y21*.8062 Y22*.8062 Y23*.8062;

X1@1;
X2@1;
Y1@.6815;
Y2@.91;

X1 WITH X2*.3;

Y1 ON X1*.35 X2*.35;
Y2 ON Y1*.3;
```

```
X11-X13*.5;
X21-X23*.45;
Y11-Y13*.4;
Y21-Y23*.35;

ANALYSIS:
estimator = ml;

MODEL:
X1 BY X11*.7071 X12*.7071 X13*.7071;
X2 BY X21*.7416 X22*.7416 X23*.7416;
Y1 BY Y11*.7746 Y12*.7746 Y13*.7746;
Y2 BY Y21*.8062 Y22*.8062 Y23*.8062;

X1@1;
X2@1;
X1 WITH X2*.3;

Y1@.6815;
Y2@.91;

Y1 ON X1*.35 X2*.35;
Y2 ON Y1*.3;

X11-X13*.5;
X21-X23*.45;
Y11-Y13*.4;
Y21-Y23*.35;

OUTPUT: res;
```

The above `MODEL POPULATION:` specifications are copied and pasted into a `MODEL:` command. Results from the SEM Monte Carlo simulation power analysis assuming lower internal consistency reliability estimates (Mplus 4.2) is shown below.

```
MODEL RESULTS

                              ESTIMATES                S. E.      M. S. E.  95%   % Sig
                  Population  Average    Std. Dev.   Average               Cover Coeff
Y1        ON
  X1                  0.350    0.3612     0.1269      0.1224      0.0162 0.952 0.871
  X2                  0.350    0.3569     0.1226      0.1190      0.0151 0.955 0.876

 Y2        ON
  Y1                  0.300    0.2983     0.1115      0.1091      0.0124 0.949 0.805
```

Likewise, in R, the changes to syntax occur only within the population model,

R Syntax for Lower Reliability SEM Power Analysis

```
PopulationModel <- "
  X1 =~ 0.7071*X11 + 0.7071*X12 + 0.7071*X13
  X2 =~ 0.7416*X21 + 0.7416*X22 + 0.7416*X23
  Y1 =~ 0.7746*Y11 + 0.7746*Y12 + 0.7746*Y13
  Y2 =~ 0.8062*Y21 + 0.8062*Y22 + 0.8062*Y23

  X1 ~~ 1*X1
  X2 ~~ 1*X2
  Y1 ~~ 0.6815*Y1
  Y2 ~~ 0.91*Y2

  X1 ~~ 0.30*X2

  Y1 ~ 0.35*X1 + 0.35*X2
  Y2 ~ 0.30*Y1

  X11 ~~ 0.50*X11
  X12 ~~ 0.50*X12
  X13 ~~ 0.50*X13
  X21 ~~ 0.45*X21
  X22 ~~ 0.45*X22
  X23 ~~ 0.45*X23
  Y11 ~~ 0.40*Y11
  Y12 ~~ 0.40*Y12
  Y13 ~~ 0.40*Y13
  Y21 ~~ 0.35*Y21
  Y22 ~~ 0.35*Y22
  Y23 ~~ 0.35*Y23
"
```

and after reevaluating the simulation power analysis with this new population model, using R code from earlier in this chapter, power estimate results for effects of interest are .8760, .8858, and .8152, which are comparable to those found in Mplus.

As shown in both the Mplus and R syntax results above, and due to the use of observed indicator variables with considerably lower internal consistency reliability estimates, a sample size of $N = 126$, a roughly 25% increase, is now needed for power $\geq .80$ to reject the null hypothesis for all three structural predictions.

Simulation Power Analysis Write-Up: SEM

An example SEM Monte Carlo simulation power analysis write-up using Mplus (but it could be modified to reflect results found from R) is shown below and consists of four sections: (1) a statement of the power analysis question; (2) a description of how power was calculated, including the data analysis model assumed, and the statistical software package and version used; (3) a clear statement of all power analysis assumptions, including specific parameter estimate values; and (4) a clear answer to the power analysis question that includes the number of simulated dataset replications requested, the effect size assumed, and the sample size needed to achieve power ≥ .80:

> "The power analysis question involves the smallest sample size needed to achieve power ≥ .80 to reject the null hypothesis for the three structural coefficients in the proposed SEM. A Monte Carlo simulation power analysis was conducted using Mplus (version 8.6) assuming: (1) a unit latent factor variance constraint was used to identify the four latent variables (X_1, X_2, Y_1, and Y_2) in the SEM, (2) the latent exogenous variables (X_1 and X_2) were correlated at $r_{X1,X2} = 0.30$, (3) reliability (R_{xx}) estimates ranging between 0.70 and 0.85 were used to specify all 12 standardized factor loadings (λ_β) for the four latent variables by $\lambda_\beta = \sqrt{R_{xx}}$, (4) reliability ($R_{xx}$) estimates were also used to specify measurement error variances (ε) by $\varepsilon = 1 - R_{xx}$, (5) standardized regression coefficient values of $\beta = 0.35$ were assumed for both latent exogenous variables (X_1 and X_2) predicting the endogenous latent variable Y_1, resulting in ($R^2 = 0.3185$) 31.85% of Y_1 variance explained by X_1 and X_2, (6) a standardized regression coefficient value of $\beta = 0.30$ was assumed for the endogenous latent variable Y_1 as a predictor of endogenous latent variable Y_2, resulting in ($R^2 = 0.09$) 9% of Y_2 variance explained by Y_1, and (7) the admissibility of the SEM specifications was verified by computing a model-reproduced correlation matrix. Monte Carlo simulation power analysis results aggregated over 5,000 replications showed power ≥ .80 to reject the null hypothesis for all three SEM structural coefficients for a sample size of $N = 99$."

SUGGESTED READINGS

- Berkout, O. V., Gross, A. M., & Young, J. (2014). Why so many arrows? Introduction to structural equation modeling for the novitiate user. *Clinical Child and Family Psychology Review, 17,* 217–229.
- Buchberger, E. S., Ngo, C. T., Peikert, A., Brandmaier, A. M., & Werkle-Bergner, M. (2024). Estimating statistical power for structural equation models in developmental cognitive science: A tutorial in R: Power simulation for SEMs. *Behavior Research Methods, 56*(7), 1–18.
- Dragan, D., & Topolšek, D. (2014, June). Introduction to structural equation modeling: Review, methodology and practical applications. In *The 11th International Conference on Logistics* (pp. 1–27).
- Goldsmith, K. A., MacKinnon, D. P., Chalder, T., White, P. D., Sharpe, M., & Pickles, A. (2018). Tutorial: The practical application of longitudinal structural equation mediation models in clinical trials. *Psychological Methods, 23,* 191–207.
- Hancock, G. R., & Mueller, R. O. (2011). The reliability paradox in assessing structural relations within covariance structure models. *Educational and Psychological Measurement, 71,* 306–324.
- Heene, M., Hilbert, S., Draxler, C., Ziegler, M., & Bühner, M. (2011). Masking misfit in confirmatory factor analysis by increasing unique variances: A cautionary note on the usefulness of cutoff values of fit indices. *Psychological Methods, 16,* 319–336.

- Hox, J. J., & Bechger, T. M. (1998). An introduction to structural equation modeling. *Family Science Review, 11*, 354–373.
- Jak, S., Jorgensen, T. D., Verdam, M. G., Oort, F. J., & Elffers, L. (2021). Analytical power calculations for structural equation modeling: A tutorial and Shiny app. *Behavior Research Methods, 53*, 1385–1406.
- Jobst, L. J., Bader, M., & Moshagen, M. (2023). A tutorial on assessing statistical power and determining sample size for structural equation models. *Psychological Methods, 28*(1), 207–221.
- Lee, T., & Shi, D. (2021). A comparison of full information maximum likelihood and multiple imputation in structural equation modeling with missing data. *Psychological Methods, 26*, 466–485.
- Lei, P. W., & Wu, Q. (2007). Introduction to structural equation modeling: Issues and practical considerations. *Educational Measurement: Issues and Practice, 26*, 33–43.
- McNeish, D., An, J., & Hancock, G. R. (2018). The thorny relation between measurement quality and fit index cutoffs in latent variable models. *Journal of Personality Assessment, 100*, 43–52.
- Moshagen, M., & Bader, M. (2024). semPower: General power analysis for structural equation models. *Behavior Research Methods, 56*(4), 2901–2922.
- Rhemtulla, M., van Bork, R., & Borsboom, D. (2020). Worse than measurement error: Consequences of inappropriate latent variable measurement models. *Psychological Methods, 25*, 30–45.
- Tarka, P. (2018). An overview of structural equation modeling: Its beginnings, historical development, usefulness and controversies in the social sciences. *Quality & Quantity, 52*, 313–354.
- Wang, Y. A., & Rhemtulla, M. (2021). Power analysis for parameter estimation in structural equation modeling: A discussion and tutorial. *Advances in Methods and Practices in Psychological Science, 4*, 1–17.
- Zhai, H., Li, Q., & Wei, X. (2022). Power analysis in structural equation modeling: Principles and methods. *Advances in Psychological Science, 30*(9), 2117–2130.

5

Logistic Regression

A Prelude to Missing Data Inclusion

The Logistical Foundation: Probabilities, Odds, and Log Odds (Logits)

All of the previous chapters have dealt with response variables measured on a continuous scale. However, many response variables of interest across a great many areas of research exist naturally as a simple indicator of whether or not an event of research interest occurred. The birth of a child or the death of a family member, getting married or divorced, being hired to or fired from a job, graduating from or dropping out of high school or college, getting arrested and convicted of a crime, or whether a patient meets diagnostic criteria for a specific disease or disorder are only a few of the response variables of potential research interest that can be measured as a binary indicator of whether (= 1) or not (= 0) the particular event occurred. Furthermore, the *mean* of a binary variable is defined as the proportion of respondents who experienced the event of interest. Proportions are bounded by values of 0 and 1, and this would appear, at first glance, to reflect a continuous measurement scale. If so, it would seem reasonable to assume a multiple regression could be used, even with a binary indicator response variable, to model probabilities (*Pr*) of event occurrence as shown in Equation (5.1)

$$Pr(Y_{i_{\text{BINARY}}} = 1) = \beta_0 + \beta_1(X_i) + \varepsilon_i \tag{5.1}$$

It would, by extension, also seem reasonable to interpret Equation (5.1) as a unit increases in the (X_i) predictor variable, indicating the expected change (β_1) in the probability of observing a response variable value of 1. The difficulty in the previous assumptions stems from the fact that multiple regression assumes a linear relationship between predictor and response variables, and this causes three specific problems when the response variable is binary:

1. Use of multiple regression with a binary response variable could produce parameter estimates that result in model-predicted proportions less than 0 or greater than 1.
2. Multiple regression further assumes *homoscedasticity*, which is defined as the expectation that the residual variance (σ_ε^2) in binary Y proportions, for each (X_i) predictor variable value, is a constant. The likelihood of this assumption being violated can be illustrated with a simple example. If age (X_i) was used to predict a binary response variable indicating the birth of a first child ($Y_{i_{\text{BINARY}}}$), it is reasonable to assume a probability at or near .50 (with greater variability) for a participant at or near 25 years of age, but a much lower probability at or near .05 (with much less variability) for a participant between 45 and 55 years of age. Stated differently, a predictor variable (X_i) could have a very different effect on the binary response, depending on where in the probability distribution the effect of a unit increase in (X_i) results in the greatest expected probability change.
3. Multiple regression also assumes that at each (X_i) predictor variable value, the response variable proportions are assumed to be normally distributed around a predicted mean probability defined by $\beta_0 + \beta_1(X_i)$. If the response variable is binary, the residual variance will be binomially distributed by definition, and not normally distributed.

What is needed is a way to model binary response probabilities such that greater probability changes per unit increase in (X_i) occur near the middle (50%) of the probability distribution versus the extremes (5% or 95%), but that also allows binary probabilities to maintain a linear relationship with predictor variables. This goal can be accomplished using a two-step process that first mathematically removes the ceiling effect, or upper bound, of 1, and then mathematically removes the floor effect, or lower bound, of 0.

First, *odds* are defined as a ratio of probabilities (*Pr*) and are computed as shown in (Equation (5.2)

$$Pr(Y_{i_{\text{BINARY}}} = 1)/1 - Pr(Y_{i_{\text{BINARY}}} = 1) \tag{5.2}$$

It can easily be seen in Equation (5.2) that, for any probability value greater than zero and less than one, the resulting odds will always be a positive value. If odds can be computed as a function of probabilities, then probabilities can also be computed as a function of odds by $Pr(Y_{i_{\text{BINARY}}} = 1) = \text{Odds}/1 + \text{Odds}$. Regardless of the magnitude of the odds value considered, the resulting probability (*Pr*) will never achieve or exceed a value of 1. Using probabilities to compute odds (or vice versa) essentially removes the upper bound, or ceiling effect, for ($Y_{i_{\text{BINARY}}} = 1$). Second, applying a natural logarithm transformation (ln) to the formula for computing odds from probabilities results in log odds, or *logits*, by Equation (5.3)

$$\text{Logit} = \text{log odds} = \ln[Pr(Y_{i_{\text{BINARY}}} = 1)/1 - Pr(Y_{i_{\text{BINARY}}} = 1)] \tag{5.3}$$

Logits, or log odds, removes the floor effect, or lower bound, for ($Y_{i_{\text{BINARY}}} = 0$) because logits have neither an upper limit nor a lower limit. More importantly, the logit measurement scale is symmetric at the middle (i.e., Pr = .50, or odds = 1) of the probability distribution for ($Y_{i_{\text{BINARY}}}$ = 1), but unit changes in probability of ($Y_{i_{\text{BINARY}}}$ = 1) result in different magnitudes of change in logits at different locations in the probability distribution. Most importantly, converting probabilities to log odds allows Equation (5.3) to be extended to Equation (5.4)

$$\text{Logit} = \text{log odds} = \ln[Pr(Y_{i_{\text{BINARY}}} = 1)/1 - Pr(Y_{i_{\text{BINARY}}} = 1)] = \beta_0 + \beta_1 X \tag{5.4}$$

Equation (5.4) shows that by applying a logit transformation to the equation to compute odds, binary response variable probabilities can now be modeled as a linear function ($\beta_0 + \beta_1 X$) of predictor variables (X_i). Specifically, as shown in in Figure 5.1, the previously stated goal of modeling binary response probabilities, such that greater probability changes per unit increase in (X_i) occur near the middle (50%) of the probability distribution versus the extremes (5% or 95%), but in a way that allows binary probabilities to maintain a linear relationship with predictor variables, has been met.

Furthermore, logits can be converted back to probabilities (Pr) by using the mathematical inverse of a natural logarithm: exponentiation, as shown in Equation (5.5)

$$Pr = \exp^{(\beta_0 + \beta_1 X)} / 1 + \exp^{(\beta_0 + \beta_1 X)} \tag{5.5}$$

Finally, logit slope estimates (β_1) can be interpreted as odds ratios, or the expected change in the odds of observing a response variable of 1 versus 0, for each unit increase in X also by exponentiation, or $\exp^{\beta_1}$. Although not readily apparent or obvious, Equation (5.5) does show the two primary pieces of information needed to perform a Monte Carlo simulation power analysis for a logistic regression: (1) researchers must specify the anticipated odds ratio effects for each predictor variable ($\beta_n X_n$) in the form of logit slope estimates and (2) researchers must specify the anticipated proportion of participants who will experience the event of interest (i.e., $Pr[Y_{i_{\text{BINARY}}} = 1]$) in the form of a logit intercept (β_0) estimate.

First, the odds ratio (OR) effects for specific predictors in a logistic regression ($OR = \exp^{\beta_n}$) can be converted back into logit slope form by a natural logarithmic transformation

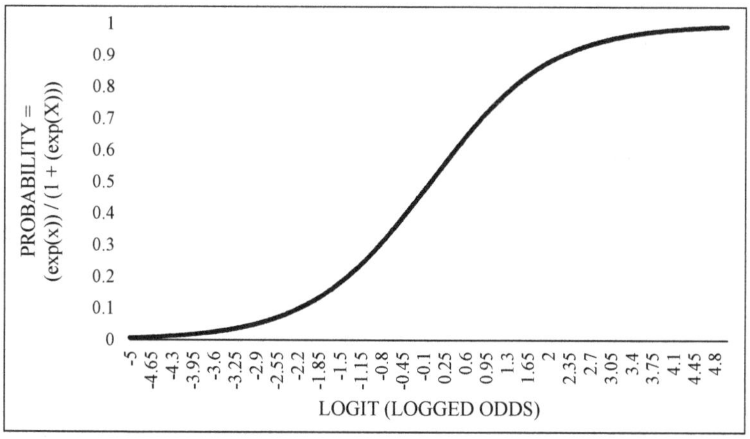

FIGURE 5.1. Probability as a function of log odds.

(ln[*OR*] = logit slope). For example, Table 5.1 shows the common odds ratio effect sizes, with small (1.75), medium (2.50), and large (3.25) odds ratio effect sizes in bold in the left column, and those same values logarithmically transformed (i.e., ln[1.75] = 0.5596) into logit slopes in the right column.

For example, as shown Table 5.1, a logit slope estimate of $\beta = 0.4055$ can interpreted as the odds are ($\exp^{0.4055} = 1.50$) 50% greater for observing a response variable value of 1 versus a value of 0 for every unit increase in the (X) predictor variable, while a logit slope estimate of $\beta = 0.6931$ means the odds are doubled ($\exp^{0.6931} = 2.00$) in favor of a response variable value of 1 versus a value of 0 per unit increase in X. As will be shown, the reason why the relationships between predictor variables and a binary response must be provided on a logit slope scale is because performing a logistic regression power analysis in Mplus requires researchers to declare a binary response variable using the 'CATEGORICAL' option of the 'VARIABLES:' command. In doing so, Mplus will, by default, apply a logistic link function to the analysis model, which means that parameter estimate information consistent with a logit link function, or on a logit scale, will need to be provided.

Second, a researcher must also specify a priori the proportion of participants expected to experience the event of interest or have a response variable value of 1 instead of 0. That anticipated proportion is determined by the logit intercept (β_0) value. To illustrate why, let's assume a logistic regression model with three predictor variables of interest as follows [Equation (5.6)]

$$\ln[Pr(Y_{i_{\text{BINARY}}} = 1)] = \beta_0 + \beta_1 X_1 + \beta_2 X_2 + \beta_3 X_3 \tag{5.6}$$

As stated previously, the odds ratios for the anticipated effects of $X1$–$X3$ are added to a Monte Carlo power analysis simulation as logit slopes after a natural logarithmic transformation is applied (i.e., $\ln[\beta_1, \beta_2, \beta_3]$). As an example, let's further assume that from a literature search or prior pilot testing, a researcher expects the following predictor variable effects: (1) a 31% increase in the odds of a response variable value of 1 versus the odds of a response variable value of 0 per unit increase in X_1 (i.e., Logit $[\beta_1] = \ln[1.31] = 0.27$), (2) an 84% increase in the odds of a response variable value of 1 versus the odds of a response variable value of 0 per unit increase in X_2 (i.e., Logit $[\beta_2] = \ln[1.84] = 0.61$), and (3) a 232% increase in the odds of a response variable value of 1 versus the odds of a response variable

TABLE 5.1. Conversion between Odds Ratio and Logit Slope

Odds rato (OR)	Logit slope (ln[OR])
1.50	0.4055
1.75	0.5596
2.00	0.6931
2.25	0.8109
2.50	0.9163
2.75	1.0116
3.00	1.0986
3.25	1.1787

value of 0 per unit increase in X_3 (i.e., Logit [β_3] = ln[2.32] = 0.84). Substituting the logit slope values into the above equation produces Equation (5.7)

$$\ln[Pr(Y_{i_{\text{BINARY}}} = 1)] = \beta_0 + (0.27)X_1 + (0.61)X_2 + (0.84)X_3 \tag{5.7}$$

When generating data for Monte Carlo simulation power analysis purposes, Mplus by default generates standardized (z-score) data with a mean of zero and a standard deviation of one. Stated differently, the mean or *expected value* of Mplus generated data is zero, which means

$$\ln[Pr(Y_{i_{\text{BINARY}}} = 1)] = \beta_0 + (0.27)0 + (0.61)0 + (0.84)0 = \beta_0 \tag{5.8}$$

on average, the proportion of response variable values of 1 versus 0 is determined by the logit intercept shown in Equation (5.8).

Logistic Regression Monte Carlo Simulation Power Analysis: Vakhitova and Alston-Knox (2018)

Vakhitova and Alston-Knox (2018; see also Vakhitova, Webster, Alston-Knox, Reynald, & Townsley, 2018) conducted an exploratory investigation into *indirect cyber-abuse targetization* by quantitatively coding the content of N = 110 Australian news media reports (the data are available at *https://doi.org/10.1371/journal.pone.0205076.s002*). Specifically, the authors tested research questions involving the presence or absence of a prior cyber-abuse perpetrator–target relationship, whether the motivation behind the cyber abuse was instrumental or expressive, and whether a relationship by motivation interaction significantly moderated indirect cyber-abuse targetization. The authors defined *direct* cyber abuse as harmful communication directed at a target's personal electronic media, such as mobile phone text messages, emails, or Facebook or other social media postings. *Indirect* cyber abuse involves posting personal, private, insulting, and/or inaccurate information on public blogs or Facebook and other social media pages in ways that do not require contact with the target. *Direct* (= 0) and *indirect* (= 1) instances of cyber abuse was the binary response variable of interest. The Relationship predictor variable was a binary indicator of whether (= 1) or not (= 0) any relationship between the perpetrator and the target existed prior to the cyber-abuse incident. The Motivation predictor variable was also a binary indicator of either instrumental (= 0) or expressive (= 1) motives behind a perpetrator's cyber abuse. An *instrumental* motive was defined broadly as a desire to bring about change; a specific example would be to initiate or re-initiate an intimate relationship with the cyber-abuse target. The authors proposed several a priori hypotheses, including a statistically significant Motivation by Relationship interaction. However, as shown in the author's original Table 5 (p. 13), the authors' logistic regression analysis produced statistically nonsignificant results, quite possibly due to inadequate statistical power.

As an illustrative example of a Monte Carlo simulation power analysis for a logistic regression, let's assume a researcher wants to replicate Vakhitova and Alston-Knox's (2018) research study and is willing to treat the authors' published results (i.e., Table 2, p. 10; Table

5, p. 13) as pilot data. The power analysis question for this example would involve the number of news media reports of cyber abuse needed to reject the null hypothesis for a relationship by motivation interaction with power ≥ .80.

As shown in Vakhitova and Alston-Knox (2018, p. 13, Table 5). the logit slopes that quantify the effects of binary relationship, motivation, and the relationship by motivation interaction are the same logit slopes discussed previously Equation (5.9)]

$$\begin{aligned} \ln[Pr(Y_{i_{\text{BINARY}}} = 1)] = &-1.25 + (0.27)\text{Relationship} + (0.61)\text{Motivation} \\ &+ (0.84)\text{Relationship} * \text{Motivation} \end{aligned} \quad (5.9)$$

Specifically, Equation (5.9) reflects a researcher's hypothesis that, compared to direct cyber abuse, the odds of indirect cyber abuse will: (1) increase ($\exp^{0.27} = 1.31$) 31% under conditions of a preexisting relationship between the perpetrator and the target compared to a lack of a preexisting relationship, (2) increase ($\exp^{0.61} = 1.84$) 84% if the motivation is expressive compared to instrumental motivation, and (3) more than double ($\exp^{0.84} = 2.32$) under conditions of both a preexisting relationship and expressive motivation. The logit intercept ($\beta_0 = -1.25$) is defined as a researcher's belief that the probability of indirect cyber abuse, absent a preexisting relationship (relationship = 0) and based on instrumental motives (motivation = 0), is $Pr(Y_{i_{\text{BINARY}}} = 1) = \exp^{-1.25} / (1 + \exp^{-1.25}) = 0.22$, or 22%.

Mplus Monte Carlo Power Analysis: Logistic Regression

The Mplus syntax needed for a Monte Carlo simulation power analysis that replicates Vakhitova and Alston-Knox's (2018) logistic regression is presented below.

```
TITLE: MPLUS 5.1 LOGISTIC REGRESSION
MONTECARLO:
NAMES = INDIRECT MOTIV RELAT MOTBYREL;
NOBSERVATIONS = 528;
NREPS = 5000;
SEED = 5684;

CUTPOINTS = RELAT (-0.1764) MOTIV (-0.6128) MOTBYREL (.07527);
CATEGORICAL = INDIRECT;
GENERATE = INDIRECT(1);
```

The '`NAMES =`' line in the above syntax includes the indirect cyber-abuse response variable ('`INDIRECT`'), the main effects for motivation ('`MOTIV`') and relationship ('`RELAT`'), as well as the motivation by relationship interaction effect ('`MOTBYREL`'). The '`NOBSERVATIONS`', '`NREPS`', and '`SEED`' specifications retain their definitions from previous analyses.

The '`CUTPOINTS`' specification is used to generate the binary *predictor* variable data in Mplus. As shown in Table 2 (p. 10) of Vakhitova and Alston-Knox (2018), the mean of the relationship predictor variable showed (0.57) 57% of indirect cyber-abuse media reports involved a preexisting perpetrator–target relationship, and the mean of the motivation predictor variable showed (0.73) 73% of indirect cyber-abuse media reports involved expressive motivations. Computing the motivation by relationship interaction from the authors' data showed that (0.47) 47% of indirect cyber-abuse media reports involved both a preexisting relationship and expressive motives. The values in parentheses after the names of the predictor variables in the 'CUTPOINTS' statement are the values under a unit normal distribution that correspond to the observed proportions of values of 1 versus 0 for each predictor variable. For example, 73% of indirect cyber-abuse media reports involved expressive motives; 73% of the unit normal distribution area occurs at values of –0.6128 and greater (*Side Note*: *This value can also be obtained by typing '= –1*normsinv(0.73)' into any cell of a Microsoft Excel spreadsheet*). Similarly, 57% of indirect cyber-abuse media reports involved a preexisting perpetrator–target relationship, so 57% of the unit normal distribution area occurs at values of ('= –1*normsinv(0.57)') –0.1764 and higher. Mplus, by default, assumes all response variables are continuous. The 'CATEGORICAL' command declares the 'INDIRECT' response variable as a categorical variable, but it is the 'GENERATE' command that specifies 'INDIRECT' as a binary response variable because the '(1)' specification indicates that the 'INDIRECT' response variable has one threshold, which indicates the probability of a response value of zero versus the probability of a response value of one.

```
MODEL POPULATION:
!Logit Intercept;
[INDIRECT$1*-1.25];

!Logit Slopes;
INDIRECT ON RELAT*0.27 MOTIV*0.61 MOTBYREL*0.84;

!Unit Predictor Variances;
MOTIV*1;
RELAT*1;
MOTBYREL*1;
```

Recall that 'MODEL POPULATION:' specifies how Monte Carlo simulation data are to be generated. The '[INDIRECT$1*-1.25];' specification again refers to the logit intercept (brackets in Mplus refer to the mean or the intercept of a response variable) for the binary 'INDIRECT' response variable, the '$1' specification refers to the threshold of the logit intercept which has been assigned the value -1.25. The next line of syntax 'INDIRECT ON RELAT*0.27 MOTIV*0.61 MOTBYREL*0.84;' specifies the logit intercept values for the effects of each variable as a predictor of 'INDIRECT' cyber abuse. Finally, unit variances ($\sigma^2 = 1$) are specified for each of the binary predictor variables because CUTPOINT values were computed from the unit normal distribution having a total area equal to one.

```
ANALYSIS:
ESTIMATOR = ML;

MODEL:
INDIRECT ON RELAT*0.27 MOTIV*0.61 MOTBYREL*0.84
```

The 'ESTIMATOR = ML;' specification for the 'ANALYSIS:' command overrides the default estimator (WLSMV) for a binary response variable that would specify a probit regression; '`ESTIMATOR = ML`' specifies a logistic regression (more on probit vs. logit distinction in Chapter 11). Finally, the '`MODEL`' command specifies how the data generated by the '`MODEL POPULATION:`' are to be analyzed, so only the logistic regression portion of the data generating model is needed. Results from the Monte Carlo power analysis for the specified logistic regression (Mplus 5.1) are shown below.

```
MODEL RESULTS

                                ESTIMATES                  S. E.      M. S. E.  95%   % Sig
                   Population   Average    Std. Dev.   Average                 Cover Coeff

 INDIRECT    ON
  RELAT             0.270       0.2692      0.2942      0.2933      0.0865 0.953 0.148
  MOTIV             0.610       0.6034      0.3128      0.3048      0.0978 0.948 0.520
  MOTBYREL          0.840       0.8636      0.3277      0.3177      0.1080 0.950 0.800
```

As shown in the syntax and results above, $N = 528$ quantitatively coded news media reports of indirect cyber abuse would be needed to reject the null hypothesis for the relationship by motivation interaction effect with power ≥ .80.

Simulation Power Analysis Write-Up: Logistic Regression

Finally, an example SEM Monte Carlo simulation power analysis write-up is shown below and consists of four sections: (1) a statement of the power analysis question; (2) a description of how power was calculated, including the data analysis model assumed, and the statistical software package and version used; (3) a clear statement of all power analysis assumptions, including specific parameter estimate values; and (4) a clear answer to the power analysis question that includes the number of simulated dataset replications requested, the effect size assumed, and the sample size needed to achieve power ≥ .80:

> "The power analysis question involves the smallest number of quantitatively coded news media reports needed to replicate the exploratory research of Vakhitova and Alston-Knox (2018) and achieve power ≥ 0.80 to reject the null hypothesis for the effect of a relationship by the motivation interaction term as a predictor of indirect cyber abuse. A Monte Carlo simulation power analysis was conducted using Mplus (version 8.6) assuming: (1) 57% of indirect cyber abuse news media reports will involve a preexisting perpetrator–target relationship, and that a preexisting relationship will increase the odds of indirect cyber abuse (odds ratio = 1.31) 31% compared to a lack of a preexisting relationship; (2) 74% of indirect cyber-abuse news media reports will involve an expressive motivation, and an expressive motivation will increase the odds of indirect cyber abuse (odds ratio = 1.84) 84% compared to instrumental motives; (3) 22% of indirect cyber-abuse news media reports will involve neither a preexisting relationship nor expressive motives; and (4) 47% of indirect cyber-abuse news media reports will involve both a prior relationship and expressive motives, and a relationship by motivation interaction will more than double (odds ratio = 2.32) the odds of indirect cyber abuse. Monte Carlo simulation power analysis results aggregated over 5,000 replica-

tions showed $N = 528$ quantitatively coded news media reports would be needed for power $\geq .80$ to reject the null hypothesis for the effect of a relationship by motivation interaction term as a predictor of indirect cyber abuse."

Problems Using R Packages lavaan or simsem for Logistic Regression Power Analysis

Although statistical power for logistic regression models can be evaluated in various R packages, they are not easily replicated in lavaan or simsem. This is not inherently problematic for research evaluating just logistic regression, yet the goal of showing logistic regression in this book is to set the stage for more complex designs in later chapters. Unfortunately, there are currently no straightforward, equivalent ways to compute a Monte Carlo simulation of a combination of binary predictors and binary outcomes using either lavaan or simsem. lavaan can impose thresholds or cutpoint variables for endogenous binary variables, and simsem can be used to create binary covariates as predictors, but the combination does not seem possible at the moment. These various issues are problematic for many types of research designs, particularly those that use end-of-study binary outcomes in the context of a binary treatment/control condition, which are relatively common in both the behavioral sciences as well as health sciences. Below, we detail what is—and is not—possible at present in lavaan and simsem with respect to a design that includes both binary predictors and binary outcomes. We also looked outside these packages but were unable to find any present approaches that could adequately deal with both binary predictors and outcomes in an SEM framework.

Here is the issue: In Mplus, CUTPOINTS are used to create binary predictor variables, and this is directly from the user guide on p. 475,

> The CUTPOINTS option is used to create binary variables from the multivariate normal independent variables generated by the program. In this example, the variable x2 is cut at the value of one which is one standard deviation above the mean because the mean and variance used for data generation are zero and one. This implies that after the cut, x2 is a 0/1 binary variable where 16 percent of the population have the value of 1. The mean and variance of x2 for data generation are specified in the MODEL POPULATION command.

In the Mplus example, we learn that the cutpoints imposed create binary predictor variables based on SDs from a normal unit distribution, or what we might also call z-values. Furthermore, Mplus uses a two-step approach to simulate and evaluate binary variables, where cutpoints are first imposed and then effects are estimated based on the known binary distribution of predictor variables (this is seemingly why cutpoints are not used for endogenous variables in Mplus).

In lavaan, when attempting to replicate the cutpoint feature, many issues emerge. First, the effect between the binary variable and any outcome is underestimated, since all data are simulated to reflect an effect where every one SD increase in X causes a B-SD change in Y. Unfortunately, this produces incorrect simulated data when the predictor is binary. Typically, in the case where a binary variable predicts a continuous outcome, the relationship between predictor and outcome is interpreted as: a **one-unit** increase in *X* causes a B-SD change in *Y*. At present, there seems to be no straightforward way to adjust the estimate in simulated data without mathematically adjusting the effect (see Olsson, Drasgow, & Dorans, 1982, in the Suggested Readings section at the end of this chapter) prior to generating data.

To specify a model that included a binary endogenous variable in lavaan, we would have used the following syntax. However, this model does not account for the binary exogenous variables.

```
PopulationModel_Ch5 <- "
 INDIRECT | -1.25*t1                                    # Logit intercept/threshold
 INDIRECT ~ .27*RELAT + .61*MOTIV + .84*MOTBYREL # Logit slopes
 MOTIV ~~ 1*MOTIV                                       # Variances
 RELAT ~~ 1*RELAT
 MOTBYREL ~~ 1*MOTBYREL
 MOTIV ~ 0*1
 RELAT ~ 0*1
 MOTBYREL ~ 0*1
 "
```

One solution we attempted in lavaan was to cut the exogenous variables after simulating data. However, this solution led to an underestimation of the logit slope estimates, due to the relationship among variables being simulated based on the unit-normal distribution, rather than the point-biserial or binomial distribution that reflects the relationship among a binary predictor with either another binary variable or a continuous variable. Although there are mathematical approaches that can be used to adjust the effects prior to data generation (see Olsson et al., 1982) and then evaluate those effects under a different analysis model, use of such an adjusted, two-step approach requires reestimating all the expected parameters of interest and opens the door to many user errors. Another way to adjust for binary predictor variables is to use a multigroup approach, as shown in previous chapters, yet this solution only works in the case of one binary or categorical predictor and becomes exponentially more complex as the estimated model becomes more complex, as happens later in this book. Thus, while lavaan can adequately handle binary outcome variables, it cannot, at the time of writing this book, appropriately handle binary predictor variables.

Using binary predictors in simsem is far more flexible than lavaan. However, simsem cannot easily incorporate binary outcome variables using threshold models. Thus, while simsem can be used to include a binary predictor, it cannot in combination be used to evaluate both a binary predictor and a binary outcome, which highlights the inability of either of these packages to account for a very common type of research design. Below, we show how to create a model that includes binary predictors using simsem, which requires using matrix notation to build the model.

We first create each matrix separately. After each relevant matrix is created, we input it appropriately into the simsem function 'model', or one of the model derivatives (e.g., 'model.cfa', 'model.path', or 'model.sem'. The matrices are created as follows:

```
#psi matrix of total (co)variance of endogenous variables
PS <- binds(free = matrix(NA, nrow=1, ncol=1), popParam = matrix(1, nrow=1, ncol=1))
```

```
#beta matrix of (co)variances among endogenous variables
BE <- bind(free = matrix(NA, nrow=1, ncol=1), popParam = matrix(0, nrow=1, ncol=1))

#phi matrix of (co)variances among exogenous variables
VYfix <- matrix(0, nrow=3, ncol = 3)
diag(VYfix) <- NA #only diagonals of the error var matrix will be freely estimated (set to NA)
VYpop <- matrix(0, nrow=3, ncol = 3)
diag(VYpop) <- 1 #fix the diagonal values to 1
VY <- bind(VYfix, VYpop)

#matrix from covariates to indicators; use GA if covariates to factors
KAfix <- matrix(NA, 1, 3) #creates a 3x1 matrix of NAs; freely estimated in the model
KApop <- matrix(NA, 1, 3) #creates a 3x1 matrix of NAs ready to populate
KApop[1:3] <- c(.27, .61, .84) #the estimated logit slopes
KA <- bind(KAfix, KApop)
```

All created matrices are then input into a model command to create a full SEM model, named here as Model_Ch5.

```
Model_Ch5 <-   model(PS = PS, BE = BE, KA = KA, VY = VY,          #matrices
               indLab=c("INDIRECT"),                              #indicator labels
               covLab = c("RELAT", "MOTIV", "MOTBYREL"),          #covariate labels
               modelType = "Path")
summary(Model_Ch5)
```

Next, create a dataframe of 0s and 1s for each covariate, or predictor variable, that is binary, ensuring that all combinations of 0/1 of all observed variables are present. Since this example uses two binary predictors, plus the interaction (product term) between the two predictors, we need to create a design matrix that has the four possible combinations of 0/1 when looking at two observed binary predictors and their interaction term.

```
designMatrix <-  expand.grid(RELAT = c(0, 1),
                 MOTIV = c(0, 1))
designMatrix$MOTBYREL <- designMatrix$RELAT * designMatrix$MOTIV
```

The total sample size must be a multiple of 4, assuming balanced groups. However, we don't have balanced groups, so this becomes more complex. Recall that the proportions for RELAT, MOTIV, and MOTBYREL were .57, .73, and .47. This is enough information to determine the design matrix, assuming all proportions sum to 1. First, we must determine the proportions assigned to each combination of variables. We know one certain combination: the proportion where all variables = 1 is .47. Second, we know that the proportion where RELAT = 1 is .57. Already, .47 of this proportion is accounted for, so we determine the difference as .57–.47 = .10. Third, we know that the proportion where MOTIV = 1 is .73. Again, .47 of this proportion is accounted for, so we determine the difference as .73–.47 = .26. Finally, we know that the total proportion of all variable combinations will equal 1. This means that we can easily calculate the proportion where RELAT, MOTIV, and MOTBYREL all equal 0 by determining a difference, 1–.47–.10–.26 = .17.

After determining the proportions, set a sample size and create the design matrix.

```
N = 528
prop111 <- .47
prop100 <- .10
prop010 <- .26
prop000 <- .17
n111 <- round(N*prop111, 0)
n100 <- round(N*prop100, 0)
n010 <- round(N*prop010, 0)
n000 <- round(N*prop000, 0)
designMatrix #here, the first row corresponds to the condition when both RELAT and MOTIV
are 1, the second is when only RELAT is 1, the third is when only MOTIV is 1, and the last is
when both RELAT and MOTIV are 0
covar <- designMatrix %>% slice(rep(1:n(), times = c(n000, n100, n010, n111)))
covar <- as.data.frame(covar)
```

If the outcome variable was continuous, we would have enough information to move forward with the simulation by creating a population model,

```
PopulationModel_Ch5 <- model(PS=PS, BE=BE, VY=VY, KA=KA, modelType="Path",
        indLab=c("INDIRECT"), #indicator labels
        covLab = c("RELAT", "MOTIV", "MOTBYREL")) #covariate labels
```

and running the simulation:

```
Output_Ch5 <- sim(PopulationModel_Ch5,
        nRep = 5000,
        n = N,
        covData = covar,
        seed = 1234,
        silent = T)
summary(Output_Ch5)
```

Yet since the outcome of interest is binary, we cannot complete the simulation.

The inability to include both binary predictors and outcomes (or correlations among binary predictors, which is relevant to later chapters) was one of the largest issues we encountered when working through power analysis examples using R packages. Although R is open source and can be an excellent resource for researchers, at the time of writing this book, it did not have the same capabilities regarding SEM statistical power as Mplus. A great deal of additional funding and development is needed for such freeware programming to be as flexible for such common research designs.

SUGGESTED READINGS

- Baranger, D. A., Finsaas, M. C., Goldstein, B. L., Vize, C. E., Lynam, D. R., & Olino, T. M. (2023). Tutorial: Power analyses for interaction effects in cross-sectional regressions. *Advances in Methods and Practices in Psychological Science, 6*(3), 1–13.
- Gambarota, F., & Altoè, G. (2024). Ordinal regression models made easy: A tutorial on parameter interpretation, data simulation and power analysis. *International Journal of Psychology, 59*(6), 1263–1292.

- Greenhouse, J. B., Bromberg, J. A., & Fromm, D. (1995). An introduction to logistic regression with an application to the analysis of language recovery following a stroke. *Journal of Communication Disorders, 28*, 229–246.
- Hosmer, D. W. Jr., Lemeshow, S., & Sturdivant, R. X. (2013). *Applied logistic regression* (3rd ed.; Vol. 398). Wiley.
- Johns, H., Campbell, B., Turc, G., & Churilov, L. (2023). Power analysis for ordinal analyses of the modified Rankin scale and an online and downloadable tool for practical use. *Stroke, 54*(7), 1750–1760.
- Lodder, P., Emons, W. H., Denollet, J., & Wicherts, J. M. (2020). Latent logistic interaction modeling: A simulation and empirical illustration of Type D personality. *Structural Equation Modeling: A Multidisciplinary Journal, 28*, 440–462.
- Olsson, U., Drasgow, F., & Dorans, N. J. (1982). The polyserial correlation coefficient. *Psychometrika, 47*, 337–347. *https://doi.org/10.1007/BF02294164*
- Pampel, F. C. (2020). *Logistic regression: A primer* (Vol. 132). Sage.

6

Missing Data in Monte Carlo Simulation Power Analyses

While earlier chapters described Monte Carlo simulation power calculations in analyses, such as a multiple regression with two predictors, univariate and multivariate two-group comparisons, path analysis, and structural equation models, these chapters all assumed continuous response variables and then Chapter 5 showed how to conduct a Monte Carlo simulation power analysis for a logistic regression with a binary response variable that may have seemed a somewhat digressive and tangential exercise. However, consider that, although not explicitly stated, all of the Monte Carlo simulation power calculations in the previous chapters assumed complete data with no missing values. Assuming an absence of missing data for statistical power calculations is unrealistic, and many grant review study sections expect not only an acknowledgment of the likelihood that some percentage of a research investigator's data (e.g., 10–20%) will likely be missing, but also expect this likelihood to be incorporated into all power analysis calculations. All the concepts, procedures, and explanations included in the previous chapter will be referred to again here to illustrate how missing data considerations can be included in Monte Carlo simulation power analysis calculations.

Both Mplus and the R simsem package have missing data commands that are very similar in both code and functionality. Across both programs, missing data can be generated using a logistic regression technique. The next two sections introduce commands used in both Mplus and R simsem that are used to compute missing data.

Missing Data in Mplus

As shown in previous chapters, the Mplus '`MODEL POPULATION:`' command allows the researcher to specify how Monte Carlo simulation datasets are to be generated, while the '`MODEL:`' command specifies how the generated data should be analyzed. By default, Mplus will generate complete data for all Monte Carlo simulation sample dataset replications if no other syntax specifications are made. A feature available in Mplus is the '`MODEL MISS-`

ING:' command which enables researchers to specify, using logistic regression techniques, specific probabilities to determine whether a generated data point remains observed (= 0) or is converted to a missing data indicator value (= 1), for all data points across all generated Monte Carlo simulation datasets. Furthermore, Mplus can generate missing data consistent with each of the three theoretical explanations to show why missing data are missing: missing completely at random (MCAR), missing at random (MAR), and missing not at random (MNAR). When researchers address missing data in statistical analyses, either using maximum likelihood estimation or multiple imputation, they are implicitly assuming the missing data are either MCAR or MAR (MNAR data are not reviewed here, but interested readers are referred to Muthén, Asparouhov, Hunter, & Leuchter, 2011; Muthén, Muthén, & Asparouhov, 2017, pp. 464–472; Peugh, Toland, & Harrison, 2023). Two simple illustrative and conceptual examples—a univariate example to demonstrate MCAR missing data generation and a simple regression example to demonstrate MAR missing data generation—can clarify how the 'MODEL MISSING:' command in Mplus works. As will be shown, the 'MODEL POPULATION:' command in Mplus generates complete data, the 'MODEL MISSING:' command determines which data points remain observed or are specified as missing values, and the 'MODEL:' command analyzes the result to produce a Monte Carlo simulation power estimate that incorporates the effects of missing data.

Missing Data in R Using simsem and lavaan Packages

Similar to Mplus, SEM packages in R can readily deal with and generate missing data based on a given missing data structure. The R package, simsem, generates complete data by default, but missingness can be imposed on the data generating or the analysis phase of the simulation analysis by specifying a missing data model using lavaan-style syntax. Although there are multiple ways to impose missingness into SEMs using simsem, this book focuses on the lavaan-style syntax approach to missing data because it is most similar to the Mplus syntax.

Much like the approach to simulating missing data in Mplus, logistic regression techniques can be used to impose missing data, where missing data are generated based on prespecified probabilities that can reflect MAR, MCAR, and MNAR (the last of which is not elaborated on further in this book). Two illustrative examples demonstrate how missing data are generated in simsem by creating and imposing MCAR and MAR missing data structures on simulated data and then evaluating how missing data mechanisms impact the Monte Carlo simulation power estimate.

A Univariate Example of MCAR

MCAR is defined as all potential observations in a dataset that: (1) have an equal probability of being a missing data point; (2) probability is unrelated to any past, present, or future predictor, covariate, or response variable, observed or missing; and (3) is also independent of the research study design (e.g., cross-sectional or longitudinal). A completely random process that is very similar to a lottery determines whether a data point is an observed value or a missing value under MCAR. Furthermore, in theory, if a given dataset is obtained using a simple random sample from a population, and any missing data are MCAR, the remaining observed data points still constitute a simple random sample from the population.

To illustrate, let's begin by assuming a researcher wants to generate $N = 40$ observations of standardized (z-score) data for a single Y variable with no missing values. An example of such data is shown in the first column of Table 6.1 and indicated by Y_{complete}. The second column of Table 6.1 shows the results of solving the equation ($Pr = \exp^{Y_{\text{complete}}} / [1 + \exp^{Y_{\text{complete}}}]$) to obtain the probabilities of observing each of the $N = 40$ generated data points. A key point warrants emphasis: If the data values shown in the Y_{complete} column were generated by a completely random process (they were), then the probabilities of observing each of the Y_{complete} values shown in the second column can also be considered completely random values. The importance of this fact can be illustrated by further assuming that a researcher wants to then specify a 0.40 probability for the values in the Y_{complete} column to be missing completely at random (MCAR). Specifically, a logistic regression equation for a 0.40 probability of MCAR data (= 1) versus observed data (= 0) would be $Pr(Y_{i_{\text{BINARY}}} = 1) = \beta_0 = (-0.40546)$, where β_0 indicates a logistic regression intercept, and the assigned value (−0.40546) specifies a probability (Pr) of $Pr = \exp^{-0.40546} / (1 + \exp^{-0.40546}) = 0.40$ for a missing value. The above equation will be revisited and expanded upon when the statistical power estimates from analysis models in previous chapters are reconsidered to include the effect of missing data.

However, at this point, a simpler way to accomplish this goal of 40% MCAR using only the information in the first two columns of Table 6.1 would be to assign probability values less than 0.60 in the second column a value of 0, indicating observed data, and probability values of 0.60 or greater in the second column (i.e., which will occur with a probability of $1 - 0.60 = 0.40$, or 40% of the time by definition) a value of 1, indicating missing data, in the third column. As shown in the fourth column (Y_{MCAR}) of Table 6.1 data points from the first Y_{complete} column showing values of 0 in the third column are retained as observed data in the fourth (Y_{MCAR}) column, but data points from the first Y_{complete} column showing values of 1 in the third column are converted to a missing data indicator value, 999 (the default in Mplus) in the fourth (Y_{MCAR}) column. The missing (999) values in the fourth column are MCAR because a completely random process produced both the observed data in the first column and the associated probabilities in the second column. By extension, this means that probabilities ≥ 0.60 could have occurred for any data point, so converting data points with probabilities ≥ 0.60 to missing data values is consistent with MCAR.

A Simple Regression MAR Example

As many have observed, the term "missing at random" (MAR) is very misleading. Defined, MAR states that missing data for a given (Y) variable is not *random*, but is instead related to one or more (X) *additional variables* that are either already included in the data analysis model or not part of the analysis model but available for possible analysis model inclusion (e.g., see Graham, 2003). A hypothetical MAR example from pediatric research could involve a scenario in which missing response variable data from adolescent participants were due to participants experiencing levels of depression that render them unable to pro-

TABLE 6.1. MCAR Probabilities

$Y_{complete}$	$Pr = exp^{Y_{complete}}/(1 + exp^{Y_{complete}})$	$Pr \geq 0.60$? (0 = NO, 1 = YES)	Y_{MCAR}
–0.17702	0.46	0	–0.17702
–1.035721	0.26	0	–1.035721
–1.027845	0.26	0	–1.027845
–0.01098	0.50	0	–0.01098
0.2725	0.57	0	0.2725
0.963418	0.72	1	999
0.562664	0.64	1	999
1.070447	0.74	1	999
–0.027743	0.49	0	–0.027743
1.84948	0.86	1	999
–0.531787	0.37	0	–0.531787
0.952217	0.72	1	999
0.028793	0.51	0	0.028793
0.717471	0.67	1	999
0.880736	0.71	1	999
1.177115	0.76	1	999
–0.263409	0.43	0	–0.263409
0.31889	0.58	0	0.31889
0.017913	0.50	0	0.017913
–1.142851	0.24	0	–1.142851
0.077237	0.52	0	0.077237
–0.4748	0.38	0	–0.4748
1.374216	0.80	1	999
–1.362725	0.20	0	–1.362725
0.149704	0.54	0	0.149704
–0.379971	0.41	0	–0.379971
–0.561758	0.36	0	–0.561758
–1.014645	0.27	0	–1.014645
–0.730314	0.33	0	–0.730314
–0.730595	0.33	0	–0.730595
0.615839	0.65	1	999
0.266221	0.57	0	0.266221
–0.093249	0.48	0	–0.093249
–0.432057	0.39	0	–0.432057
0.33101	0.58	0	0.33101
1.16032	0.76	1	999
–0.049821	0.49	0	–0.049821
–0.152913	0.46	0	–0.152913
0.735992	0.68	1	999
–0.904647	0.29	0	–0.904647

vide response variable data. If the primary investigator of the hypothetical study also collected Child Depression Inventory (CDI) responses, and CDI scores were included in the data analysis model, the missing response variable data could be assumed to be MAR. To illustrate further, let's assume a researcher generates $N = 40$ data values based on the simple regression model shown in Figure 6.1.

An example of randomly generated and standardized data, based on the simple regression model above, is shown in the first two columns of Table 6.2. Furthermore, a logistic regression equation for a 0.40 probability of missing data (= 1) versus observed data (= 0) that is conditional upon, or related to, values of the X predictor variable consistent with MAR could be [Equation (6.1)]

$$Pr(Y_{i_{\mathrm{BINARY}}} = 1) = \beta_0 + \beta_1(X) = -0.40546 + 0.69315(X) \tag{6.1}$$

where the logit intercept value still specifies a probability of $Pr = \exp^{-0.40546} / (1 + \exp^{-0.40546}) = 0.40) = 0.40$ for observing a missing value, but Equation (6.1) also specifies that, per unit increase in X, the odds of observing a missing value double (odds ratio = $\exp^{0.69315} = 2$) consistent with MAR. The third column in Table 6.2 shows the probabilities (Pr) of observing a missing data value that result from solving the following extension of the above probability equation [Equation (6.2)]

$$Pr = \exp^{Y_{\mathrm{complete}} + (0.69315 * X_{\mathrm{complete}})} / (1 + \exp^{Y_{\mathrm{complete}} + (0.69315 * X_{\mathrm{complete}})}) \tag{6.2}$$

The fourth column of Table 6.2 is a binary indicator of probability values ≥ 0.60 consistent with the previous MCAR example. The last column in Table 6.2 (Y_{MAR}) retains data from the first column (Y_{complete}) for binary indicator values of zero, but changes observed data in first column to missing data for binary indicator values of one. The missing values (999) in the fifth column (Y_{MAR}) are MAR because they depend not only on observed (Y_{complete}) response variable data, but also on the relationship between the response variable and the predictor (X) variable: Unit increases in X double the odds of a missing value for Y.

Monte Carlo Simulation Power Estimates and Missing Data

Many researchers proceed under the erroneous assumption that, because missing data-handling methods such as maximum likelihood estimation preserve the intended sample size for statistical analysis, missing data need not be a concern when estimating statistical

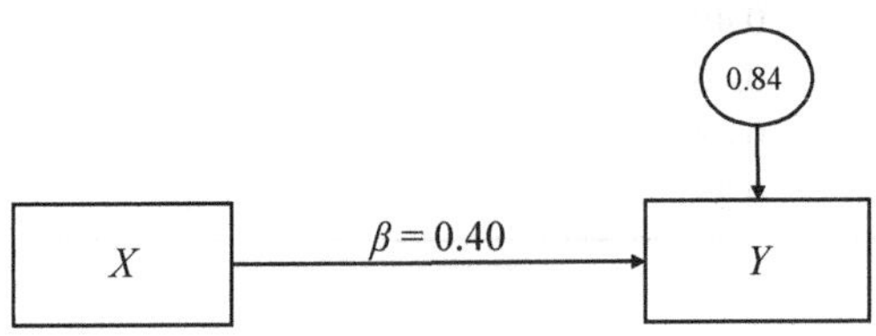

FIGURE 6.1. A bivariate MAR example.

TABLE 6.2. MAR Probabilities

$Y_{complete}$		$X_{complete}$	$Pr = \exp^{Y_{complete}+(0.69315*X_{complete})} / (1 + \exp^{Y_{complete}+(0.69315*X_{complete})})$	$Pr > 0.60$? (0 = NO, 1 = YES)	Y_{MAR}
–0.435117	–0.610749	–0.17702	0.36	0	–0.435117
–0.173083	0.246113	–1.027845	0.29	0	–0.173083
–0.043774	–1.303686	0.2725	0.54	0	–0.043774
0.518679	–0.685904	0.562664	0.71	1	999
1.75894	0.767542	–0.027743	0.85	1	999
0.889533	–0.445051	–0.531787	0.63	1	999
1.620328	–0.227598	0.028793	0.84	1	999
2.01016	2.05385	0.880736	0.93	1	999
–0.634448	0.791943	–0.263409	0.31	0	–0.634448
1.883001	0.581448	0.017913	0.87	1	999
–2.283296	0.380335	0.077237	0.10	0	–2.283296
–1.134242	–0.671942	1.374216	0.45	0	–1.134242
–0.109897	0.215621	0.149704	0.50	0	–0.109897
–1.491531	0.070168	–0.561758	0.13	0	–1.491531
–0.115758	–1.210733	–0.730314	0.35	0	–0.115758
–1.669048	–0.33721	0.615839	0.22	0	–1.669048
–1.306272	–1.501953	–0.093249	0.20	0	–1.306272
0.655667	0.88526	0.33101	0.71	1	999
–1.261045	–1.75055	–0.049821	0.21	0	–1.261045
–0.084813	1.161781	0.735992	0.60	1	999
–1.180731	–1.631316	0.615505	0.32	0	–1.180731
0.031798	–0.905067	0.371092	0.57	0	0.031798
1.203419	1.661313	–0.839547	0.65	1	999
–1.327085	–0.99394	–1.266743	0.10	0	–1.327085
–0.565021	0.93277	–0.268787	0.32	0	–0.565021
–0.361821	0.582304	–0.69689	0.30	0	–0.361821
–0.394609	0.141276	1.368852	0.64	1	999
–1.006822	–0.900724	0.800331	0.39	0	–1.006822
0.563818	1.03774	–1.669014	0.36	0	0.563818
1.57927	1.103484	0.677802	0.89	1	999
1.764579	–0.404925	0.640928	0.90	1	999
–0.156883	–1.421539	–0.618053	0.36	0	–0.156883
1.200416	1.200164	–0.18104	0.75	1	999
–1.286833	–0.592197	–1.060587	0.12	0	–1.286833
1.553904	1.394381	0.78901	0.89	1	999
–1.609581	–0.709861	0.293955	0.20	0	–1.609581
1.679958	0.284466	–1.158491	0.71	1	999
2.289054	–0.290423	–0.28024	0.89	1	999
–0.065445	–0.191466	0.875712	0.63	1	999
–0.295959	0.124878	–0.357614	0.37	0	–0.295959

power despite much evidence to the contrary (e.g., Enders, 2010; Graham, 2012; Little & Rubin, 2019). Recall that all Monte Carlo simulation power analyses performed up to this point in this book have assumed that complete data would be available for analysis. One way to demonstrate the effect of missing data on statistical power estimates would be to revisit previous Monte Carlo simulation power calculations, incorporate reasonable amounts of anticipated missing data, and examine the effects on the sample sizes needed for power ≥ .80 for the same effect size assumptions.

Multivariate Two-Group Power Analysis Using Mplus

Recall that, in Chapter 2, the Monte Carlo simulation power analysis under consideration involved a two-group (treatment vs. control assuming random assignment) multivariate comparison of mean differences on adherence (ADH), disease activity (DA), functional activity (FA), and health-related quality of life (HRQ) at posttest with pretest versions of the same variables serving a control covariates. The analysis model (Figure 6.2), the Monte Carlo simulation power analysis syntax, and the results are all given again below.

```
MONTECARLO:
NAMES ARE
ADH_pre   DA_pre   FA_pre   HRQ_pre
ADH_post DA_post FA_post HRQ_post;
NOBSERVATIONS = 66 66;
NGROUPS = 2;
NREPS = 5000;
SEED = 10127;

!IV: Control Group;
MODEL POPULATION:

[ADH_pre*0];
[DA_pre*0];
[FA_pre*0];
[HRQ_pre*0];
ADH_pre*1;
DA_pre*1;
FA_pre*1;
HRQ_pre*1;

[ADH_post*0.16];
[DA_post*0.16];
[FA_post*0.16];
[HRQ_post*0.16];

ADH_post*.84;
DA_post*.84;
FA_post*.84;
HRQ_post*.84;

ADH_post DA_post FA_post WITH DA_post*0.3 FA_post*0.3 HRQ_post*0.3;
ADH_pre DA_pre FA_pre WITH DA_pre*0.3 FA_pre*0.3 HRQ_pre*0.3;
```

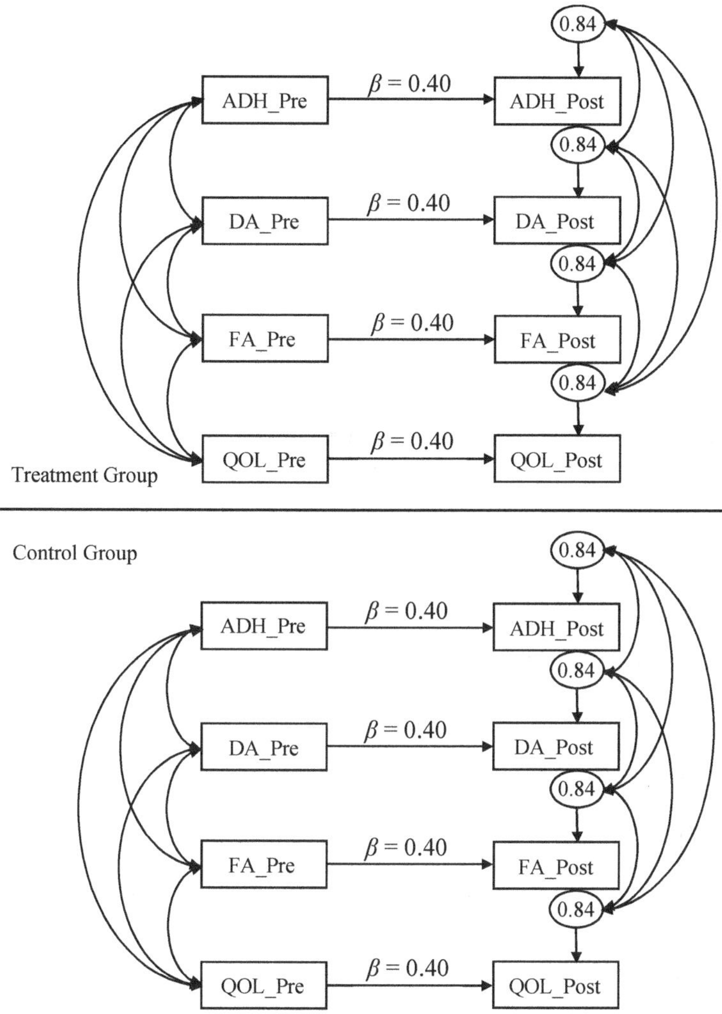

FIGURE 6.2. Multivariate two-group comparison model.

```
ADH_post ON ADH_pre*.4(1);
DA_post ON DA_pre*.4(2);
FA_post ON FA_pre*.4(3);
HRQ_post ON HRQ_pre*.4(4);

!IV: Treatment Group;
MODEL POPULATION-g2:

[ADH_pre*0];
[DA_pre*0];
[FA_pre*0];
[HRQ_pre*0];
```

```
ADH_pre*1;
DA_pre*1;
FA_pre*1;
HRQ_pre*1;

[ADH_post*0.61];
[DA_post*0.61];
[FA_post*0.61];
[HRQ_post*0.61];

ADH_post*.84;
DA_post*.84;
FA_post*.84;
HRQ_post*.84;

ADH_post DA_post FA_post WITH DA_post*0.3 FA_post*0.3 HRQ_post*0.3;
ADH_pre DA_pre FA_pre WITH DA_pre*0.3 FA_pre*0.3 HRQ_pre*0.3;

ADH_post ON ADH_pre*.4(1);
DA_post ON DA_pre*.4(2);
FA_post ON FA_pre*.4(3);
HRQ_post ON HRQ_pre*.4(4);

MODEL: !IV: Control Group;
ADH_post DA_post FA_post WITH DA_post*0.3 FA_post*0.3 HRQ_post*0.3;

ADH_post ON ADH_pre*.4(1);
DA_post ON DA_pre*.4(2);
FA_post ON FA_pre*.4(3);
HRQ_post ON HRQ_pre*.4(4);

[ADH_post*0.16](E);
[DA_post*0.16](F);
[FA_post*0.16](G);
[HRQ_post*0.16](H);

ADH_post*.84;
DA_post*.84;
FA_post*.84;
HRQ_post*.84;

MODEL g2: !IV: Treatment Group;
ADH_post DA_post FA_post WITH DA_post*0.3 FA_post*0.3 HRQ_post*0.3;

ADH_post ON ADH_pre*.4(1);
DA_post ON DA_pre*.4(2);
FA_post ON FA_pre*.4(3);
HRQ_post ON HRQ_pre*.4(4);

[ADH_post*0.61](A);
[DA_post*0.61](B);
[FA_post*0.61](C);
[HRQ_post*0.61](D);
```

```
ADH_post*.84;
DA_post*.84;
FA_post*.84;
HRQ_post*.84;

MODEL CONSTRAINT:
NEW (ADH_DIFF*.45 DA_DIFF*.45 FA_DIFF*.45 HRQ_DIFF*.45);
ADH_DIFF = A-E;
DA_DIFF = B-F;
FA_DIFF = C-G;
HRQ_DIFF = D-H;
```

```
MODEL RESULTS

                               ESTIMATES                S. E.      M. S. E.  95%   % Sig
                  Population   Average    Std. Dev.   Average              Cover  Coeff

New/Additional Parameters
  ADH_DIFF           0.450      0.4476      0.1576      0.1582      0.0248 0.949 0.808
  DA_DIFF            0.450      0.4509      0.1600      0.1581      0.0256 0.943 0.809
  FA_DIFF            0.450      0.4482      0.1594      0.1580      0.0254 0.947 0.804
  HRQ_DIFF           0.450      0.4474      0.1584      0.1580      0.0251 0.946 0.808
```

As shown in both the syntax and results, $N = 132$ ($n = 66$ in both the treatment and control groups) is needed to detect a treatment effect of $d = 0.45$. However, the above power analysis also assumes that a sample of $N = 132$ can be collected with no missing data on any of the pretest or posttest measures, which is unrealistic. To incorporate a reasonable amount of anticipated missing data into the simulation power estimate, the above syntax would need to be changed in two ways.

```
TITLE: MPLUS 6.1 Multivariate Two-Group with Missing Data

MONTECARLO:
NAMES ARE
ADH_pre ADH_post DA_pre DA_post
FA_pre FA_post HRQ_pre HRQ_post;
NOBSERVATIONS = 81 81;
NGROUPS = 2;
NREPS = 5000;
SEED = 9693674;

MISSING =
ADH_post DA_post FA_post HRQ_post;
```

First, the '`MISSING = ADH_post DA_post FA_post HRQ_post;`' statement is required within the '`MONTECARLO:`' command and specifies a researcher's intent that data generated for the posttest response variables include missing data. Second, the '`MODEL MISSING:`' command is necessary to describe how missingness will be generated.

```
MODEL MISSING:
[ADH_post*-1.3861943];
[DA_post*-1.3862943];
[FA_post*-1.3862943];
[HRQ_post*-1.3862943];

ADH_post ON
ADH_pre*-0.336472 DA_pre*0.336472 FA_pre*-0.336472 HRQ_pre*-0.336572;

DA_post ON
ADH_pre*-0.336472 DA_pre*0.336472 FA_pre*-0.336472 HRQ_pre*-0.336572;

FA_post ON
ADH_pre*-0.336472 DA_pre*0.336472 FA_pre*-0.336472 HRQ_pre*-0.336572;

HRQ_post ON
ADH_pre*-0.336472 DA_pre*0.336472 FA_pre*-0.336472 HRQ_pre*-0.336572;
```

The '`MODEL MISSING:`' command allows the researcher the opportunity to specify and include a specific probability of missing data for all four of the posttest response variables based on a logistic regression equation. The value in brackets (`-1.3862943`) beside each of the four posttest response variables specifies a $Pr = \exp^{-1.3862943} / (1 + \exp^{-1.3862943}) = 0.20$ probability (Pr) of missing data. If those four statements in brackets were the only statements listed in the '`MODEL MISSING:`' command, a probability of 0.20 for MCAR missing data would be specified. (*Side Note: Notice how the '`$1`' specification needed in Chapter 5 for a logistic regression power analysis is not needed here. This is because the '`MODEL MISSING:`' command is based solely on logistic regression specifications, but a multinomial logistic regression power analysis could have been performed also in the previous chapter. If a multinomial logistic regression power analysis involved an ordinal response variable with three levels, the multinomial logistic intercepts would be specified with separate '`$1`' and a '`$2`' specifications.*) The inclusion of the next four '`ON`' statements specify MAR data. Specifically, the value listed in the '`ON`' statements (`0.336472`) specify a (odds ratio $= \exp^{0.336472} = 1.40$) 40% change in the odds of a generated data value being converted to a missing value per unit changes in each of the pretest variables. Specifically, the odds of a generated data value being converted to a missing data value will increase 40% for unit increases in disease activity pretest (`DA_pre`) scores and unit decreases in adherence (`ADH_pre`), functional activity (`FA_pre`), and health-related quality-of-life (`HRQ_pre`) pretest scores.

Before examining the power analysis results for the above syntax, the flexibility of the '`MODEL MISSING:`' command in a multigroup Monte Carlo simulation power analysis, and missing data patterns and covariance coverage matrices both warrant mention. First, use of a single '`MODEL MISSING:`' command, such as was done above, means that the same missing data model is specified for both the treatment and control groups. However, different missing data models could be specified for both the control and treatment conditions separately under '`MODEL MISSING:`' and '`MODEL MISSING:-g2`' commands, respectively. Specifying different missing data models separately for the treatment and control groups would also be consistent with MAR because missing data would then also be related to random assignment. Second, output files for Mplus Monte Carlo simulations using the '`MODEL`

MISSING:' command will, by default, contain both a missing data patterns illustration and a covariance coverage matrix. The missing data patterns that result from the above Mplus syntax are shown below.

```
 MISSING DATA PATTERN FREQUENCIES FOR G1

Pattern    Frequency       Pattern    Frequency       Pattern    Frequency
      1           25             5           13             9            8
      2            7             6            3            10            3
      3            7             7            3            11            6
      4            4             8            1            12            1

    MISSING DATA PATTERNS FOR G2 (x = not missing)
            1  2  3  4  5  6  7  8  9  10  11  12
ADH_POST    x  x  x  x  x  x
DA_POST     x  x  x  x        x  x  x  x
FA_POST     x  x        x     x  x          x
HRQ_POST    x     x     x  x  x     x       x   x

 MISSING DATA PATTERN FREQUENCIES FOR G2
Pattern    Frequency       Pattern    Frequency       Pattern    Frequency
      1           30             5            7             9            3
      2           10             6            1            10            1
      3            8             7            7            11            7
      4            3             8            3            12            1
```

For the above output, G1 represents the control condition, G2 represents the treatment condition. In these patterns matrices, an 'x' indicates observed data while a blank indicates missing data. Taken together, the missing data pattern matrices and frequency counts can be interpreted as $n = 25$ records in the control group, and $n = 30$ records in the treatment group show missing data pattern #1, which is complete data for all four posttest response variables, while $n = 4$ records in the control group, and $n = 3$ records in the treatment group show missing data pattern #4, which indicates observed data for adherence (ADH_POST) and disease activity (DA_POST) posttest scores, but missing values for posttest functional activity (FA_POST) and health-related quality-of-life (HRQ_POST).

The covariance coverage matrices that also result from the above Mplus syntax are shown below.

```
    PROPORTION OF DATA PRESENT FOR G1

         Covariance Coverage
           ADH_POST      DA_POST       FA_POST       HRQ_POST
ADH_POST     0.778
DA_POST      0.531         0.753
FA_POST      0.593         0.531         0.728
HRQ_POST     0.593         0.568         0.568         0.765
ADH_PRE      0.778         0.753         0.728         0.765
DA_PRE       0.778         0.753         0.728         0.765
FA_PRE       0.778         0.753         0.728         0.765
HRQ_PRE      0.778         0.753         0.728         0.765
```

```
PROPORTION OF DATA PRESENT FOR G2

          Covariance Coverage
             ADH_POST       DA_POST       FA_POST       HRQ_POST
ADH_POST     0.728
DA_POST      0.630          0.802
FA_POST      0.580          0.617         0.790
HRQ_POST     0.568          0.593         0.630         0.790
ADH_PRE      0.728          0.802         0.790         0.790
DA_PRE       0.728          0.802         0.790         0.790
FA_PRE       0.728          0.802         0.790         0.790
HRQ_PRE      0.728          0.802         0.790         0.790
```

`G1` and `G2` again represent the control and treatment groups, respectively. Covariance coverage matrices show the proportion of data *present* for all possible pairs of analysis variables. Pretest data were generated with no missing values; the pairwise covariance coverage proportion values between pretest variables is 1 by definition and are not included here. For illustration purposes, the covariance coverage matrices for both the control and treatment groups have been partitioned by rectangles into upper and lower portions. As shown in the lower portion of both matrices, missing data for pairwise comparisons of pretest and posttest variables varied between (1 – 0.778 = 0.222) 22.2% and (1 – 0.728 = 0.272) 27.2% for the control (`G1`) group, and between (1 – 0.802 = 0.198) 19.8% and (1 – 0.728 = 0.272) 27.2% for the treatment (`G2`) group. However, as shown in the upper portion of both matrices, missing data for pairwise comparisons among posttest variables varied between (1 – 0.778 = 0.222) 22.2% and (1 – 0.531 = 0.469) 46.9% for the control (`G1`) group, and between (1 – 0.802 = 0.198) 19.8% and (1 – 0.58 = 0.42) 42% for the treatment (`G2`) group. Recall that the '`MODEL MISSING:`' syntax lines specified the generation of 20% MAR missing data; those values can be revisited and adjusted as needed.

The Monte Carlo simulation power analysis results for a multivariate two-group comparison incorporating an expected 20% of MAR missing data for the posttest response variables is shown below.

```
                   ESTIMATES              S. E.     M. S. E.  95%   % Sig
            Population   Average   Std. Dev.   Average           Cover Coeff
ADH_DIFF       0.450      0.4490     0.1586     0.1578    0.0251 0.948 0.809
DA_DIFF        0.450      0.4477     0.1594     0.1580    0.0254 0.946 0.809
FA_DIFF        0.450      0.4521     0.1582     0.1577    0.0250 0.950 0.809
HRQ_DIFF       0.450      0.4523     0.1590     0.1579    0.0253 0.947 0.815
```

As shown in both the Mplus syntax and power analysis results above, $N = 162$ ($n = 81$ per group) is now needed for power ≥ .80 to detect the same treatment effect ($\Delta d = 0.45$), as specified in Chapter 2 (recall $N = 132$ was needed for adequate statistical power assuming no missing data). The inclusion of an expected 20% of MAR missing data on all posttest response variables increased the sample size requirement (162 – 132) / 132 = 22.72% in order to maintain adequate statistical power. Finally, the Monte Carlo simulation power analysis write-up from Chapter 2 that now has the missing data specifications included is given next.

Multivariate Two-Group Power Analysis Using R

The analysis model from Chapter 2 involved a treatment versus control multivariate comparison of mean differences across four pretest and posttest variables: adherence (ADH), disease activity (DA), functional activity (FA), and health-related quality of life (HRQ). The R code to specify the population model, analysis model, run the simulation, and obtain power analysis estimates from Chapter 2 analysis are provided here:

```
library(simsem)
library(lavaan)

PopulationModel_Ch2 <- "
  ADH_pre ~ 0                          # means are set to 0 for documentation
  DA_pre ~ 0
  FA_pre ~ 0
  HRQ_pre ~ 0
  ADH_pre ~~ 1*ADH_pre                 # variances are constrained to 1
  DA_pre ~~ 1*DA_pre
  FA_pre ~~ 1*FA_pre
  HRQ_pre ~~ 1*HRQ_pre

  ADH_post ~ c(0.16, 0.61)*1           # mean values differ across populations
  DA_post ~ c(0.16, 0.61)*1
  FA_post ~ c(0.16, 0.61)*1
  HRQ_post ~ c(0.16, 0.61)*1
  ADH_post ~~ 0.84*ADH_post            # residual variances are constrained to .84
  DA_post ~~ 0.84*DA_post
  FA_post ~~ 0.84*FA_post
  HRQ_post ~~ 0.84*HRQ_post

  ADH_post ~~ 0.3*DA_post + 0.3*FA_post + 0.3*HRQ_post
  DA_post ~~ 0.3*FA_post + 0.3*HRQ_post
  FA_post ~~ 0.3*HRQ_post
  ADH_pre ~~ 0.3*DA_pre + 0.3*FA_pre + 0.3*HRQ_pre
  DA_pre ~~ 0.3*FA_pre + 0.3*HRQ_pre
  FA_pre ~~ 0.3*HRQ_pre

  ADH_post ~ 0.4*ADH_pre + a1*ADH_pre # constrain parameters equal across groups
  DA_post ~ 0.4*DA_pre + a2*DA_pre
  FA_post ~ 0.4*FA_pre + a3*FA_pre
  HRQ_post ~ 0.4*HRQ_pre + a4*HRQ_pre

  ADH_DIFF := .45 # set population value mean difference
  DA_DIFF := .45
  FA_DIFF := .45
  HRQ_DIFF := .45 "

  AnalysisModel_Ch2 <- "
  ADH_pre ~~ ADH_pre
  DA_pre ~~ DA_pre
  FA_pre ~~ FA_pre
  HRQ_pre ~~ HRQ_pre
```

```
  ADH_post ~ c(E, A)*1          # mean label across groups
  DA_post ~ c(F, B)*1
  FA_post ~ c(G, C)*1
  HRQ_post ~ c(H, D)*1
  ADH_post ~~ ADH_post
  DA_post ~~ DA_post
  FA_post ~~ FA_post
  HRQ_post ~~ HRQ_post

  ADH_post ~~ DA_post + FA_post + HRQ_post
  DA_post ~~ FA_post + HRQ_post
  FA_post ~~ HRQ_post
  ADH_pre ~~ DA_pre + FA_pre + HRQ_pre
  DA_pre ~~ FA_pre + HRQ_pre
  FA_pre ~~ HRQ_pre

  ADH_post ~ a1*ADH_pre    # label parameter and constrain equal across groups
  DA_post ~ a2*DA_pre
  FA_post ~ a3*FA_pre
  HRQ_post ~ a4*HRQ_pre

  #Creating mean difference values
  ADH_DIFF := A-E
  DA_DIFF := B-F
  FA_DIFF := C-G
  HRQ_DIFF := D-H "

SampleDatasets_Ch2 <- simulateDataSets(PopulationModel_Ch2,
                          nIterations = 5000,
                          nObservations = c(66, 66),
                          seed = 10127)
output_Ch2 <- sim(model = AnalysisModel_Ch2,
                  rawData = SampleDatasets_Ch2,
                  group = "group",
                  silent = TRUE)

getPower(output_Ch2)[c("ADH_DIFF ", "DA_DIFF", "FA_DIFF", "HRQ_DIFF")]
ADH_DIFF  DA_DIFF   FA_DIFF   HRQ_DIFF
0.82      0.82      0.86      0.83
```

The above analysis assumes no missing data, implying that a sample size of $N = 132$ can be collected using pre- and posttest measures without any missing responses. This is a highly unrealistic assumption. Incorporation of a reasonable amount of anticipated missing data is needed to understand the effective sample size necessary to obtain the expected estimates. In R, a missing data model can be specified and imposed on the sample datasets generated from the population model. Although multiple ways to impose missing data are available using simsem, this book only uses the lavaan-style syntax approach. The missing model can be specified as follows using logit values:

```
MissingData_Ch2 <- "
  ADH_post ~ -1.3862943 + -0.336472*ADH_pre + 0.336472*DA_pre
             + -0.336472*FA_pre + -0.336472*HRQ_pre
```

```
    DA_post ~   -1.3862943 + -0.336472*ADH_pre + 0.336472*DA_pre
                + -0.336472*FA_pre + -0.336472*HRQ_pre
    FA_post ~   -1.3862943 + -0.336472*ADH_pre + 0.336472*DA_pre
                + -0.336472*FA_pre + -0.336472*HRQ_pre
    HRQ_post ~ -1.3862943 + -0.336472*ADH_pre + 0.336472*DA_pre
                + -0.336472*FA_pre + -0.336472*HRQ_pre
"
MissingModel_Ch2 <- miss(logit=MissingData_Ch2)
```

The intercept values (–1.3862943) reflect the logit value associated with the probability of MCAR for each of the posttest variables. To check what probability this logit value is associated with, input the following into the R console:

```
prob <- function(logval){exp(logval)/(1+exp(logval))}
prob(-1.3862943)
```

which results in output of 0.2. The next part of the equation includes slope values, which is the method for generating MAR data. These values, –0.336472, are multiplied by each of the pretest scores and reflect the change in missing conditional values on pretest values. The interpretation of these values is most easily thought of in terms of an odds ratio, where the exponentiated slope value ($\exp^{-0.336472} = 1.40$) reflects a change in the odds of the generated data value being converted to a missing value per unit changes in each of the pretest variables. In other words, the odds of a generated data value being converted to a missing data value will increase 40% for unit increases in disease activity pretest (DA_pre) scores and unit decreases in adherence (ADH_pre), functional activity (FA_pre), and health-related quality-of-life (HRQ_pre) pretest scores.

The power analysis can now be conducted the same way as in prior chapters, but including an additional line of code, miss = MissingModel_Ch2, to incorporate the missing data model. For this first analysis, the missing data model will be imposed on the simulated datasets.

```
SampleDataMiss_Ch2 <- simulateDataSets(PopulationModel_Ch2,
                      nIterations = 5000,
                      nObservations = c(81, 81),
                      miss = MissingModel_Ch2,
                      seed = 9693674)
```

Once the data are simulated, a summary of the first dataset can be examined to determine if the model imposed missingness as expected.

```
summary(SampleDataMiss_Ch2[[1]])

ADH_post            DA_post             FA_post             HRQ_post            ADH_pre
Min.   :-2.2727     Min.   :-2.2218     Min.   :-2.3764     Min.   :-2.4569     Min.   :-3.13399
1st Qu.:-0.1896     1st Qu.:-0.3490     1st Qu.:-0.3237     1st Qu.:-0.3064     1st Qu.:-0.59305
Median : 0.4902     Median : 0.4169     Median : 0.5146     Median : 0.3791     Median : 0.18803
Mean   : 0.4538     Mean   : 0.3784     Mean   : 0.4843     Mean   : 0.4038     Mean   : 0.08595
3rd Qu.: 1.1655     3rd Qu.: 0.9861     3rd Qu.: 1.2847     3rd Qu.: 1.0225     3rd Qu: 0.78573
Max.   : 3.1933     Max.   : 3.3491     Max.   : 2.9079     Max.   : 2.5343     Max.   : 2.04944
NA's   :35          NA's   :31          NA's   :41          NA's   :33
```

```
DA_pre               FA_pre               HRQ_pre              group          iteration
Min.   :-2.76103    Min.   :-3.61076    Min.   :-3.12837    Min.   :1.0    Min.   :1
1st Qu.:-0.74076    1st Qu.:-0.63255    1st Qu.:-0.63174    1st Qu.:1.0    1st Qu.:1
Median : 0.14926    Median :-0.01127    Median : 0.12618    Median :1.5    Median :1
Mean   : 0.03251    Mean   : 0.03295    Mean   : 0.04189    Mean   :1.5    Mean   :1
3rd Qu.: 0.77695    3rd Qu.: 0.71294    3rd Qu.: 0.72203    3rd Qu.:2.0    3rd Qu.:1
Max.   : 2.23761    Max.   : 2.72264    Max.   : 2.49077    Max.   :2.0    Max.   :1
```

As shown in the summary of the first dataset, missingness is imposed on all posttest scores, such that 31 to 41 observations are missing on posttest scores. To ensure that the missing data mechanism includes some randomness across observations, examine summaries of the second dataset.

```
summary(SampleDataMiss_Ch2[[2]])

ADH_post           DA_post            FA_post             HRQ_post            ADH_pre
Min.   :-2.3281   Min.   :-2.2608   Min.   :-3.14731   Min.   :-2.50360   Min.   :-2.67165
1st Qu.:-0.1681   1st Qu.:-0.2000   1st Qu.:-0.06528   1st Qu.:-0.09268   1st Qu.:-0.65511
Median : 0.5446   Median : 0.4258   Median : 0.44804   Median : 0.46641   Median : 0.10065
Mean   : 0.5482   Mean   : 0.4677   Mean   : 0.47511   Mean   : 0.51236   Mean   : 0.05843
3rd Qu.: 1.2685   3rd Qu.: 1.1357   3rd Qu.: 1.15810   3rd Qu.: 1.17489   3rd Qu.: 0.81459
Max.   : 2.5884   Max.   : 2.8505   Max.   : 3.34397   Max.   : 3.28084   Max.   : 2.55199
NA's   :38        NA's   :26        NA's   :34         NA's   :34

DA_pre              FA_pre             HRQ_pre            group          iteration
Min.   :-2.58973   Min.   :-2.2819   Min.   :-2.0042   Min.   :1.0    Min.   :2
1st Qu.:-0.63885   1st Qu.:-0.4561   1st Qu.:-0.4569   1st Qu.:1.0    1st Qu.:2
Median : 0.15012   Median : 0.1970   Median : 0.1665   Median :1.5    Median :2
Mean   : 0.08331   Mean   : 0.1459   Mean   : 0.1642   Mean   :1.5    Mean   :2
3rd Qu.: 0.85257   3rd Qu.: 0.8000   3rd Qu.: 0.8040   3rd Qu.:2.0    3rd Qu.:2
Max.   : 2.79627   Max.   : 2.4851   Max.   : 2.7461   Max.   :2.0    Max.   :2
```

Missingness differs for the second dataset so an examination of missingness summaries for the full sample of simulated datasets is required. In the final step of the simulation power analysis, covariance coverage aggregating missingness across all datasets will be evaluated.

Unlike in Mplus, obtaining aggregate missing data patterns and covariance coverage in simsem is not automatically provided with the model output. Instead one relatively straightforward approach to assess missingness is to examine the covariance coverage of the model using the outfun option in simsem. This outfun option can be used to estimate additional output from every iteration of simsem. Below, the outfun option equal cov_coverage, which is a function specifically developed to inspect covariance coverage from each output in lavaan.

```
cov_coverage <- function(fit) {coverage <- lavInspect(fit, "coverage")}
```

To use the outfun option to obtain additional lavaan output, functions should be developed beforehand and then included in the final sim function of the Monte Carlo simulation analysis.

```
outputMiss_Ch6 <-  sim(model = AnalysisModel_Ch2,
                   rawData = SampleDataMiss_Ch2, # datasets with missing
                   group = "group",
                   silent = TRUE,
                   outfun = cov_coverage)
```

Overall, the covariance coverage can be evaluated according to group membership by creating a new function called groupavg_cov_coverage.

```
groupavg_cov_coverage <- function(output, group) {
round(tril(apply(simplify2array(simplify2array(getExtraOutput(output))[group,]), 1:2, mean)), 3)
}
```

The function can then be called for group 1,

```
groupavg_cov_coverage(outputMiss_Ch6, 1)
```

or group 2,

```
groupavg_cov_coverage(outputMiss_Ch6, 2)
```

resulting in almost equivalent covariance coverage output matrices across groups, where group 1 covariance coverage is:

```
8 x 8 Matrix of class "dtrMatrix"
         ADH_post DA_post FA_post HRQ_post ADH_pre DA_pre FA_pre HRQ_pre
ADH_post    0.781       .       .        .       .      .      .       .
DA_post     0.622   0.781       .        .       .      .      .       .
FA_post     0.622   0.622   0.781        .       .      .      .       .
HRQ_post    0.621   0.622   0.621    0.781       .      .      .       .
ADH_pre     0.781   0.781   0.781    0.781   1.000      .      .       .
DA_pre      0.781   0.781   0.781    0.781   1.000  1.000      .       .
FA_pre      0.781   0.781   0.781    0.781   1.000  1.000  1.000       .
HRQ_pre     0.781   0.781   0.781    0.781   1.000  1.000  1.000   1.000
```

and group 2 covariance coverage is:

```
8 x 8 Matrix of class "dtrMatrix"
         ADH_post DA_post FA_post HRQ_post ADH_pre DA_pre FA_pre HRQ_pre
ADH_post    0.782       .       .        .       .      .      .       .
DA_post     0.623   0.782       .        .       .      .      .       .
FA_post     0.623   0.623   0.782        .       .      .      .       .
HRQ_post    0.621   0.622   0.622    0.780       .      .      .       .
ADH_pre     0.782   0.782   0.782    0.780   1.000      .      .       .
DA_pre      0.782   0.782   0.782    0.780   1.000  1.000      .       .
FA_pre      0.782   0.782   0.782    0.780   1.000  1.000  1.000       .
HRQ_pre     0.782   0.782   0.782    0.780   1.000  1.000  1.000   1.000
```

Recall that covariance coverage matrices show the proportion of data that are not missing for all pairs of analysis variables. Pretest data were generated with no missing values. Missing data for pairwise comparisons of pretest and posttest variables approximated (1 – 0.781 = 0.219) 21.9% for the control group (Group 1), and between (1 – 0.782 = 0.218) 21.8% and (1 – 0.780 = 0.220) 22.0% for the treatment group (Group 2). However, as shown in the upper portion of both matrices, missing data for pairwise comparisons among posttest variables varied between (1 – 0.782 = 0.218) 21.8% and (1 – 0.621 = .379) 37.9% for the control group, and between (1 – 0.802 = 0.198) 19.8% and (1 – 0.621 = 0.379) 37.9% for the treatment group.

Now that missing data have been imposed and assessed for accuracy, the Monte Carlo simulation power analysis results for a multivariate two-group comparison incorporating approximately 20% MAR missing data for the posttest response variables is shown:

```
getPower(outputMiss_Ch6)[c("ADH_DIFF ", "DA_DIFF", "FA_DIFF", "HRQ_DIFF")]

ADH_DIFF      DA_DIFF      FA_DIFF      HRQ_DIFF
0.80          0.76         0.81         0.78
```

Note that these results do not perfectly mimic the results from Mplus, with some power estimates lower than .80. Further analysis using a larger sample size is needed. An analysis increasing the sample size to $n = 86$ per group, for a total sample size of $N = 172$ was evaluated.

```
SampleDataMiss2_Ch2 <- simulateDataSets(PopulationModel_Ch2,
                    nIterations = 5000,
                    nObservations = c(86, 86),
                    miss = MissingModel_Ch2,
                    seed = 9693674)

outputMiss2_Ch6 <- sim(model = AnalysisModel_Ch2,
                    rawData = SampleDataMiss2_Ch2, # datasets with missing
                    group = "group",
                    silent = TRUE,
                    outfun = cov_coverage)
```

The model output now shows that statistical power estimates are acceptable across all difference variables.

```
getPower(outputMiss2_Ch6)[c("ADH_DIFF ", "DA_DIFF", "FA_DIFF", "HRQ_DIFF")]
ADH_DIFF      DA_DIFF      FA_DIFF      HRQ_DIFF
0.82          0.80         0.84         0.80
```

Multivariate Two-Group Simulation Power Analysis with Missing Data Write-Up

"The power analysis question involved the smallest sample size needed to achieve power ≥ .80 to detect a posttest mean effect size difference (Δd) between the treatment and control conditions of $\Delta d = 0.45$ after controlling for pretest scores as covariates. A Monte Carlo simulation power analysis was conducted using Mplus (version 8.6) assuming: (1) the SEM equivalent of a multivariate analysis of covariance (MANCOVA) data analysis model where pretest response variables are included as covariates for each of their respective posttest variables (adherence, disease activity, functional activity, and health-related quality of life), (2) standardization of all pretest and posttest response variables, (3) random assignment results in equivalent groups across the four response variables at the pretest assessment, (4) the control condition will experience a minimal pretest to posttest difference ($\Delta d = 0.16$; Kahana, Drotar, & Frazier, 2008), (5) the treatment condition will experience a pretest to posttest difference of ($\Delta d = 0.61$), resulting in a treatment versus control group difference of ($\Delta d = 0.61 - 0.16 = 0.45$) at posttest, (6) the MANCOVA assumption of homogeneity of covariate regression slopes (i.e., the effect of each posttest response variable regressed onto their respective pretest counterparts is equal across the treatment and control groups) will be ensured using parameter estimate equality constraints, (7) the use of pretest scores as covariates will explain ($R^2 = 0.16$) 16% of response variable error variance, (8) 20% of posttest data was specified to be missing at random, such that the odds of a missing value increased 40% per unit increase in disease activity pretest scores and per unit decreases in treatment adherence, functional activity, and health-related quality-of-life pretest scores, and (9) all four response variables will be correlated at a medium effect size (i.e., $r_{\text{Pearson}} = 0.30$) at both the pretest and posttest assessments. Monte Carlo simulation power analysis results aggregated over 5,000 replications showed power ≥ .80 for the anticipated treatment versus control posttest difference ($\Delta d = 0.45$) if $N = 162$ ($n_{\text{Treatment}} = n_{\text{Control}} = 81$) is available for analysis."

Structural Equation Model

Recall that, in Chapter 4, the Monte Carlo simulation power analysis under consideration involved combining 12 observed variables into four latent variables: two exogenous (X_1 and X_2) and two endogenous (Y_1 and Y_2). The specific power analysis question involved the sample size needed for power ≥ .80 for all three latent variable predictions, as shown in Figure 6.3.

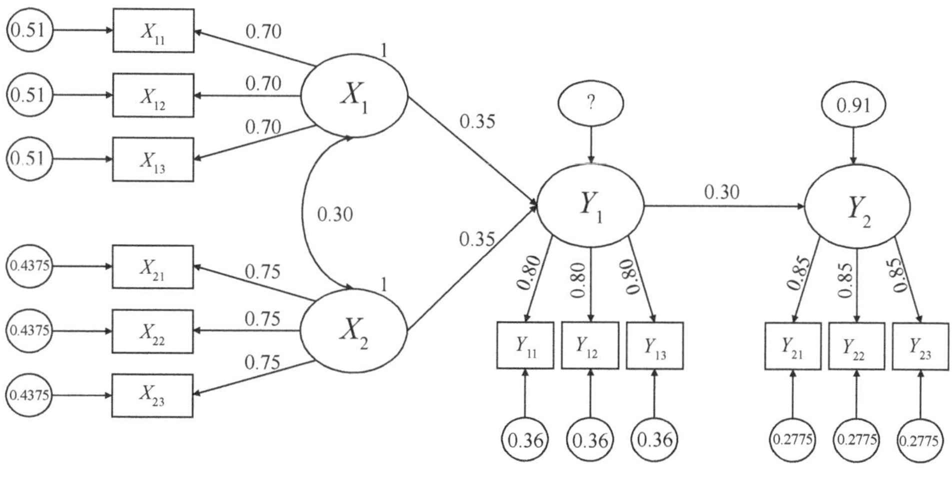

FIGURE 6.3. Structural equation model.

Structural Equation Modeling Power Analysis Using Mplus

The analysis model, Monte Carlo simulation power analysis syntax, and results from Mplus are all reprinted below.

```
MONTECARLO:
NAMES ARE
X11 X12 X13 X21 X22 X23
Y11 Y12 Y13 Y21 Y22 Y23;

NOBSERVATIONS = 99;

NREPS = 5000;

MODEL POPULATION:
X1 BY X11*.8367 X12*.8367 X13*.8367;
X2 BY X21*.866 X22*.866 X23*.866;
Y1 BY Y11*.8944 Y12*.8944 Y13*.8944;
Y2 BY Y21*.922 Y22*.922 Y23*.922;

X1@1;
X2@1;
Y1@.6815;
Y2@.91;

X1 WITH X2*.3;

Y1 ON X1*.35 X2*.35;
Y2 ON Y1*.3;

X11-X13*.30;
X21-X23*.25;
Y11-Y13*.20;
Y21-Y23*.15;

ANALYSIS:
estimator = ml;

MODEL:
X1 BY X11*.8367 X12*.8367 X13*.8367;
X2 BY X21*.866 X22*.866 X23*.866;
Y1 BY Y11*.8944 Y12*.8944 Y13*.8944;
Y2 BY Y21*.922 Y22*.922 Y23*.922;

X1@1;
X2@1;
Y1@.6815;
Y2@.91;

X1 WITH X2*.3;

Y1 ON X1*.35 X2*.35;
Y2 ON Y1*.3;
```

```
X11-X13*.30;
X21-X23*.25;
Y11-Y13*.20;
Y21-Y23*.15;

OUTPUT: res;
```

MODEL RESULTS

		ESTIMATES		S. E.	M. S. E.	95%	% Sig
	Population	Average	Std. Dev.	Average		Cover	Coeff
Y1 ON							
X1	0.350	0.3592	0.1153	0.1120	0.0134	0.950	**0.916**
X2	0.350	0.3556	0.1138	0.1101	0.0130	0.946	**0.917**
Y2 ON							
Y1	0.300	0.2992	0.1115	0.1084	0.0124	0.951	**0.807**

As shown in both the syntax and results, $N = 99$ is needed to reject the null hypotheses for the three latent variable predictions. But again, the above power analysis also assumes that 12 observed variables can be collected from a sample of $N = 99$ with no missing data on any of the 12 variables, which again is unrealistic. Incorporating a reasonable estimate of anticipated missing data into the simulation power estimate would again involve adding `MODEL MISSING:` and related specifications to the above syntax.

```
TITLE: MPLUS 6.2 SEM with MISSING

MONTECARLO:
NAMES ARE
X11 X12 X13 X21 X22 X23
Y11 Y12 Y13 Y21 Y22 Y23;

NOBSERVATIONS = 99;
NREPS = 5000;

MISSING =
Y11 Y12 Y13 Y21 Y22 Y23;
```

The addition of the `MISSING =` specification to the `MONTECARLO:` command indicates that missing data will be generated for the six observed endogenous variables.

```
MODEL MISSING:
[Y11-Y23*-2.1972];
Y11 ON X11*0.18232 X12*-0.3365 X13*0.18232;
Y12 ON X11*0.18232 X12*-0.3365 X13*0.18232;
Y13 ON X11*0.18232 X12*-0.3365 X13*0.18232;
Y21 ON X21*0.18232 X22*-0.3365 X23*0.18232;
Y22 ON X21*0.18232 X22*-0.3365 X23*0.18232;
Y23 ON X21*0.18232 X22*-0.3365 X23*0.18232;
```

The first line of syntax below the `MODEL MISSING:` statement specifies a ($\exp^{-2.1972} / (1 + \exp^{-2.1972}) = 1/(1 + \exp^{-1*-2.1972}) = 0.10$) 10% probability of missing data for any of the observed endogenous ($Y_{11} - Y_{23}$) variables. If this were the only syntax line included in the `MODEL MISSING:` statement, this would specify MCAR missing data. The last six lines of syntax below the `MODEL MISSING:` statement makes missing data on observed endogenous variables conditional on values for the exogenous observed variables, which now means, by definition, the generated missing data will be MAR. Specifically, missing on two of the three endogenous variables is expected to result in a ($\exp^{0.18232} = 1.20$) 20% per unit increase in the corresponding exogenous variables, and result in a ($\exp^{-0.3365} = 0.7143$; $1/0.7143 = 1.40$) 40% per unit decrease in the corresponding exogenous variable. Unlike the multivariate two-group comparison example, the missing data specifications here are arbitrary because no intuitive hypotheses regarding missing data can be made for generic observed variables. However, this SEM with the above missing data specifications will be expanded upon to demonstrate a Monte Carlo simulation power analysis for latent variable moderation in Appendix A in the online supplemental material (at *www.guilford.com/peugh-materials*). The modified SEM Monte Carlo simulation power analysis syntax that includes missing data is provided below, followed by simulation results.

```
TITLE: MPLUS 6.2 SEM with MISSING

MONTECARLO:
NAMES ARE
X11 X12 X13 X21 X22 X23
Y11 Y12 Y13 Y21 Y22 Y23;

NOBSERVATIONS = 101;
NREPS = 5000;
MISSING = Y11-Y23;

MODEL POPULATION:
X1 BY X11*.8367 X12*.8367 X13*.8367;
X2 BY X21*.866 X22*.866 X23*.866;
Y1 BY Y11*.8944 Y12*.8944 Y13*.8944;
Y2 BY Y21*.922 Y22*.922 Y23*.922;

X1@1;
X2@1;
Y1@.6815;
Y2@.91;

X1 WITH X2*.3;

Y1 ON X1*.35 X2*.35;
Y2 ON Y1*.3;

X11-X13*.30;
X21-X23*.25;
Y11-Y13*.20;
Y21-Y23*.15;

MODEL MISSING:
[Y11-Y23*-2.1972];
```

```
Y11 ON X11*0.18232 X12*-0.3365 X13*0.18232;
Y12 ON X11*0.18232 X12*-0.3365 X13*0.18232;
Y13 ON X11*0.18232 X12*-0.3365 X13*0.18232;
Y21 ON X21*0.18232 X22*-0.3365 X23*0.18232;
Y22 ON X21*0.18232 X22*-0.3365 X23*0.18232;
Y23 ON X21*0.18232 X22*-0.3365 X23*0.18232;

MODEL:
X1 BY X11*.8367 X12*.8367 X13*.8367;
X2 BY X21*.866 X22*.866 X23*.866;
Y1 BY Y11*.8944 Y12*.8944 Y13*.8944;
Y2 BY Y21*.922 Y22*.922 Y23*.922;

X1@1;
X2@1;
Y1@.6815;
Y2@.91;

X1 WITH X2*.3;

Y1 ON X1*.35 X2*.35;
Y2 ON Y1*.3;

X11-X13*.30;
X21-X23*.25;
Y11-Y13*.20;
Y21-Y23*.15;
```

			ESTIMATES		S. E.	M. S. E.	95%	% Sig
		Population	Average	Std. Dev.	Average		Cover	Coeff
Y1	ON							
X1		**0.350**	0.3586	0.1156	0.1120	0.0134	0.947	**0.914**
X2		**0.350**	0.3563	0.1120	0.1101	0.0126	0.950	**0.922**
Y2	ON							
Y1		**0.300**	0.2987	0.1115	0.1088	0.0124	0.949	**0.802**

Structural Equation Modeling Power Analysis Using R

The R code to specify the population model, analysis model, run the simulation, and obtain power analysis estimates from the analysis in Chapter 4 are repeated below.

```
library(simsem)
library(lavaan)

PopulationModel_Ch4 <- "
  X1 =~ 0.8367*X11 + 0.8367*X12 + 0.8367*X13
  X2 =~ 0.866*X21 + 0.866*X22 + 0.866*X23
  Y1 =~ 0.8944*Y11 + 0.8944*Y12 + 0.8944*Y13
  Y2 =~ 0.922*Y21 + 0.922*Y22 + 0.922*Y23

  X1 ~~ 1*X1
```

```
  X2 ~~ 1*X2
  Y1 ~~ 0.6815*Y1
  Y2 ~~ 0.91*Y2

  X1 ~~ 0.30*X2

  Y1 ~ 0.35*X1 + 0.35*X2
  Y2 ~ 0.30*Y1

  X11 ~~ 0.30*X11
  X12 ~~ 0.30*X12
  X13 ~~ 0.30*X13
  X21 ~~ 0.25*X21
  X22 ~~ 0.25*X22
  X23 ~~ 0.25*X23
  Y11 ~~ 0.20*Y11
  Y12 ~~ 0.20*Y12
  Y13 ~~ 0.20*Y13
  Y21 ~~ 0.15*Y21
  Y22 ~~ 0.15*Y22
  Y23 ~~ 0.15*Y23"

AnalysisModel_Ch4 <- "
  X1 =~ X11 + X12 + X13
  X2 =~ X21 + X22 + X23
  Y1 =~ Y11 + Y12 + Y13
  Y2 =~ Y21 + Y22 + Y23

  X1 ~~ 1*X1 #constrain all factor variances to freely estimate the factor loadings
  X2 ~~ 1*X2
  Y1 ~~ 0.6815*Y1
  Y2 ~~ 0.91*Y2

  X1 ~~ X2

  Y1 ~ X1 + X2
  Y2 ~ Y1

  X11 ~~ X11
  X12 ~~ X12
  X13 ~~ X13
  X21 ~~ X21
  X22 ~~ X22
  X23 ~~ X23
  Y11 ~~ Y11
  Y12 ~~ Y12
  Y13 ~~ Y13
  Y21 ~~ Y21
  Y22 ~~ Y22
  Y23 ~~ Y23
"

output_Ch4 <-    sim( nRep = 5000,
                 n = 99,
                 model = AnalysisModel_Ch4
```

```
            generate = PopulationModel_Ch4
            std.lv = FALSE,
            seed = 35170,
            silent = TRUE)

getPower(output_Ch4)[c("Y1~X1", "Y1~X2", "Y2~Y1")]
Y1~X1       Y1~X2       Y2~Y1
0.9122      0.9286      0.8046
```

This output shows that $N = 99$ would provide sufficient power to detect the expected three latent variable predictions. However, this sample size assumes that all 12 observed variables can be collected from the sample with no missing data, which is unrealistic. Incorporating a reasonable estimate of anticipated missing data into the simulation power estimate involves creating another missing data model.

```
MissingData_Ch4 <- "
Y11 ~ -2.1972 + 0.18232*X11 -0.3365*X12 0.18232*X13;
Y12 ~ -2.1972 + 0.18232*X11 -0.3365*X12 0.18232*X13;
Y13 ~ -2.1972 + 0.18232*X11 -0.3365*X12 0.18232*X13;
Y21 ~ -2.1972 + 0.18232*X21 -0.3365*X22 0.18232*X23;
Y22 ~ -2.1972 + 0.18232*X21 -0.3365*X22 0.18232*X23;
Y23 ~ -2.1972 + 0.18232*X21 -0.3365*X22 0.18232*X23;
"
MissingModel_Ch4 <- miss(logit=MissingData_Ch4)
```

The intercept values in each equation reflects a ($\exp^{-2.1972}/(1 + \exp^{-2.1972}) = 1/(1 + \exp^{-1*-2.1972}) = 0.10$) 10% probability of MCAR data for any of the observed endogenous variables. The next components of each equation reflect the probability of MAR data, or missing data that are conditional on values for the exogenous observed variables. Specifically, missing on two of the three endogenous variables is expected to result in a ($\exp^{0.18232} = 1.20$) 20% per unit increase in the corresponding exogenous variables, and result in a ($\exp^{-0.3365} = 0.7143$; $1/0.7143 = 1.40$) 40% per unit decrease in the corresponding exogenous variable. Unlike the multivariate two-group comparison example, the missing data specifications here are arbitrary because no intuitive hypotheses regarding missing data can be made for generic observed variables, unless other information from prior studies is previously known. The modified SEM Monte Carlo simulation power analysis with missing data can now be computed and examined as follows:

```
OutputMiss2_Ch6 <- sim(nRep = 5000,
                       n =  101,
                            model = AnalysisModel_Ch4,
                            generate = PopulationModel_Ch4,
                            miss = MissingModel_Ch4,
                            std.lv = FALSE,
                            seed = 35170,
                            silent = TRUE)
getPower(outputMiss2_Ch6)[c("Y1 ~ X1", "Y1 ~ X2", "Y2 ~ Y1")]
Y1~X1       Y1~X2       Y2~Y1
0.9128      0.9242      0.7952
```

Rounded to the second decimal place, all power estimates equal .80 or greater. Because much time-intensive computation was completed in R in this chapter, one last step to lessen future computation time is to save the Monte Carlo simulation power analysis results to an external .R or .Rmd file in the current working directory (or elsewhere). This can be done by saving the environment image, using:

```
save.image("mcpower_Ch6.R")
```

which can then be called back into the environment later by loading the previously saved file.

```
load("mcpower_Ch6.R")
```

Structural Equation Modeling Simulation Power Analysis with Missing Data Write-Up

"The power analysis question involves the smallest sample size needed to achieve power ≥ .80 to reject the null hypothesis for the three structural coefficients in the proposed SEM. A Monte Carlo simulation power analysis was conducted using Mplus (version 8.6) assuming: (1) a unit latent factor variance constraint was used to identify the four latent variables (X_1, X_2, Y_1 and Y_2) in the SEM; (2) the latent exogenous variables (X_1 and X_2) were correlated at $r_{X1,X2} = 0.30$; (3) reliability (R_{xx}) estimates ranging between 0.70 and 0.85 were used to specify all 12 standardized factor loadings (λ_β) for the four latent variables by $\lambda_\beta = \sqrt{R_{xx}}$; (4) reliability ($R_{xx}$) estimates were also used to specify measurement error variances (ε) by $\varepsilon = 1 - R_{xx}$; (5) standardized regression coefficient values of $\beta = 0.35$ were assumed for both latent exogenous variables (X_1 and X_2) predicting the endogenous latent variable Y_1, resulting in ($R^2 = 0.3185$) 31.85% of Y_1 variance explained by X_1 and X_2; (6) a standardized regression coefficient value of $\beta = 0.30$ was assumed for the endogenous latent variable Y_1 as a predictor of endogenous latent variable Y_2, resulting in ($R^2 = 0.09$) 9% of Y_2 variance explained by Y_1; (7) missing data were expected to be 20% MAR for the endogenous (Y_{11}–Y_{23}) variables, and was expected to result in a 20% per unit increase in four of the six exogenous variables and a 40% per unit decrease in the remaining two exogenous variables; and (8) the admissibility of the SEM specifications was verified by computing a model-reproduced correlation matrix. Monte Carlo simulation power analysis results aggregated over 5,000 replications showed power ≥ .80 to reject the null hypothesis for all three SEM structural coefficients if proper missing data handling makes a sample size of $N = 101$ available for analysis."

Missing Data Concluding Remarks

Missing data are a reality that can be expected in research, no matter how tightly controlled the research design may be. As shown in both the multivariate two-group comparison and the structural equation model examples, the effect of missing data on power analysis estimates can vary by analysis type as well as across statistical programs. Overall, missingness does have an effect on statistical power estimates, where larger sample sizes are often needed to detect an effect in the presence of missing data. From this point forward, all Monte Carlo simulation power analysis examples will include a consideration of missing data.

SUGGESTED READINGS

- Enders, C. K. (2010). *Applied missing data analysis.* Guilford Press.
- Enders, C. K. (2017). Multiple imputation as a flexible tool for missing data handling in clinical research. *Behaviour Research and Therapy, 98,* 4–18.
- Enders, C. K. (2022). *Applied missing data analysis* (2nd ed.). Guilford Press.
- Enders, C. K., Du, H., & Keller, B. T. (2020). A model-based imputation procedure for multilevel regression models with random coefficients, interaction effects, and nonlinear terms. *Psychological Methods, 25,* 88–112.
- Enders, C. K., Hayes, T., & Du, H. (2018). A comparison of multilevel imputation schemes for random coefficient models: Fully conditional specification and joint model imputation with random covariance matrices. *Multivariate Behavioral Research, 53,* 695–713.
- Enders, C. K., Keller, B. T., & Levy, R. (2018). A fully conditional specification approach to multilevel imputation of categorical and continuous variables. *Psychological Methods, 23,* 298–317.
- Gomila, R., & Clark, C. S. (2020). Missing data in experiments: Challenges and solutions. *Psychological Methods, 27*(2), 143–155.
- Graham, J. W. (2003). Adding missing-data-relevant variables to FIML-based structural equation models. *Structural Equation Modeling, 10,* 80–100.
- Graham, J. W. (2012). *Missing data: Analysis and design.* Springer.
- Lee, T., & Shi, D. (2021). A comparison of full information maximum likelihood and multiple imputation in structural equation modeling with missing data. *Psychological Methods, 26*(4), 466–485.
- Little, R. J. A., & Rubin, D. B. (2020). *Statistical analysis with missing data* (3rd ed.). Wiley.
- Mistler, S. A., & Enders, C. K. (2017). A comparison of joint model and fully conditional specification imputation for multilevel missing data. *Journal of Educational and Behavioral Statistics, 42,* 432–466.
- Molenberghs, G., Fitzmaurice, G., Kenward, M. G., Tsiatis, A., & Verbeke, G. (Eds.). (2020). *Handbook of missing data methodology.* CRC Press.
- Shin, T., Davison, M. L., & Long, J. D. (2017). Maximum likelihood versus multiple imputation for missing data in small longitudinal samples with nonnormality. *Psychological Methods, 22,* 426–449.
- van Ginkel, J. R., Linting, M., Rippe, R. C., & van der Voort, A. (2020). Rebutting existing misconceptions about multiple imputation as a method for handling missing data. *Journal of Personality Assessment, 102,* 297–308.

Part II

Longitudinal Power Analyses

7

Unconditional Latent Growth Curve

An observational pediatric study conducted by Carmody et al. (2019) tracked *medication adherence* (defined as medical patients consistently taking the prescribed amount of medication at the prescribed frequency) in the months following an ulcerative colitis diagnosis. The mean medication adherence percentages, with 95% error bars, for the first 5 months of data collection are shown in Figure 7.1.

Two conclusions can quickly be drawn from Figure 7.1. First, medication adherence in the first 5 months postdiagnosis appears to decline in a somewhat linear trend. Second, a notable amount of variation exists in the average rate of adherence across participants, as shown by the width of the error bars at each assessment time point.

Modeling the longitudinal mean adherence data shown in Figure 7.1 could begin with the simplest latent growth curve model, an "intercept only" model, as shown in Figure 7.2.

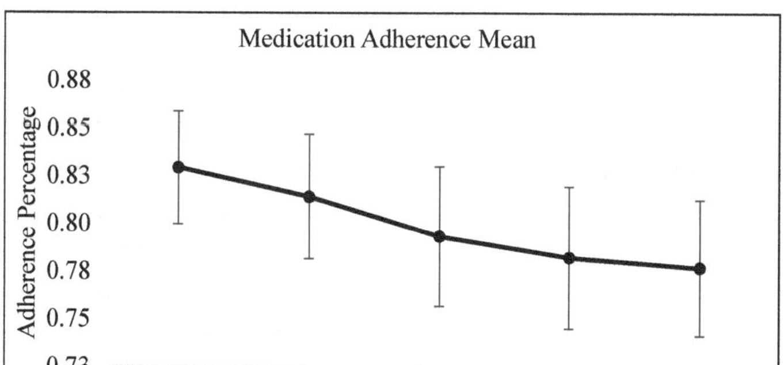

FIGURE 7.1. Medication adherence error bars. Data from Carmody et al. (2019).

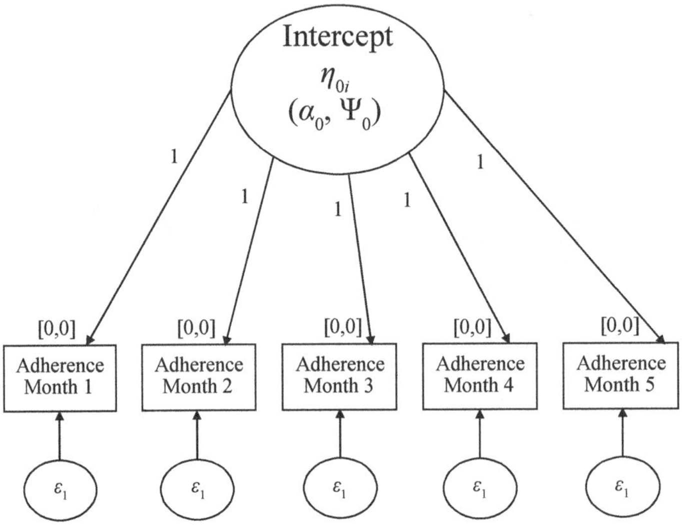

FIGURE 7.2. An intercept-only longitudinal SEM.

The rectangles shown in Figure 7.2 represent the observed adherence data for all N = 268 participants at all five monthly assessment time points. The circle at the top of the figure represents the Intercept (η_{0i}), or how the adherence data at all five assessment time points for all $i = N = 268$ participants will be summarized. The zeros in brackets ([0,0]) above each of the five adherence variables represent, by default in most SEM programs, the means and the variances of the observed longitudinal variables that are fixed at zero. First, this default, together with the loadings (regression arrows from the Intercept [η_{0i}] to each of the observed adherence variables) fixed at values of one, indicates that the means of the observed adherence variables at all five measurement occasions are weighted equally and estimated as a grand mean adherence value across all participants and measurement time points (α_0). Second, the zeros in brackets also indicate that the variances in the observed adherence data at all five measurement occasions is fixed at zero, and essentially gets split into an estimate of the amount of variance explained by the grand mean estimate (Ψ_0), and the amount of adherence variance at each time point left unexplained ($\varepsilon_1 - \varepsilon_5$).

An "intercept-only" model, as shown in Figure 7.2, would likely be a poor model for the adherence data shown in the error bar figure. For example, if the "intercept-only" model estimated grand mean adherence to be α_0 = 80%, such an estimate would underestimate the observed adherence averages at the first 2 months of assessment and would overestimate adherence at the final 2 months of assessment. What is needed in an addition to the "intercept-only" model is an estimate that captures a linear change, and in the case of the adherence data, a linear decline over time.

A linear latent growth curve model that allows for the estimation of average linear change over time is shown in Figure 7.3. The linear latent growth curve model shown in Figure 7.3 differs from the "intercept-only" model shown previously with the addition of a second latent variable, slope (η_{1i}), that allows for average change over time to be estimated. The loadings from the slope latent variable to the observed adherence responses are fixed at sequential integer values beginning with zero. Sequential integer value slope loadings are needed because they match the assessment schedule: participant data were collected over 5 consecutive months. Furthermore, fixing the loading from the latent slope to the first observed adherence variable changes the interpretation of the intercept: The intercept is now defined as the average level of medication adherence (α_0), and the variation around the average adherence (Ψ_0), assessed at month 1. The latent slope mean (α_1) quantifies the average change in adherence per unit change (i.e., per month) in the time metric. The slope variance (Ψ_1) quantified the variation, on average, in the rate of adherence change per month across participants. The intercept/slope covariance ($\Psi_{0,1}$) answers the question of whether a participant's adherence value at the first assessment time point (month 1) will have any relationship to how their adherence is likely to change over time. A statistically significant and positive intercept/slope covariance estimate means individual adherence trajectories would look more dissimilar (i.e., would show a "fan spread" over time). Individuals with higher initial response variable scores will show more rapid response variable score increases over time if the slope mean is positive or will show a slower response variable decrease over time if the slope mean is negative. A statistically significant and negative intercept/slope covariance estimate means individual adherence trajectories would look more similar (i.e., would show a "convergence" over time). Individuals with higher initial response variable scores will show slower response variable score increases over time if the slope mean is positive or will show a more rapid response variable decrease over time if the slope mean is negative. *Residual variances* ($\varepsilon_1 - \varepsilon_5$) are now defined as the amount of variation in adherence observed scores not explained by the linear trend.

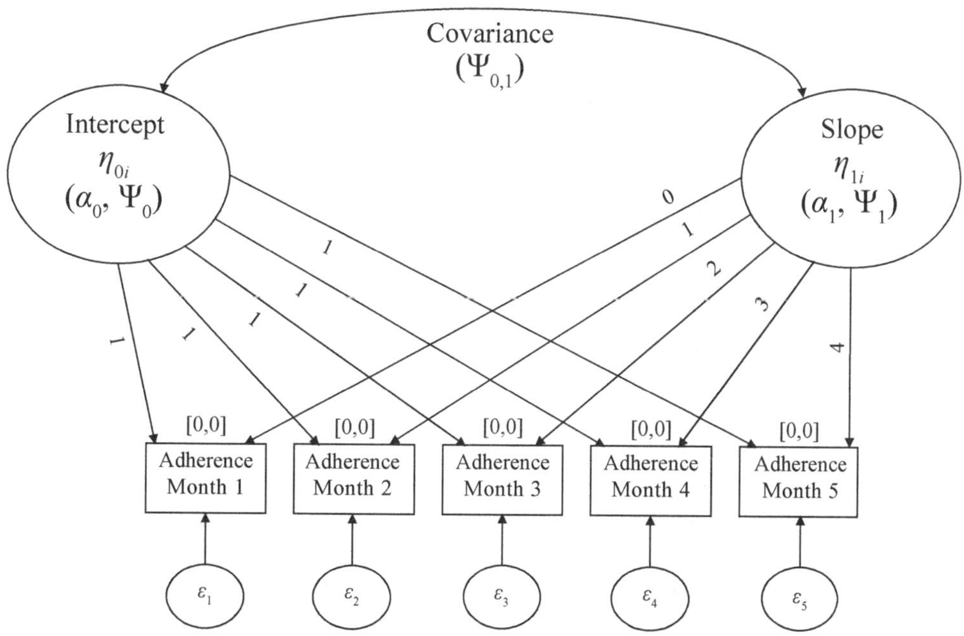

FIGURE 7.3. A linear longitudinal SEM.

The Metric of Time: Scaling and Centering

In any longitudinal study, the metric of time used to capture response variable changes must be clearly specified. Using only the information contained in the error bar graph, the only metric of time available would be an ordinal indication of assessment month. Other popular ordinal metrics of time could include grade in school for academic achievement research in education. However, continuous metrics of time, such as decimal age and time in days, weeks, months, or years since receiving a medical diagnosis, are often used in longitudinal developmental and health care studies. Previous publications have shown (Singer & Willett, 2003a, pp. 140–146; see also Biesanz, Deeb-Sossa, Papadakis, Bollen, & Curran, 2004) that the measurement scale used in longitudinal analysis for the metric of time directly impacts model fit and parameter estimate precision. The measurement scale for the metric of time used for a longitudinal study should be consistent with the research question and as accurate as possible.

In the above example, the slope loadings (0, 1, 2, 3, 4) are centered such that the intercept is defined as the expected adherence percentage at the first assessment occasion: month 1. For ordinal scales of time, such as assessment time point or month of assessment, the slope loadings can be specified to center the intercept at the study midpoint (–2, –1, 0, 1, 2) or endpoint (–4, –3, –2, –1, 0), depending on the research question. For continuous time metrics, such as decimal age or time in days, months, or years since receiving a medical diagnosis, four centering options are available: (1) raw metric inclusion (uncentered time), (2) centering around a meaningful value, (3) grand mean centering, and (4) participant mean centering (or centering within participants; Mehta & West, 2000; Blozis & Cho, 2008).

For example, if decimal age, calculated as the difference between assessment date and participant birth date at each *t* assessment time point for all *i* individual participants (Age_{ti}), is used as the metric of time, inclusion of the decimal age in a raw and uncentered metric would center the intercept at birth. If the longitudinal study involved an investigation of adolescent participants, centering decimal age around a meaningful constant value, (e.g., $\text{Age}_{ti} - 12$) would result in the intercept being interpreted as the expected response variable value for a participant age 12. However, in other research studies involving athletic performance, where the metric of time is measured by speed, in milliseconds, grand mean (e.g., $\text{Age}_{ti} - \overline{\text{Age}}$) or participant mean (e.g., $\text{Age}_{ti} - \overline{\text{Age}_i}$) centering could prove to be better centering options, depending on the research question. Which would seem to beg an obvious question: If a longitudinal research study has a metric of time available on a continuous measurement scale, but the continuous metric of time shows considerable variation across a cohort sample of participants, what is the optimal method for centering time?

Blozis and Cho (2008) examined meaningful constant centering, grand mean centering, and participant mean centering of decimal age in a longitudinal study of adolescent antisocial behavior, and number of years since receiving a multiple sclerosis diagnosis in a longitudinal study of physical incapacity. Results showed that either meaningful constant centering or grand mean centering of decimal age produced the best fitting model in the adolescent antisocial behavior study, but person mean centering produced the best fitting model in the physical incapacity due to a multiple sclerosis (MS) diagnosis study. Perhaps most interesting is the reason given by the authors for the difference in optimal model fit due to centering: The antisocial behavior study was limited to adolescents, so the admissible range of ages was limited relative to the ranges of years since the MS diagnosis. As a result, the variance, in years, since the MS diagnosis was more than 12 times larger than the variance in decimal age for adolescent antisocial behavior. To summarize, both the measurement scale available for the metric of time used to capture the response variable changes and the method used to center it both directly impact parameter estimates and longitudinal model fit.

An Unconditional Latent Growth Curve Model Power Analysis

Returning to the longitudinal adherence data shown in the error bar graph (Figure 7.1), let's assume a researcher studying adolescent medication adherence wants to conduct an unconditional latent growth curve model power analysis, but has only two reliable pieces of longitudinal information based on the published literature, previous experience, or both. First, assume that based on previous experience and absent parental monitoring, adolescents are initially at an 80% medication adherence level, that is, most adolescents take most of their medication most of the time as prescribed. Second, let's also assume that, based on the published literature or professional guidelines, a 5% change in adherence per assessment time point is deemed to be of clinical significance for treatment purposes. So, the researcher can assume that, absent parental monitoring, adolescent medication adherence would likely decrease 5% per month on average. If the adherence researcher's power analysis question involved the sample size needed to detect a 5% decrease in medication adherence per assessment time point (e.g., monthly for 5 months) with power ≥ .80, several additional questions immediately arise: (1) How much *variation* in medication adherence per assessment time point across participants should be assumed? (2) Repeated measures collected from multiple participants over several assessment time points are correlated, but at what assumed magnitude? and (3) Missing data are to be expected in longitudinal studies, so how much missing data should be assumed? Answering these three questions would seem to be a very daunting task at this point, yet they can be answered using either Mplus or R by conducting a statistical power analysis.

Mplus Monte Carlo Simulation Power Analysis

Recall that in Mplus, the `MODEL POPULATION:` command specifies how Monte Carlo simulation data are to be *generated*, the `MODEL:` command specifies how the generated data should be *analyzed*. Let's focus first on how to generate (`MODEL POPULATION:`) the data needed to answer the power analysis question: the data needed to answer a power analysis research question can be generated from descriptive information if three quantities are known or can be reasonably inferred—means, variances, and covariances. Beginning with the response variable means, and assuming medication adherence is measured on a proportional scale where zero indicates complete nonadherence and one represents perfect adherence, adolescent adherence is initially assumed to be .80. Furthermore, assuming five monthly adherence assessments, adolescent medication adherence is assumed to decrease 5% in the absence of parental monitoring. Using Mplus syntax, these average adherence (ADH) proportion assumptions can be specified as (recall that means or intercepts are specified in Mplus using brackets)

```
MODEL POPULATION:
[ADH_1*0.80];
[ADH_2*0.75];
[ADH_3*0.70];
[ADH_4*0.65];
[ADH_5*0.60];
```

where _1 through _5 indicate the five monthly adherence assessments, and the assumed adherence proportions decrease by .05 (5%) at each subsequent assessment time point. Consistent with the theme of this book, *standardization simplifies*, unit variances for medication adherence proportions at each assessment time point can be assumed and specified in Mplus "shortcut" syntax by

```
ADH_1 - ADH_5*1;
```

At this point, only the information regarding assumed covariances among the monthly adherence assessments remains. If variances are assumed to be one based on the assumption of standardization, then correlations among the monthly adherence assessments need to be specified, but this is information a researcher is very unlikely to have, so invoking reasonable logic can help. For example, it is reasonable to assume that adjacent monthly adherence assessments would be more highly correlated than monthly adherence assessments separated by one or more months. Furthermore, because longitudinal data are known to be highly correlated, it seems reasonable to assume a high correlation between adjacent monthly adherence assessments and decreasing correlations as pairs of monthly adherence assessments are separated by one or more months. These assumptions can be specified in Mplus syntax as

```
ADH_1 WITH ADH_2*0.50;
ADH_2 WITH ADH_3*0.50;
ADH_3 WITH ADH_4*0.50;
ADH_4 WITH ADH_5*0.50;
```

which shows that immediately adjacent adherence measures correlated at a large effect size, or $r_{\text{Pearson}} = .50$.

```
ADH_1 WITH ADH_3*0.40;
ADH_2 WITH ADH_4*0.40;
ADH_3 WITH ADH_5*0.40;
```

Monthly adherence assessments separated by 1 month are correlated at a lower value, $r_{\text{Pearson}} = .40$.

```
ADH_1 WITH ADH_4*0.30;
ADH_2 WITH ADH_5*0.30;
ADH_1 WITH ADH_5*0.20;
```

Monthly adherence assessments separated by 2 months or more are correlated at still lower values, $r_{\text{Pearson}} = .30$ and $r_{\text{Pearson}} = .20$. Stated differently, a *band diagonal* (or *first-order autoregressive*) correlation structure is assumed for the longitudinal adherence data, as shown in matrix form below, where the rectangles enclose bands of identical correlations and correlations decrease as distance from the main diagonal increases.

	ADH_1	ADH_2	ADH_3	ADH_4	ADH_5
ADH_1	1				
ADH_2	0.50	1			
ADH_3	0.40	0.50	1		
ADH_4	0.30	0.40	0.50	1	
ADH_5	0.20	0.30	0.40	0.50	1

The next question to address is missing data, which can be expected in almost all longitudinal studies. The specific question of how much missing data to assume again bears on the issue of reasonableness. If study participant recruitment goals have been met, it is reasonable to assume no missing data at the initial assessment, but that missing data will likely increase at each monthly assessment over the course of the study. Furthermore, given that the time frame of the study is only 5 months long, it is also reasonable to assume, barring an incident, that missing data would not likely accelerate to problematic levels. For example, a researcher could reasonably assume: (1) no missing data at the initial assessment time point, (2) missing data will be minimal beginning at the first postbaseline assessment, (3) missing data will increase monotonically at each subsequent assessment month, and (4) missing data will be no more than 20% of the sample at the final assessment time point. These missing data assumptions can be specified in Mplus syntax as follows

```
MODEL MISSING:
[ADH_2*-2.9444]; !5%;
[ADH_3*-2.1972]; !10%;
[ADH_4*-1.7346]; !15%;
[ADH_5*-1.3862]; !20%;

ADH_2 ON ADH_1*-0.4055;
ADH_3 ON ADH_2*-0.4055 ADH_1*-0.4055;
ADH_4 ON ADH_3*-0.4055 ADH_2*-0.4055 ADH_1*-0.4055;
ADH_5 ON ADH_4*-0.4055 ADH_3*-0.4055 ADH_2*-0.4055 ADH_1*-0.4055;
```

Immediately following the `MODEL MISSING:` command, and contained within brackets, are logit intercept values that specify 5% missing data at the first postbaseline assessment time point (`ADH_2`; i.e., $\exp^{-2.9444}/[1 + \exp^{-2.9444}] = 0.05$) that increases in 5% increments to 20% missing data at the final assessment time point. As seen in previous chapters, if the first four lines of syntax following the `MODEL MISSING:` command were the only syntax, this would imply a missing completely at random (MCAR) assumption. However, the next four lines of Mplus syntax are `ON` statements that relate missing data at a postbaseline assessment time point to observed adherence values at one or more previous time points. Specifically, the last four lines of syntax in the `MODEL MISSING:` command state that unit decreases in medication adherence at any assessment time point increase the odds of a missing data point at a subsequent assessment time point by 50% (i.e., $\exp^{-0.4055} = 0.667$; $1/0.667 = 1.50$). This assumption makes intuitive sense: A decreased likelihood to take medication as prescribed increases the likelihood of needing a medical intervention (hospitalization) that can result in missing data. Finally, missing data are now assumed to be missing at random (MAR) because missing adherence data at a given assessment time point is now conditional on observed adherence data at one or more previous time points.

Now that Monte Carlo data generation and missing data assumptions have been specified, the last step is data analysis, which consists of a single line of syntax in Mplus.

```
MODEL:
I S | ADH_1@0 ADH_2@1 ADH_3@2 ADH_4@3 ADH_5@4;
```

The above line of syntax is an Mplus "shorthand" specification for a growth curve model analysis. Specifically, the above line specifies a linear growth curve model, consisting of a latent intercept (`I`) and a latent slope (`S`) that are both "measured by" (|) each of the five longitudinal adherence assessments. Notice also, following the "at" (@) symbols, there are ascending integer values (0, 1, 2, 3, 4), which represent slope loadings that indicate an ordinal metric of time (assessment month) centered such that the intercept is interpreted as the average adherence proportion at the first assessment time point (`ADH_1`). Mplus will specify intercept loadings at a value of one for each adherence assessment by default.

Shown below is the combined Mplus Monte Carlo syntax for a linear growth curve power analysis. The only additions made are shown at the top, including the standard `MONTECARLO:` command that initializes the power analysis estimation algorithms, and lines that allow for: (1) names to be specified for the medication adherence proportion variables (`NAMES = ADH_1 – ADH_5`), (2) a specific sample size to be tested for adequate statistical power (`NOBS = 297`), (3) the number of simulated dataset replications to be specified (`NREPS = 5000`), and (4) the syntax that specifies missing data only occurring at the postbaseline assessment time points (`MISSING = ADH_2 ADH_3 ADH_4 ADH_5`).

```
TITLE: MPLUS 7.1 Unconditional LGM

MONTECARLO:
NAMES = ADH_1-ADH_5;
NOBS = 297;
NREPS = 5000;
MISSING =
ADH_2 ADH_3 ADH_4 ADH_5;

MODEL POPULATION:

[ADH_1*0.80];
[ADH_2*0.75];
```

```
[ADH_3*0.70];
[ADH_4*0.65];
[ADH_5*0.60];

ADH_1 - ADH_5*1;

ADH_1 WITH ADH_2*0.50;
ADH_2 WITH ADH_3*0.50;
ADH_3 WITH ADH_4*0.50;
ADH_4 WITH ADH_5*0.50;

ADH_1 WITH ADH_3*0.40;
ADH_2 WITH ADH_4*0.40;
ADH_3 WITH ADH_5*0.40;

ADH_1 WITH ADH_4*0.30;
ADH_2 WITH ADH_5*0.30;

ADH_1 WITH ADH_5*0.20;

MODEL MISSING:
[ADH_2*-2.9444]; !5%;
[ADH_3*-2.1972]; !10%;
[ADH_4*-1.7346]; !15%;
[ADH_5*-1.3862]; !20%;

ADH_2 ON ADH_1*-0.4055;
ADH_3 ON ADH_2*-0.4055 ADH_1*-0.4055;
ADH_4 ON ADH_3*-0.4055 ADH_2*-0.4055 ADH_1*-0.4055;
ADH_5 ON ADH_4*-0.4055 ADH_3*-0.4055 ADH_2*-0.4055
ADH_1*-0.4055;

MODEL:
I S | ADH_1@0 ADH_2@1 ADH_3@2 ADH_4@3 ADH_5@4;
```

Results from running the Monte Carlo syntax above are shown below, beginning with the results of the missing data syntax specifications.

Covariance Coverage

	ADH_1	ADH_2	ADH_3	ADH_4	ADH_5
ADH_1	1.000				
ADH_2	0.956	0.956			
ADH_3	0.933	0.896	0.933		
ADH_4	0.869	0.828	0.811	0.869	
ADH_5	0.919	0.882	0.859	0.815	0.919

The proportions of observed data for all possible pairwise considerations for the five adherence response variables are shown above. Notice how the proportion of data present at the first assessment time point is one, indicating complete data. Notice also that at no point does the proportion of observed data drop below .80, or 80%, indicating that missing data did not exceed 20% at any time point consistent with MAR missing data syntax specifications.

```
        MISSING DATA PATTERNS (x = not missing)
              1   2   3   4   5   6   7   8   9  10  11  12
AOH 1         x   x   x   x   x   x   x   x   x   x   x   x
AOH-2         x   x   x   x   x   x   x   x
ADH-3         x   x   x   x                   x   x   x
AOH-4         x   x           x   x           x   x       x
ADH=S         x       x       x       x       x           x

      MISSING DATA PATTERN FREQUENCIES
      Pattern     Frequency        Pattern     Frequency        Pattern     Frequency
            1           217              5            14              9             9
            2            14              6             1             10             1
            3            29              7             2             11             1
            4             6              8             1             12             2
```

Also shown above are the resulting missing data patterns and their associated frequencies. Specifically, most of the generated data (217/297 = 73%) showed pattern #1, indicating no missing data at any of the five monthly assessment time points. Missing data patterns #3, 5, 7, 9, and 12 show *intermittent missing data*, defined as participants who completed the longitudinal study and did not drop out, but are missing adherence observations for one or more intervening assessment time points. Missing data patterns #2, 4, 6, 8, 10, and 11 indicate dropout missing data, defined as a participant leaving the longitudinal study prior to completion. Taken together, the missing data coverage matrix, patterns, and frequencies specify roughly 20% MAR data, but also specifies (24/297 = .08) 8% of the specified missing data are due to participant dropout.

Monte Carlo statistical power estimates resulting from the Mplus syntax (Mplus 7.1) are shown below.

```
MODEL RESULTS
                                    ESTIMATES                  S. E.     M. S. E.   95%   % Sig
                    Population    Average     Std. Dev.     Average                Cover Coeff
Means
 S                    -0.050      -0.0507      0.0179        0.0180       0.0003 0.950 0.799

Residual Variances
 ADH_1                 0.500       0.4500      0.0661        0.0659       0.0069 0.858 1.000
 ADH_2                 0.500       0.5035      0.0542        0.0540       0.0029 0.950 1.000
 ADH_3                 0.500       0.5298      0.0542        0.0541       0.0038 0.941 1.000
 ADH_4                 0.500       0.5018      0.0569        0.0562       0.0032 0.948 1.000
 ADH_5                 0.500       0.4469      0.0702        0.0695       0.0077 0.852 1.000
```

As shown in the results, a sample size of $N = 297$ is needed for statistical power $\geq .80$ to detect a mean slope estimate of –.05, indicating a 5% decrease in adolescent medication adherence per month in the absence of parental monitoring. Also shown above are the results for the residual variance estimates. As shown in the second column, even though the residual variances across adherence time points ranged between .47 and .55 (47% to 55%), the residual variances indicate that roughly 50% of observed adherence variance, on average, is explained by linear growth. Following the example Monte Carlo simulation power in R and an analysis write-up shown below, the issue of linear model specification, standardization simplification, and observed variable proportions of variance explained will be explored in greater detail.

R Monte Carlo Simulation Power Analysis

Using R, recall that the first step in evaluating a power analysis is specifying the population model. Similar to Mplus, data can be generated from descriptive information if the means, variances, and covariances are known or can be inferred. Beginning with the response variable means, and assuming medication adherence is measured on a proportional scale where zero indicates complete nonadherence and one represents perfect adherence, adolescent adherence is initially assumed to be .80. Furthermore, assuming five monthly adherence assessments, adolescent medication adherence is assumed to decrease 5% in the absence of parental monitoring. After loading simsem, lavaan, and a source file with additional functions relevant for this book, the full population model is shown below and then discussed.

```
library(simsem)
library(lavaan)
source("simsemTools.R")

PopulationModel_Ch7 <- "
  ADH_1 ~ 0.80*1
  ADH_2 ~ 0.75*1
  ADH_3 ~ 0.70*1
  ADH_4 ~ 0.65*1
  ADH_5 ~ 0.60*1
  ADH_1 ~~ 1*ADH_1
  ADH_2 ~~ 1*ADH_2
  ADH_3 ~~ 1*ADH_3
  ADH_4 ~~ 1*ADH_4
  ADH_5 ~~ 1*ADH_5

  ADH_1 ~~ 0.5*ADH_2
  ADH_2 ~~ 0.5*ADH_3
  ADH_3 ~~ 0.5*ADH_4
  ADH_4 ~~ 0.5*ADH_5

  ADH_1 ~~ 0.4*ADH_3
  ADH_2 ~~ 0.4*ADH_4
  ADH_3 ~~ 0.4*ADH_5

  ADH_1 ~~ 0.3*ADH_4
  ADH_2 ~~ 0.3*ADH_5

  ADH_1 ~~ 0.2*ADH_5
  slopemean := -.05
"
```

First, the mean values range from .80 to .60 across five assessments. The ~ combined with *1 reflects mean values, while the value before *1 is the population mean at each time point. Continuing with the population model, and continuing with the theme of this book, standardization simplifies, variances for medication adherence proportions at each assessment are set to 1.

The ~~ reflects a covariance, and a variable that covaries with itself is the variance of that variable. The 1* sets the values to 1. The next pieces of information in the population model that need to be specified are the covariances among monthly adherence assessments. Although the means and variances are easily obtained, it is a bit more difficult to determine adequate values for the covariance matrix from prior literature reviews. One alternative method is to use logical reasoning to infer what expected correlations should be across time. For example, it is reasonable to assume that adjacent monthly adherence assessments would be more highly correlated than monthly adherence assessments separated by one or more months. Furthermore, because longitudinal data are known to be highly correlated, it seems reasonable to assume a high correlation between adjacent monthly adherence assessments, as well as decreasing correlations as pairs of monthly adherence assessments are separated by one or more months.

Finally, the last piece of information needed in the R version of the population model is the population parameter that will be estimated in the sample model but *is not* directly specified in the means, variance, and covariances. This chapter deals with generating data from descriptive statistics yet evaluating that data using a more complex model. Later, in the analysis section, a growth model will be specified, and the parameter of interest will be compared to zero, unless otherwise specified in the population model. For this reason, in order to evaluate the sample model against a specific value, it is necessary to create a new variable name using ':=' and to provide the appropriate value for comparison.

Before moving forward, assess the accuracy of the covariance matrix and mean vector,

```
fitted(sem(PopulationModel_Ch7)),
```

which shows the following result, confirming that the population model is correct.

```
$cov
       ADH_1  ADH_2  ADH_3  ADH_4  ADH_5
ADH_1  1.0
ADH_2  0.5    1.0
ADH_3  0.4    0.5    1.0
ADH_4  0.3    0.4    0.5    1.0
ADH_5  0.2    0.3    0.4    0.5    1.0

$mean
ADH_1     ADH_2     ADH_3     ADH_4     ADH_5
0.80      0.75      0.70      0.65      0.60
```

After the population model is verified as correct, the next question to address is missing data, which is practically inevitable in longitudinal studies. The question of missingness bears on issues of reasonableness. Typically, at the first time point, it is reasonable to assume no—or very little—missing data, but missingness is likely to increase at each assessment over the course of the study, and missingness may depend on a variety of factors. In the present study being examined, the time frame of the study is 5 months long and is not expected to accelerate to problematic levels. For example, a researcher could reasonably assume: (1) no missing data at the initial assessment time point, (2) missing data will be minimal beginning at the first postbaseline assessment, (3) missing data will increase monotonically at each subsequent assessment month, and (4) missing data will be no more than 20% of the sample at the final assessment time point. These missing data assumptions can be easily implemented in R using lavaan-style syntax. There are other methods for imposing missingness (see simsem package details), but we will use this style throughout the book.

```
MissingModel_Ch7 <- "
    ADH_2 ~ -2.9444 + -0.4055*ADH_1
    ADH_3 ~ -2.1972 + -0.4055*ADH_2 + -0.4055*ADH_1
    ADH_4 ~ -1.7346 + -0.4055*ADH_3 + -0.4055*ADH_2 + -0.4055*ADH_1
    ADH_5 ~ -1.3862 + -0.4055*ADH_4 + -0.4055*ADH_3 + -0.4055*ADH_2 + -0.4055*ADH_1
"
MissingModel_Ch7 <- miss(logit = MissingModel_Ch7)
```

The missing completely at random logit intercept values are combined with the missing at random logit slope values to form an equation of missingness for each adherence time point beyond baseline. ADH_2 has 5% data missing completely at random, yet the unit decreases in medication adherence at any assessment point increase the odds of missing data at a subsequent assessment time point by 50% ($\exp^{-0.4055} = 0.667$; $1/0.667 = 1.50$). This assumption makes intuitive sense: A decreased likelihood to take medication as prescribed increases the likelihood of needing a medical intervention (hospitalization) that can result in missing data. Finally, missing data are now assumed to be MAR because missing adherence data at a given assessment time point is now conditional on observed adherence data at one or more previous time points.

Now that the population data-generation model and missing data assumptions have been specified, the last step is analysis. Unlike Mplus, this requires a few lines of code in R. First, we must specify the analysis model.

```
AnalysisModel_Ch7 <- "
  I =~ 1*ADH_1 + 1*ADH_2 + 1*ADH_3 + 1*ADH_4 + 1*ADH_5
  S =~ 0*ADH_1 + 1*ADH_2 + 2*ADH_3 + 3*ADH_4 + 4*ADH_5
  S ~ slope*1

  slopemean := slope
  "
```

Note the addition of two pieces of code here. First, the line `S ~ slope*1`; this piece of code *names* the slope mean value. Next, the line `slopemean := slope` names the slope mean as slopemean, which will be compared to the population-specified value of –.05.

After specifying the population and sample models, the Monte Carlo simulation was evaluated using the package using the ‘`sim()`’ command.

```
output_Ch7 <-   sim(nRep = 5000,
                n = 297,
                model = AnalysisModel_Ch7,
                generate = PopulationModel_Ch7,
```

```
          miss = MissingModel_Ch7,
          std.lv = FALSE,
          seed = 35170,
          silent = TRUE,
          lavaanfun = "growth",
          outfun = cov_coverage)
```

Because missing data were imposed, the covariance coverage and missing data patterns should first be assessed. For this reason, the 'sim()' command includes the new line of code 'outfun = cov_coverage'. The cov_coverage function in the additional output pulls in all the covariance coverages for every iteration in the simulation. To examine the average and SD of covariance coverage, the following functions can be developed and used:

```
avg_cov_coverage <- function(output) {
  round(tril(apply(simplify2array(simplify2array(getExtraOutput(output))), 1:2, mean)), 3)
}
avg_cov_coverage(output_Ch7)
```

which result in the covariance coverage matrix. The covariance coverage matrix shows the proportions of observed data for all possible pairwise considerations for the five adherence response variables. Notice how the proportion of data present at the first assessment time point is one, indicating complete data. Notice also that at no point does the proportion of observed data drop below .80, or 80%, indicating that missing data did not exceed 20% at any time point consistent with MAR missing data syntax specifications. This step is crucial to determine that the missing data are not overly sparse.

```
        ADH_1     ADH_2     ADH_3     ADH_4     ADH_5
ADH_1  1.000
ADH_2  0.960     0.960
ADH_3  0.927     0.892     0.927
ADH_4  0.902     0.868     0.837     0.902
ADH_5  0.877     0.844     0.818     0.803     0.877
```

Now that missing data have been assessed, the summary of model results can be examined. This overall summary contains two elements: (1) a summary of the model fit and convergence and (2) a dataframe which contains the Monte Carlo simulation model estimate(s). There is a column called Power, which reflects the power estimates for all parameters in the model. The power estimate for any specific parameter can be obtained by calling the parameter's name. Here, that parameter name is 'slopemean'.

```
getPower(output)[["slopemean"]]
```

which results in the power estimate of .798, or approximately .80, showing that a sample size of $N = 297$ is needed to obtain adequate statistical power to detect a mean slope estimate of –.05, indicating a 5% decrease in adolescent medication adherence per month in the absence of parental monitoring.

Unconditional Latent Growth Curve Model Simulation Power Analysis Write-Up

"The power analysis question involved the smallest sample size needed to achieve power $\geq .80$ to detect an anticipated 5% monthly decrease (i.e., slope mean = –.05) in adolescent medication adherence from an initial .80 (80%) adherence rate in the absence of parental monitoring across a 5-month study. A Monte Carlo simulation power analysis was conducted using Mplus version 8.6 (or R packages simsem and lavaan) assuming: (1) standardization of all adherence proportion variables at all five study months, (2) correlations across the five monthly adherence variables are best captured via a band-diagonal correlation structure, where adjacent adherence measurements assumed more highly correlated (r = .50) than adherence measurements separated by one (r = .40), two (r = .30), or three (r = .20) assessment months, (3) linear trend explained 50% of observed adherence response variable variance, on average, and (4) missing data is assumed to be (a) 0% at the initial assessment, (b) 5% at the first postbaseline assessment, (c) monotonically increasing in 5% increments to 20% at the final assessment, (d) missing at random, such that unit decreases in adherence at any previous assessment time point are assumed to result in a 50% increase in the odds of missing data, and (e) up to 8% of the specified missing data is assumed to be due to participant dropout. Monte Carlo simulation power analysis results aggregated over 5,000 dataset replications showed power $\geq .80$ to detect a slope mean of –.05 if proper missing data make a sample size of N = 297 available for analysis."

Latent Growth Curve Models: Moving Forward

As shown in the residual variances portion of the Monte Carlo simulation power analysis results, the previous data generation specifications, when analyzed with a linear latent growth curve, resulted in an assumption that 50% of adherence response variable variance, on average, was explained by linear growth. Figure 7.4 shows a linear latent growth curve model that uses standardized parameter estimates (based on standardized estimates obtained from a modified version of a latent growth curve model shown in Bauer & Curran, 2004, p. 14) and assumes that 50% of response variable variance is explained by linear growth.

The assumption that the linear latent growth model in Figure 7.4 explains 50% of observed response variable variance can easily be verified by computing the model-reproduced correlation matrix ($\mathbf{\Sigma\theta}$) as a model admissibility check with the following matrix equation [Equation (7.1)]:

$$\mathbf{\Sigma\theta} = \mathbf{\Lambda\Phi\Lambda}^T + \mathbf{\Psi} \tag{7.1}$$

Recall that the Equation (7.1) was first introduced in Chapter 4 as the needed model-reproduced equation for a confirmatory factor analysis (CFA) model. A linear longitudinal growth curve model is a two-factor confirmatory factor analysis model with fixed rather than estimated factor loadings. Recall that the dimensions of the lambda ($\mathbf{\Lambda}$) matrix are

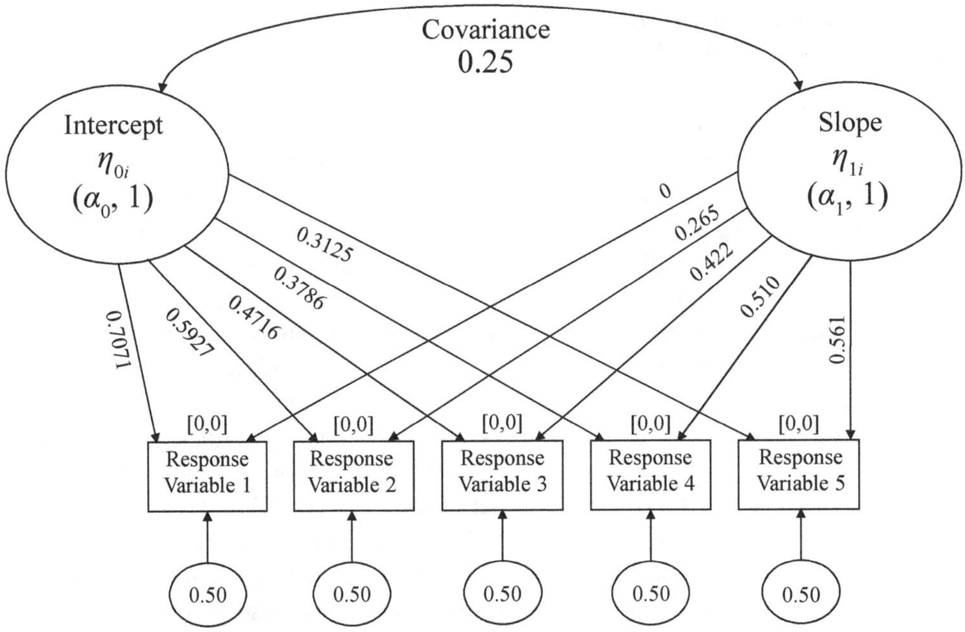

FIGURE 7.4. A longitudinal growth model specifying 50% of response variable variance explained.

defined as the number of rows equal to the number of observed analysis variables (five repeated response variable measures), the number of columns equals to the number of latent factors (two, Intercept and Slope), and the cells contain the constrained factor loading values, as shown in Equation (7.2).

$$\begin{array}{r|cc|} & \text{Intercept} & \text{Slope} \\ \text{Response Variable 1} & 0.7071 & 0 \\ \text{Response Variable 2} & 0.5927 & 0.265 \\ \Lambda = \quad \text{Response Variable 3} & 0.4716 & 0.422 \\ \text{Response Variable 4} & 0.3786 & 0.510 \\ \text{Response Variable 5} & 0.3125 & 0.561 \end{array} \tag{7.2}$$

The dimensions of the phi ($\boldsymbol{\Phi}$) matrix are defined as the number of rows and columns that are both equal to the number of latent factors (two, Intercept and Slope), and the cells of the matrix contain the latent intercept and slope variances and correlation, as shown in Equation (7.3).

$$\begin{array}{r|cc|} & \text{Intercept} & \text{Slope} \\ \boldsymbol{\Phi} = \text{Intercept} & 1 & 0.25 \\ \text{Slope} & 0.25 & 1 \end{array} \tag{7.3}$$

The dimensions of the psi (**Ψ**) matrix are defined as the number of rows and columns that are both equal to the number of observed response variables and the cells on the main diagonal contain the residual variances for the observed response variables, as shown in Equation (7.4).

$$\boldsymbol{\Psi} = \begin{array}{c|ccccc|} & Y1 & Y2 & Y3 & Y4 & Y5 \\ Y1 & 0.50 & 0 & 0 & 0 & 0 \\ Y2 & 0 & 0.50 & 0 & 0 & 0 \\ Y3 & 0 & 0 & 0.50 & 0 & 0 \\ Y4 & 0 & 0 & 0 & 0.50 & 0 \\ Y5 & 0 & 0 & 0 & 0 & 0.50 \end{array} \quad (7.4)$$

The model-reproduced correlation matrix equation can be solved using the information contained in the above matrices using R syntax.

```
Lambda <- matrix(c(.7071, 0, .5927, .265, .4716, .422, .3786, .51, .3125, .561),
ncol = 2, byrow = TRUE)
Phi <- matrix(c(1, .25, .25, 1), nrow = 2, byrow = TRUE)
Psi <- matrix(c(0.50, 0, 0, 0, 0, 0, 0.50, 0, 0, 0, 0, 0, .50, 0, 0, 0, 0, 0, .50, 0, 0, 0, 0, 0, 0.50),
      nrow = 5, byrow = TRUE)
corr_matrix <- (Lambda %*% Phi %*% t(Lambda)) + Psi
corr_matrix
```

Solving the matrix results in a model-reproduced correlation matrix, shown below.

	Response Variable 1	Response Variable 2	Response Variable 3	Response Variable 4	Response Variable 5
Response Variable 1	1	0.4659	0.4081	0.3579	0.3201
Response Variable 2	0.4659	1	0.4851	0.4602	0.4377
Response Variable 3	0.4081	0.4851	1	0.4938	0.4832
Response Variable 4	0.3579	0.4602	0.4938	1	0.4974
Response Variable 5	0.3201	0.4377	0.4832	0.4974	1

Furthermore, two additional longitudinal linear growth curve models, which explain between 60 and 70% of the response variable variance, respectively, are also shown below and followed immediately by their respective model-reproduced correlation matrix calculations to confirm their admissibility (Figures 7.5 and 7.6).

```
Lambda <- matrix(c(.7746, 0, .6527, .265, .5352, .422, .4498, .51, .3917, .561),
ncol = 2, byrow = TRUE)
Phi <- matrix(c(1, .30, .30, 1), nrow = 2, byrow = TRUE)
Psi <- matrix(c(0.40, 0, 0, 0, 0, 0, 0.40, 0, 0, 0, 0, 0, .40, 0, 0, 0, 0, 0, .40, 0, 0, 0, 0, 0, 0.40),
      nrow = 5, byrow = TRUE)
corr_matrix <- (Lambda %*% Phi %*% t(Lambda)) + Psi
corr_matrix
```

Solving the matrix results in a model-reproduced correlation matrix, shown below.

	Response Variable 1	Response Variable 2	Response Variable 3	Response Variable 4	Response Variable 5
Response Variable 1	1	0.5672	0.5126	0.4669	0.4338
Response Variable 2	0.5672	1	0.5863	0.5644	0.5453
Response Variable 3	0.5126	0.5863	1	0.5948	0.586
Response Variable 4	0.4669	0.5644	0.5948	1	0.5979
Response Variable 5	0.4338	0.5453	0.586	0.5979	1

```
Lambda <- matrix(c(.8367, 0, .7063, .265, .5897, .422, .5084, .51, .4547, .561),
ncol = 2, byrow = TRUE)
Phi <- matrix(c(1, .35, .35, 1), nrow = 2, byrow = TRUE)
Psi <- matrix(c(0.30, 0, 0, 0, 0, 0, 0.30, 0, 0, 0, 0, 0, .30, 0, 0, 0, 0, 0, .30, 0, 0, 0, 0, 0, 0.30),
      nrow = 5, byrow = TRUE)
corr_matrix <- (Lambda %*% Phi %*% t(Lambda)) + Psi
corr_matrix
```

Solving the matrix results in a model-reproduced correlation matrix, shown below.

	Response Variable 1	Response Variable 2	Response Variable 3	Response Variable 4	Response Variable 5
Response Variable 1	1	0.6686	0.6170	0.5747	0.5447
Response Variable 2	0.6686	1	0.6874	0.6675	0.6507
Response Variable 3	0.617	0.6874	1	0.6954	0.6878
Response Variable 4	0.5747	0.6675	0.6954	1	0.6983
Response Variable 5	0.5447	0.6507	0.6878	0.6983	1

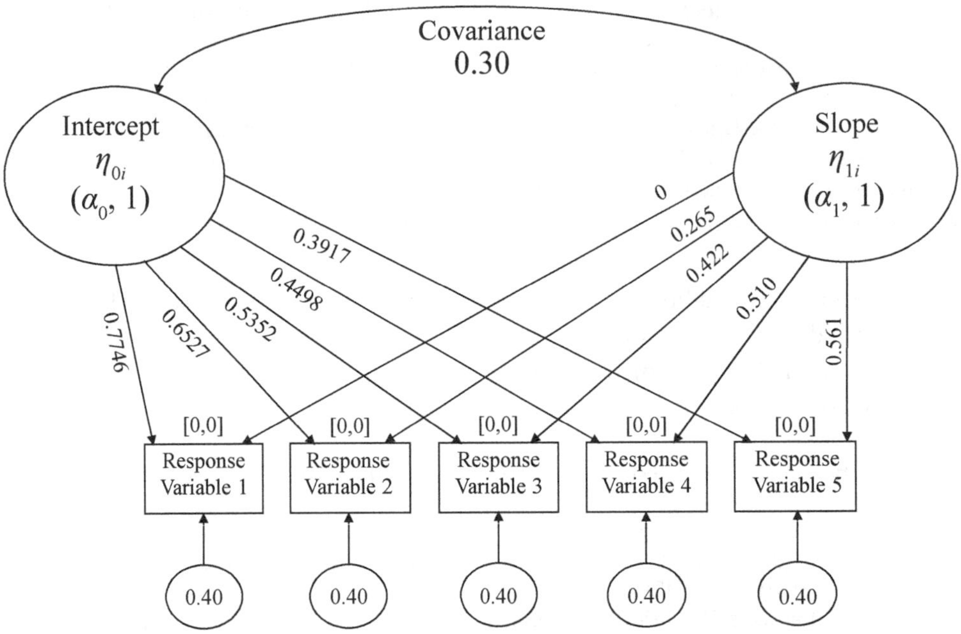

FIGURE 7.5. A longitudinal growth model specifying 60% of response variable variance explained.

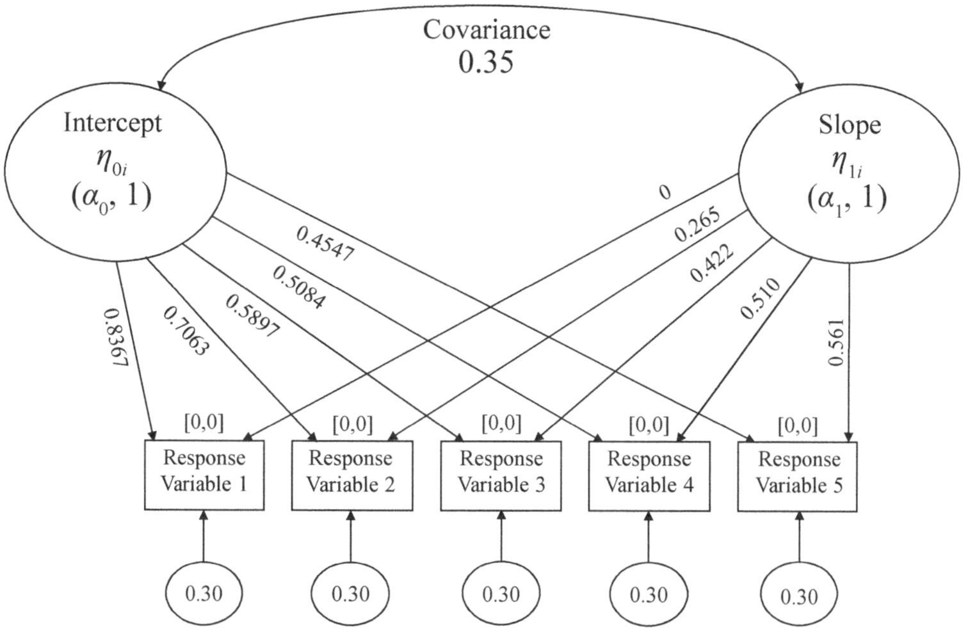

FIGURE 7.6. A longitudinal growth model specifying 70% of response variable variance explained.

A litany of longitudinal research has shown that linear latent growth models tend to explain, on average, between 50 and 70% of observed response variable variance. So the question becomes: Which model would be most appropriate for a given longitudinal power analysis? As always, model assumptions should be based primarily on a researcher's experience with the subject matter under investigation, published research, and the specifics of the longitudinal research design proposed. For example, a research design consideration could be the length of time specified between consecutive response variable assessments. Notice how, as the amount of variance explained increases from 50 to 70%, the correlations in the model-reproduced correlation matrices increase in magnitude. It makes intuitive sense, for example, to assume a greater amount of variance explained and greater correlations among the response variables for consecutive assessments planned to occur very closely in time (e.g., weekly or monthly) versus consecutive assessments planned to occur much farther apart in time (e.g., yearly). Notice also how, in all three linear growth models, there was no specification of either an intercept mean (α_0) or a slope mean (α_1). However, this will change when moving from an unconditional model in this chapter to a conditional latent growth model that includes one or more time invariant covariates in the next chapter.

Finally, for the linear models that explained 50, 60, and 70% of response variable variance, each of the three models was checked for admissibility with the same model-reproduced correlation matrix ($\boldsymbol{\Sigma\theta}$) formula used in previous chapters to verify the admissibility of the CFA model shown in Chapter 4. This is because an unconditional growth curve model is equivalent to a two-factor CFA with loadings constrained to fixed values rather than freely estimated [Equation (7.1) as shown again here

$$\boldsymbol{\Sigma\theta} = \boldsymbol{\Lambda\Phi\Lambda}^T + \boldsymbol{\Psi}$$

Another model-reproduced correlation matrix, from Bollen and Curran (2006, pp. 218–225), can also be used to verify model admissibility [Equation (7.5)]

$$\boldsymbol{\Sigma\theta} = \mathbf{P}(\mathbf{I} - \mathbf{B})^{-1}\boldsymbol{\Psi}(\mathbf{I} - \mathbf{B})^{-1\mathrm{T}}\mathbf{P}^{\mathrm{T}} \tag{7.5}$$

The linear growth model that explains 50% of response variable variance can be used to illustrate the matrices in the Bollen and Curran equation. First, the two different model admissibility equations share an element in common: the psi (**Ψ**) matrix. Recall that while the previous formula specified that the psi matrix contain only response variable (Y) residual variances [see Equation (7.4) shown again here],

Ψ =

	Response Variable 1	Response Variable 2	Response Variable 3	Response Variable 4	Response Variable 5
Response Variable 1	0.50	0	0	0	0
Response Variable 2	0	0.50	0	0	0
Response Variable 3	0	0	0.50	0	0
Response Variable 4	0	0	0	0.50	0
Response Variable 5	0	0	0	0	0.50

the number of rows and columns for the psi matrix in Bollen and Curran's equation are equal to the number of observed variables plus the number of latent variables as follows [Equation (7.6)]:

Ψ =

	$Y1$	$Y2$	$Y3$	$Y4$	$Y5$	Intercept	Slope
$Y1$	0.50	0	0	0	0	0	0
$Y2$	0	0.50	0	0	0	0	0
$Y3$	0	0	0.50	0	0	0	0
$Y4$	0	0	0	0.50	0	0	0
$Y5$	0	0	0	0	0.50	0	0
Intercept	0	0	0	0	0	1	0.25
Slope	0	0	0	0	0	0.25	1

(7.6)

Notice how the psi matrix for the Bollen and Curran equation can be viewed as a more general variance/covariance (or, correlation) matrix because it contains not only observed variable residual variances (.50) on the main diagonal, but also shows unit (1) variances for the intercept and slope on the lower main diagonal, and the intercept/slope covariance (correlation) on the lower off-diagonal elements (.25).

The beta (**B**) matrix also has several rows and columns equal to the number of observed variables plus the number of latent variables, and the cell values contain the predictive or regression relationships between the observed and latent variables. For an unconditional latent growth curve model, the beta matrix contains the loadings for the latent intercept and slope [Equation (7.7)].

B =

	*Y*1	*Y*2	*Y*3	*Y*4	*Y*5	Intercept	Slope	
*Y*1	0	0	0	0	0	0.7071	0	*Y*1
*Y*2	0	0	0	0	0	0.5927	0.265	*Y*2
*Y*3	0	0	0	0	0	0.4716	0.422	*Y*3
*Y*4	0	0	0	0	0	0.3785	0.510	*Y*4
*Y*5	0	0	0	0	0	0.3125	0.561	*Y*5
Intercept	0	0	0	0	0	0	0	Intercept
Slope	0	0	0	0	0	0	0	Slope

(7.7)

The identity (**I**) matrix also has a number of rows and columns equal to the number of observed variables plus the number of latent variables and contains only values of one (1) on the main diagonal by definition [Equation (7.8)].

I =

	*Y*1	*Y*2	*Y*3	*Y*4	*Y*5	Intercept	Slope	
*Y*1	**1**	0	0	0	0	0	0	*Y*1
*Y*2	0	**1**	0	0	0	0	0	*Y*2
*Y*3	0	0	**1**	0	0	0	0	*Y*3
*Y*4	0	0	0	**1**	0	0	0	*Y*4
*Y*5	0	0	0	0	**1**	0	0	*Y*5
Intercept	0	0	0	0	0	**1**	0	Intercept
Slope	0	0	0	0	0	0	**1**	Slope

(7.8)

Finally, the **P** matrix can be thought of as a "pick" matrix because it has columns equal to the number of observed variables plus the number of latent variables, but the number of rows is equal only to the number of observed response variables [Equation (7.9)].

I =

	*Y*1	*Y*2	*Y*3	*Y*4	*Y*5	Intercept	Slope	
*Y*1	1	0	0	0	0	0	0	*Y*1
*Y*2	0	1	0	0	0	0	0	*Y*2
*Y*3	0	0	1	0	0	0	0	*Y*3
*Y*4	0	0	0	1	0	0	0	*Y*4
*Y*5	0	0	0	0	1	0	0	*Y*5

(7.9)

As will be shown below, these last two columns filled with zeros will "pick out" only the response variables and will effectively drop the latent variables from the final result.

The Bollen and Curran model equation reproduced here can be solved using the information contained in the four matrices above using the following R syntax [Equation (7.10)].

```
P <- matrix(c(1, 0, 0, 0, 0, 0, 0, 0, 1, 0, 0, 0, 0, 0, 0, 0, 1, 0, 0, 0, 0, 0, 0, 0, 1, 0, 0, 0, 0, 0, 0, 0,
        1, 0, 0), ncol = 7, byrow = TRUE)

I <- matrix(c(1, 0, 0, 0, 0, 0, 0, 0, 1, 0, 0, 0, 0, 0, 0, 0, 1, 0, 0, 0, 0, 0, 0, 0, 1, 0, 0, 0, 0, 0, 0, 0,
        1, 0, 0, 0, 0, 0, 0, 0, 1, 0, 0, 0, 0, 0, 0, 0, 1), ncol = 7, byrow = TRUE)

Beta <- matrix(c(0, 0, 0, 0, 0, 0.7071, 0, 0, 0, 0, 0, 0, 0.5927, 0.265, 0, 0, 0, 0, 0, 0.4716, 0.422,
        0, 0, 0, 0, 0, 0.3786, 0.510, 0, 0, 0, 0, 0, 0.3125, 0.561, 0, 0, 0, 0, 0, 0, 0, 0, 0, 0, 0, 0, 0,
        0), ncol = 7, byrow = TRUE)

Psi <- matrix(c(0.5, 0, 0, 0, 0, 0, 0, 0, 0.5, 0, 0, 0, 0, 0, 0, 0, 0.5, 0, 0, 0, 0, 0, 0, 0, 0.5, 0, 0, 0,
        0, 0, 0, 0, 0.5, 0, 0, 0, 0, 0, 0, 1, 0.246, 0, 0, 0, 0, 0, 0.246, 1), ncol = 7, byrow = TRUE)

corr_matrix <- P %*% (solve(I-Beta)) %*% Psi %*%t(solve(I-Beta)) %*%t(P)
corr_matrix
```

$$\Sigma\theta = \begin{array}{c|ccccc|} & Y1 & Y2 & Y3 & Y4 & Y5 \\ \hline Y1 & 1.00 & 0.47 & 0.41 & 0.36 & 0.32 \\ Y2 & 0.47 & 1.00 & 0.49 & 0.46 & 0.44 \\ Y3 & 0.41 & 0.49 & 1.00 & 0.49 & 0.48 \\ Y4 & 0.36 & 0.46 & 0.49 & 1.00 & 0.50 \\ Y5 & 0.32 & 0.44 & 0.48 & 0.50 & 1.00 \end{array} \quad (7.10)$$

As will be shown in the chapters that follow, both model-reproduced equations can be expanded to accommodate both time-invariant and time-varying predictor variables. However, as will also be shown in the chapters that follow, familiarity with both model-reproduced equations will prove advantageous.

SUGGESTED READINGS

- Baker, D. H., Vilidaite, G., Lygo, F. A., Smith, A. K., Flack, T. R., Gouws, A. D., & Andrews, T. J. (2020). Power contours: Optimising sample size and precision in experimental psychology and human neuroscience. *Psychological Methods, 26*(3), 295–314.
- Bollen, K. A., & Curran, P. J. (2006). *Latent curve models: A structural equation perspective.* Wiley.
- Curran, P. J., Obeidat, K., & Losardo, D. (2010). Twelve frequently asked questions about growth curve modeling. *Journal of Cognition and Development, 11,* 121–136.
- Estrada, E., Hamagami, F., & Ferrer, E. (2020). Estimating age-based developmental trajectories using latent change score models based on measurement occasion. *Multivariate Behavioral Research, 55,* 454–477.
- Geiser, C. (2021). *Longitudinal structural equation modeling with Mplus: A latent state-trait perspective.* Guilford Press.
- Ghisletta, P., & McArdle, J. J. (2012). Latent curve models and latent change score models estimated in R. *Structural Equation Modeling: A Multidisciplinary Journal, 19,* 651–682.
- Grimm, K. J., Ram, N., & Estabrook, R. (2017). *Growth modeling: Structural equation and multilevel modeling approaches.* Guilford Press.

- Johnson, T. L., & Hancock, G. R. (2019). Time to criterion latent growth models. *Psychological Methods, 24,* 690–707.
- Little, T. D. (2024). *Longitudinal structural equation modeling* (2nd ed.). Guilford Press.
- Liu, S., Rovine, M. J., & Molenaar, P. (2012). Selecting a linear mixed model for longitudinal data: Repeated measures analysis of variance, covariance pattern model, and growth curve approaches. *Psychological Methods, 17,* 15–30.
- Mainzer, R., Apajee, J., Nguyen, C. D., Carlin, J. B., & Lee, K. J. (2021). A comparison of multiple imputation strategies for handling missing data in multi-item scales: Guidance for longitudinal studies. *Statistics in Medicine, 40*(21), 4660–4674.
- Miller, M. L., & Ferrer, E. (2017). The effect of sampling-time variation on latent growth curve models. *Structural Equation Modeling: A Multidisciplinary Journal, 24,* 831–854.
- Raudenbush, S. W. (1993). Hierarchical linear models and experimental design. In L. K. Edwards (Ed.), *Applied analysis of variance in behavioral science* (pp. 459–496). Marcel Dekker.
- Rovine, M. J., & McDermott, P. A. (2018). Latent growth curve and repeated measures ANOVA contrasts: What the models are telling you. *Multivariate Behavioral Research, 53,* 90–101.
- Rovine, M. J., & Molenaar, P. C. (1998). A LISREL model for the analysis of repeated measures with a patterned covariance matrix. *Structural Equation Modeling: A Multidisciplinary Journal, 5,* 318–343.
- Singer, J. D., & Willett, J. B. (2003). *Applied longitudinal data analysis: Modeling change and event occurrence.* Oxford.
- Vera, J. D., & Enders, C. K. (2021). Is item imputation always better? An investigation of wave-missing data in growth models. *Structural Equation Modeling: A Multidisciplinary Journal, 28*(4), 506–517.
- Voelkle, M. C., Gische, C., Driver, C. C., & Lindenberger, U. (2018). The role of time in the quest for understanding psychological mechanisms. *Multivariate Behavioral Research, 53,* 782–805.
- Yuan, K. H., Zhang, Z., & Deng, L. (2019). Fit indices for mean structures with growth curve models. *Psychological Methods, 24,* 36–53.

8

Time-Invariant Covariates

Chapter 7 concluded by showing two different equations to compute a model-reproduced correlation matrix (assuming standardization) for an unconditional (no predictors) longitudinal structural equation model. Both equations will again be used to consider how to conduct power analyses in longitudinal structural equation models that include predictors of change over time. Unconditional longitudinal structural equation models are rarely sufficient, in and of themselves, to answer research questions. It is far more likely that longitudinal structural equation models that contain predictors of change over time, and the parameter estimates and significance tests for the predictors, are required to answer research questions.

Time-invariant predictors are defined as variables whose values will not change over the course of the longitudinal study. Education level, income, and IQ are examples of common time-invariant covariates measured on a continuous scale. Common binary time-invariant covariates include sex and randomization to either a treatment condition (= 1) or a control condition (= 0). To illustrate the procedures needed to obtain a power estimate for a longitudinal structural equation model that includes a time-invariant covariate, this chapter will begin with the simplest power analysis example that assumes a researcher wishes to replicate a pilot longitudinal clinical trial. Longitudinal clinical trial replications are the easiest power analyses to conduct because a great deal of needed information is known. Acknowledging that many longitudinal clinical trials are not replications but rather are novel investigations, we will show how the clinical trial replication example and the model-reproduced correlation matrix formulas from Chapter 7 can be combined with reasonable logic to conduct a power analysis for a novel study. We then extend the longitudinal structural equation model to include a continuous time-invariant covariate and conclude the chapter with an example of a power analysis that involves moderation, or an interaction between a binary treatment randomization variable and a continuous time-invariant covariate.

A Tauber et al. (2021) Replication Power Analysis

Tauber et al. (2021) conducted a longitudinal randomized clinical pilot trial to test the efficacy of a group therapy-based intervention (ConquerFear) to treat *fear of cancer recur-*

rence (FCR), which is defined as negative, anxious, and persistent threat-monitoring meta-cognitions in patients who have undergone previous cancer treatment, but who fear a worsening recurrence. FCR has been associated with higher levels of anxiety and depression and lower quality of life. ConquerFear is a cognitive-behavioral treatment specifically designed to target the negative meta-cognitions associated with FCR via teaching a combination of cognitive reframing and behavioral stress-reduction techniques. Originally designed as an individual therapeutic intervention, the authors suspected ConquerFear could be a cost-effective group therapeutic intervention that decreases loneliness and increases skill acquisition and mutual support.

To test these hypotheses, $N = 27$ participants were randomly assigned to either ConquerFear ($n = 14$) or a progressive behavioral relaxation control condition ($n = 13$), and response variable data were collected at baseline, 1 week posttreatment, and at 3-month and 6-month follow-ups. Although the scores on the Fear of Cancer Recurrence Inventory were of primary interest in this study, our interest here will focus on the scores from the Depression and Anxiety Stress Scale (DASS-21) at all assessments for both groups shown in Table 8.1 (data from Tauber et al., 2021, p. 6).

Although Tauber et al. reported insignificant DASS-21 score differences between the two groups (p-values = .12–.27) over time, the effect size estimates for the DASS-21 differences between the two groups were noteworthy. (Hedges $g = 0.41–0.61$; *Side Note: Hedges g values are interpreted in the same way as Cohen's d values, but are viewed by some as a more appropriate effect size estimate under small sample size conditions.*) If a researcher wanted to replicate Tauber's study, it would be helpful to conduct a Monte Carlo simulation power analysis to determine the sample size needed to reject the null hypothesis for treatment randomization predicting DASS-21 change over time with power ≥ .80. While it is very helpful to have estimates of how both the ConquerFear and Behavioral relaxation groups and their average DASS-21 scores changed over time, a first step toward conducting a replication power analysis should be an indication of the extent to which DASS-21 scores are correlated over time, and these are also shown in Table 8.2.[1]

It is helpful to have the means, standard deviations, and correlations among the DASS-21 scores for both the ConquerFear and Behavioral relaxation groups, but if we had the

TABLE 8.1. Depression and Anxiety Stress Scale Assessments-21 (DASS-21)

	ConquerFear group		Behavioral relaxation	
	Mean	SD	Mean	SD
Baseline	18.38	13.67	19.57	9.26
1 Week	11.91	10.39	17.30	12.31
3 Month	8.82	8.12	17.90	14.71
6 Month	8.82	9.12	15.20	11.93

[1] Special thanks to Dr. Nina Tauber and colleagues at Aarhus University in Denmark for allowing us to use their study and for providing the needed correlation matrices.

TABLE 8.2. DASS-21 Correlation over Time

	Behavioral relaxation			
	Baseline	1 Week	3 Month	6 Month
Baseline	1			
1 Week	0.838	1		
3 Month	0.805	0.853	1	
6 Month	0.738	0.868	0.711	1
	ConquerFear group			
	Baseline	1 Week	3 Month	6 Month
Baseline	1			
1 Week	0.588	1		
3 Month	0.705	0.888	1	
6 Month	0.775	0.900	0.811	1

Note. Data from Tauber et al. (2021).

means for both groups over time (also referred to as the *mean structure*) and the *covariance matrices* for both groups, then we would have the mean structures and the covariance matrices that constitute the minimum sufficient information needed to either generate or analyze longitudinal data in any structural equation modeling statistical analysis software program. The second step toward conducting a replication power analysis is to use the available data to compute covariance matrices for both groups, as shown in Table 8.3.

As shown in Table 8.3 for both groups, using standard deviations and correlations to compute covariance matrices is a straightforward, two-step process. In the first step, computing variances on the matrix main diagonal for both groups involves squaring the

TABLE 8.3. DASS-21 Covariance Matrices

	Behavioral relaxation			
	Baseline	1 Week	3 Month	6 Month
Baseline	$(9.26)^2$			
1 Week	(9.26)(12.31)0.838	$(12.31)^2$		
3 Month	(9.26)(14.71)0.805	(12.31)(14.71)0.853	$(14.71)^2$	
6 Month	(9.26)(11.93)0.738	(12.31)(11.93)0.868	(14.71)(11.93)0.711	$(11.93)^2$
	ConquerFear group			
	Baseline	1 Week	3 Month	6 Month
Baseline	$(13.67)^2$			
1 Week	(13.67)(10.39)0.588	$(10.39)^2$		
3 Month	(13.67)(8.12)0.705	(10.39)(8.12)0.888	$(8.12)^2$	
6 Month	(13.67)(9.12)0.775	(10.39)(9.12)0.90	(8.12)(9.12)0.811	$(9.12)^2$

Note. Data from Tauber et al. (2021).

TABLE 8.4. DASS-21 Covariance Matrices

	Behavioral relaxation			
	Baseline	1 Week	3 Month	6 Month
Baseline	85.748			
1 Week	95.524	151.536		
3 Month	109.653	154.461	216.384	
6 Month	81.528	127.473	124.774	142.325
	ConquerFear group			
	Baseline	1 Week	3 Month	6 Month
Baseline	186.869			
1 Week	83.514	107.952		
3 Month	78.255	74.918	65.934	
6 Month	96.620	85.281	60.058	83.174

Note. Data from Tauber et al. (2021).

standard deviations for the DASS-21 scores at all time points. In the second step, multiplying the correlation between any two variables by the standard deviations of both variables produces covariances on the matrix off-diagonal elements, resulting in the following covariance matrices for both groups shown in Table 8.4.

With the mean structures for both groups, as well as their respective covariance matrices, for DASS-21 scores over time, data consistent with these values can be generated for further analysis in either Mplus or R.

Mplus Monte Carlo Power Analysis: Longitudinal RCT Pilot

The Monte Carlo simulation power analysis in Mplus can be conducted with the following syntax:

```
TITLE: MPLUS 8.1 Tauber, Part 1

MONTECARLO:
NAMES ARE
DASS_B DASS_W1 DASS_M3 DASS_M6;
NGROUPS = 2;
NOBSERVATIONS = 71 71;
NREPS = 5000;
SEED = 13171;
MISSING = DASS_W1 DASS_M3 DASS_M6;
REPSAVE = ALL;
SAVE = TAUBER_*.DAT;
```

The initial syntax commands specify generating data (MONTECARLO:) for DASS-21 scores assessed at baseline (DASS_B), 1 week posttreatment (DASS_W1), and at 3-month

(DASS_M3) and 6-month (DASS_6M) follow-up assessments for both the ConquerFear and Behavioral relaxation groups (i.e., `NGROUPS = 2;`). The (`NOBSERVATIONS = 71 71;`) command specifies generating $n = 71$ observations per group ($N = 142$) to test for adequate statistical power. The number of dataset replications (`NREPS = 5000;`) remains the same as in previous power analyses, and the (`SEED = 13171;`) specification provides a random number from which Mplus begins data generation. In keeping with previous Monte Carlo simulation power analyses, data will be generated assuming missing data at each of the postbaseline assessment time points (`MISSING = DASS_W1 DASS_M3 DASS_M6;`). The final two lines of code output all generated datasets (`REPSAVE = ALL;`) and name them `TAUBER_*.DAT;`, where the asterisk is replaced by integer values from 1 to 5,000 for all datasets.

```
MODEL POPULATION: !BEHAVIORAL RELAXATION;

 [DASS_B*19.57];
 [DASS_W1*17.30];
 [DASS_M3*17.90];
 [DASS_M6*15.20];

 DASS_B*85.748;
 DASS_W1*151.536;
 DASS_M3*216.384;
 DASS_M6*142.325;

 DASS_B WITH DASS_W1*95.524 DASS_M3*109.653 DASS_M6*81.528;
 DASS_W1 WITH DASS_M3*154.461 DASS_M6*127.473;
 DASS_M3 WITH DASS_M6*124.774;

MODEL POPULATION-g2: !CONQUER FEAR;

 [DASS_B*18.38];
 [DASS_W1*11.91];
 [DASS_M3*8.82];
 [DASS_M6*8.82];

 DASS_B*186.869;
 DASS_W1*107.952;
 DASS_M3*65.934;
 DASS_M6*83.174;

 DASS_B WITH DASS_W1*83.514 DASS_M3*78.255 DASS_M6*96.62;
 DASS_W1 WITH DASS_M3*74.918 DASS_M6*85.281;
 DASS_M3 WITH DASS_M6*60.058;
```

The next two sections of syntax code generate data for both the Behavioral relaxation (`MODEL POPULATION:`) and ConquerFear (`MODEL POPULATION-g2:`) groups consistent with their respective means and covariances shown above. Specifically, within both groups, the first four lines of code in brackets [] assign mean values to the DASS scores over time consistent with Tauber et al.'s (2021, p. 6) tabled results shown earlier. The next four lines assign DASS-21 score variances consistent with the main diagonal values computed above for both groups, and the final three `WITH` statements assign covariances to pairs of DASS-21 values consistent with the off-diagonal values also computed above.

The line (`MISSING = DASS_W1 DASS_M3 DASS_M6;`) from the first block of Mplus code shown above states that missing data is expected for all postbaseline DASS-21 assessments.

```
MODEL MISSING:
[DASS_W1*-3.17805]; !4% missing MCAR;
[DASS_M3*-2.58667]; !7% missing MCAR;
[DASS_M6*-2.19715]; !10% missing MCAR;

DASS_W1 ON DASS_B*0.04879;
DASS_M3 ON DASS_W1*0.09531;
DASS_M6 ON DASS_M3*0.139762;
!5%-15% increase in missing data per unit DASS increase;
```

The first three statements in brackets following the `MODEL MISSING:` command specifies missing completely at random (MCAR) missing data from ($exp^{-3.17805}/1 + exp^{-3.17805} = 0.04$) 4% at the week 1 assessment that increases to ($exp^{-2.19715}/1 + exp^{-2.19715} = 0.10$) 10% at the 6-month assessment. The inclusion of the next four lines of code turns the MCAR missing data to missing at random (MAR) missing data by specifying unit increases in DASS-21 scores at a previous assessment time point increases the proportion of missing data at any subsequent time point from ($exp^{0.04779} = 0.05$) 5% to ($exp^{0.139762} = 0.15$) 15% as participants progress in the study.

Running the Mplus code shown above will generate 5,000 replications of data saved to external files named `TAUBER_1.DAT`, `TAUBER_2.DAT`, . . . `TAUBER_5000.DAT`. Based on the summary statistics from the data-generating output file, the generated DASS-21 data can be shown in error bars, as seen in Figure 8.1.

As shown in previous examples, researchers can inspect both the missing data patterns and covariance coverage statistics in the output for the data-generating file and adjust the missing data specifications as needed. The following Mplus syntax is needed to read in and analyze the 5,000 dataset replications to obtain a statistical power estimate.

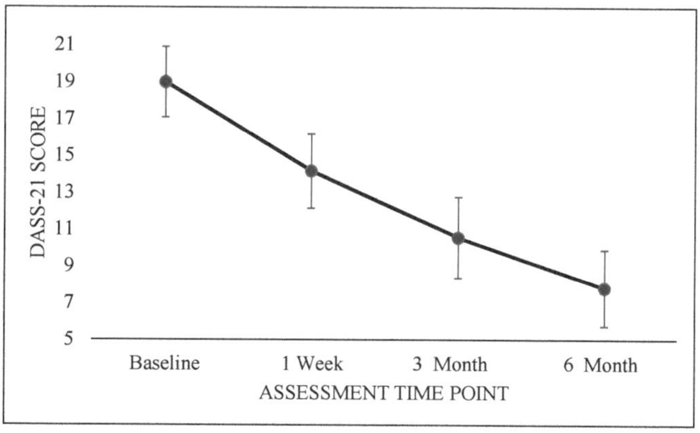

FIGURE 8.1. Error bar graph; data from Tauber et al. (2021).

```
TITLE: MPLUS 8.1 Tauber, Part 2

DATA:
File = TAUBER_list.dat;
Type = MONTECARLO;
```

Recall that when Monte Carlo dataset replications are saved, a 'list' file that contains the names of all replication files

```
TAUBER_1.dat;
TAUBER_2.dat;
...
TAUBER_5000.dat;
```

is saved also by default in Mplus. The 'File = TAUBER_list.dat;' line, together with the 'Type = MONTECARLO;' specification, essentially instructs Mplus to analyze all dataset replications in the 'list' file and summarize the results as follows:

```
VARIABLE:
NAMES =
DASS_B
DASS_W1
DASS_M3
DASS_M6
GROUP;

Missing = all (999);
```

Recall also that when Monte Carlo dataset replications are saved, the order in which the variables were saved is listed at the bottom of the data-generating output file. Missing data were specified for all assessments following baseline, so Mplus lists the missing data indicator value as 999, which is also found at the bottom of the data-generating output file.

```
DEFINE:
GROUP = GROUP - 1;
```

Notice in the 'VARIABLE: NAMES =' specification above, the last variable included in all Monte Carlo datasets is a 'GROUP' variable. Data were generated from the mean structures and covariance matrices of both treatment groups; the Behavioral relaxation group first, followed by the ConquerFear group. The variable 'GROUP' will show values of 1 to indicate Behavioral relaxation group data, and values of 2 to indicate ConquerFear group data in all replications. The 'DEFINE:' command is used to subtract a value of 1 from the 'GROUP' variable, which will result in a binary variable with the Behavioral relaxation group (= 0) as the reference group and the ConquerFear group (= 1) as the group of interest.

```
MODEL:
I S Q | DASS_B@0 DASS_W1@.25 DASS_M3@3 DASS_M6@6;
I S Q ON GROUP;
```

Recall from Chapter 7 that the first syntax line following the 'MODEL:' command is the Mplus shorthand syntax for the specification of a longitudinal growth model. Unlike the linear growth model example from Chapter 7, the longitudinal growth model syntax above specifies not only a latent 'I'ntercept and linear 'S'lope, but also 'Q'uadratic change over time. As shown in the error bar graph (Figure 8.1), DASS-21 scores decrease rapidly from baseline to week 1, and then decrease more slowly after week 1 to month 6, a trend best captured by a quadratic growth model. Recall also from Chapter 7, that following the "at" '@' symbols, are values (0, 0.25, 3, and 6) are loadings that are centered such that the intercept mean is interpreted as the expected DASS-21 score at baseline (DASS_B). The second loading (0.25) reflects that the second assessment occurs 1 week (month/4) after baseline, and subsequent assessments occur at 3- and 6-month follow-ups, consistent with Tauber et al. (2021). These loading specifications allow the slope mean to be interpreted as the expected DASS-21 score change per month increase in time. By default, Mplus will square (0^2, 0.25^2, 3^2, and 6^2) each linear slope loading to properly specify quadratic change. Although the syntax line 'I S Q ON GROUP;' specifies the binary group indicator variable as a predictor of intercept, linear slope, and quadratic change variance, the effect of treatment group as a predictor of linear slope variance is of primary interest for power analysis purposes.

```
DASS_B;
DASS_W1;
DASS_M3(1);
DASS_M6(1);
```

Finally, listing each of the DASS-21 scores in syntax refers to their respective residual variances. As shown, the DASS-21 scores assessed at the 3- and 6-month follow-ups are constrained to equality, as indicated by the (1) specifications. These specifications were needed to avoid a negative variance estimate (which can occur from estimates based on small pilot sample sizes) and obtain admissible Monte Carlo power analysis estimates. Although some may find this a questionable methodological practice, two considerations warrant mention. First, such a practice underscores the importance of transparency in the power analysis write-up: If power analyses are to be judged on both the *plausibility* of the assumptions upon which they are based and the *reproducibility* of the procedures used to obtain the power estimate(s), a completely transparent write-up that includes a detailed description of both is needed. Second, such a residual variance equality constraint highlights an important step in the modeling of longitudinal data following successful replication of Tauber et al.'s (2021) study: Proper specification and modeling of the residual variances (and possibly covariances) prior to conducting the analysis needed to answer the research question has important statistical power implications. The complete syntax needed to read in and analyze the Monte Carlo data is shown below, and is immediately followed by annotated power analysis results (from MPlus 8.1, parts 1 and 2).

```
TITLE: MPLUS 8.1 Tauber, Part 2
DATA:
File = TAUBER_list.dat;
Type = MONTECARLO;
```

```
VARIABLE:
NAMES =
DASS_B
DASS_W1
DASS_M3
DASS_M6
GROUP;

missing = all (999);

DEFINE:
GROUP = GROUP - 1;

MODEL:
I S Q | DASS_B@0 DASS_W1@.25 DASS_M3@3 DASS_M6@6;

I S Q ON GROUP;

DASS_B;
DASS_W1;
DASS_M3(1);
DASS_M6(1);
```

	Population	ESTIMATES Average	Std. Dev.	S. E. Average	M. S. E.	95% Cover	% Sig Coeff
I |							
DASS_B	1.000	1.0000	0.0000	0.0000	0.0000	1.000	0.000
DASS_W1	1.000	1.0000	0.0000	0.0000	0.0000	1.000	0.000
DASS_M3	1.000	1.0000	0.0000	0.0000	0.0000	1.000	0.000
DASS_M6	1.000	1.0000	0.0000	0.0000	0.0000	1.000	0.000
S |							
DASS_B	0.000	0.0000	0.0000	0.0000	0.0000	1.000	0.000
DASS_W1	0.250	0.2500	0.0000	0.0000	0.0000	1.000	0.000
DASS_M3	3.000	3.0000	0.0000	0.0000	0.0000	1.000	0.000
DASS_M6	6.000	6.0000	0.0000	0.0000	0.0000	1.000	0.000
Q |							
DASS_B	0.000	0.0000	0.0000	0.0000	0.0000	1.000	0.000
DASS_W1	0.062	0.0625	0.0000	0.0000	0.0000	1.000	0.000
DASS_M3	9.000	9.0000	0.0000	0.0000	0.0000	1.000	0.000
DASS_M6	36.000	36.0000	0.0000	0.0000	0.0000	1.000	0.000
S ON							
GROUP	0.000	**-2.5869**	0.9577	0.9125	7.6093	0.196	**0.804**

As shown in the first column (`Population`) for the first three distinct sections of results above, from a single line of syntax (`I S Q | DASS_B@0 DASS_W1@.25 DASS_M3@3 DASS_M6@6;`), Mplus will by default specify the growth curve loadings for the intercept (all values of 1), linear slope (0, 0.25, 3, and 6), and quadratic change (0, 0.0625 [= 0.25^2], 9 [= 3^2], and 36 [= 6^2]). For the parameter estimate of interest (`S ON GROUP;`), the value in the first column is 0, meaning that no a priori assumptions were made regarding the sign or magnitude of this estimate. Rather, as shown in the second column (`Average`), this value was estimated within, and averaged across, all 5,000 dataset replications. The results show that, assuming a sample size of $N = 142$ ($n = 71$ for both the Behavioral relaxation and ConquerFear groups) and proper missing data handling, power ≥ .80 to detect any unstandardized (b) linear "slope on group" estimate of $b \geq -2.58$.

R Monte Carlo Power Analysis: Longitudinal RCT Pilot

The simulation power analysis can be conducted similarly in R using the packages simsem and lavaan. To begin, lavaan, simsem, and source code developed for this book are loaded, and the multigroup population model is specified as:

```
library(simsem)
library(lavaan)
source("simsemTools.R")

PopulationModel_Ch8 <- "
 DASS_B ~ c(19.57, 18.38)*1
 DASS_W1 ~ c(17.30, 11.91)*1
 DASS_M3 ~ c(17.90, 8.82)*1
 DASS_M6 ~ c(15.20, 8.82)*1

 DASS_B ~~ c(85.748, 186.869)*DASS_B
 DASS_W1 ~~ c(151.536, 107.952)*DASS_W1
 DASS_M3 ~~ c(216.384, 65.934)*DASS_M3
 DASS_M6 ~~ c(142.325, 83.174)*DASS_M6

 DASS_B ~~ c(95.524, 83.514)*DASS_W1 + c(109.653, 78.255)*DASS_M3 + c(81.528,
    96.62)*DASS_M6
 DASS_W1 ~~ c(154.461, 74.918)*DASS_M3 + c(127.473, 85.281)*DASS_M6
 DASS_M3 ~~ c(124.774, 60.058)*DASS_M6
"
```

The first four lines of syntax specify the population mean values for each of DASS-21 scores assessed at baseline, 1 week posttreatment, 3 months posttreatment, and 6 months posttreatment. In these four lines of code, the notation c() is included in combination with *1. In lavaan-style syntax, *1 reflects the estimation of a mean or intercept for a given variable, whereas the notation c() is a base R function that is used to combine arguments, and is often used to create lists; in the present context, the list reflects the presence and population values of two groups. The means of DASS-21 in group 1 (the Behavioral relaxation group) are set to 19.57, 17.30, 17.90, and 15.20 at baseline, 1 week posttreatment, 3 months posttreatment, and 6 months posttreatment. The means in group 2 (the ConquerFear group) are 18.38, 11.91, 8.82, and 8.82 at the same assessment time points.

The next four lines of syntax show the group-specific variances for each of the DASS-21 scores over time. The last three lines of syntax reflect the group-specific covariances among DASS-21 scores over time, consistent with the prespecified population model implied covariance matrix.

Similar to Mplus, a missing data model can be specified.

```
MissingModel_Ch8 <- "
  #MCAR intercepts, which is based on known probabilities of missingness
  #MAR slopes, which is based on computed logit values from missingness at prior time
     points
    DASS_W1 ~ -3.17805 + 0.04879*DASS_B
    DASS_M3 ~ -2.58667 + 0.09531*DASS_W1
    DASS_M6 ~ -2.19715 + 0.139762*DASS_M3 "

MissingModel_Ch8 <- miss(logit = MissingModel_Ch8)
```

Each line of code in the missing data model reflects the logits associated with MCAR and MAR data mechanisms for each DV. The intercept value, or the first value in the equation (–3.17805, –2.58667, and –2.19715) reflects the *odds* associated with the proportion of MCAR data at each time point. Specifically, MCAR missing data ranges from ($\exp^{-3.17805}/1 + \exp^{-3.17805} = 0.04$) 4% at the week 1 assessment to ($\exp^{-2.19715}/1 + \exp^{-2.19715} = 0.10$) 10% at the 6-month assessment. The next term in each equation reflects the logits associated with the proportion of MAR data at each time point, contingent on prior time point assessments.

Replicating Mplus's `SAVE` feature in R is nearly automatic with the approaches shown in most chapters of this book. In prior chapters, simulated datasets were given the name "SampleDatasets_ChX." Up until this point, no data have been manipulated prior to analysis, but manipulating the dataset is possible and very simple.

First, create simulated datasets.

```
SampleDatasets_Ch8 <- simulateDataSets(PopulationModel_Ch8,
                      nIterations = 5000,
                      nObservations = c(71, 71),
                      miss = MissingModel_Ch8, # missingness in the data gen phase
                      seed = 13171)
```

Next, examine the summaries for a subset of datasets. Here, that subset reflects the first two datasets, using the lapply()function in combination with summary() and head().

```
lapply(head(SampleDatasets_Ch8, 2), summary)
DASS_B          DASS_W1          DASS_M3          DASS_M6          group          iteration
Min.    : -9.67  Min.    : -11.31  Min.    : -10.94  Min.    : -7.296  Min.    : 1   Min.    : 1
1st Qu. : 11.7   1st Qu. : 7.546   1st Qu. : 2.955   1st Qu. : 0.7804  1st Qu. : 1   1st Qu. : 1
Median  : 18     Median  : 13.72   Median  : 8.921   Median  : 8.1443  Median  : 2   Median  : 1
Mean    : 18.2   Mean    : 13.47   Mean    : 9.925   Mean    : 8.6486  Mean    : 2   Mean    : 1
3rd Qu. : 25.8   3rd Qu. : 20.43   3rd Qu. : 15.344  3rd Qu. : 13.799  3rd Qu. : 2   3rd Qu. : 1
Max.    : 46.3   Max.    : 48.51   Max.    : 37.416  Max.    : 40.503  Max.    : 2   Max.    : 1
                 NA's    : 19      NA's    : 37      NA's    : 67

DASS_B          DASS_W1          DASS_M3          DASS_M6          group          iteration
Min.    : -13.8  Min.    : -21.3   Min.    : -16.65  Min.    : -18.76  Min.    : 1   Min.    : 2
1st Qu. : 10.5   1st Qu. : 6.505   1st Qu. : 0.9596  1st Qu. : 0.7226  1st Qu. : 1   1st Qu. : 2
Median  : 20.2   Median  : 12.85   Median  : 8.0535  Median  : 6.7932  Median  : 2   Median  : 2
Mean    : 18.8   Mean    : 13.22   Mean    : 9.8478  Mean    : 6.6994  Mean    : 2   Mean    : 2
3rd Qu. : 26.4   3rd Qu. : 21.05   3rd Qu. : 16.902  3rd Qu. : 12.21   3rd Qu. : 2   3rd Qu. : 2
Max.    : 50.7   Max.    : 41.14   Max.    : 44.1    Max.    : 26.121  Max.    : 2   Max.    : 2
                 NA's    : 13      NA's    : 36      NA's    : 63
```

In the data output, DASS_B contains no missing data, and each consecutive time point contains more missing than the prior time points. When briefly examining the observed data values, the group variable takes on the values of 1 and 2. When using the group variable in analyses, researchers often want the data to have values of 0 and 1, which can be easily completed for all datasets by subtracting 1 from 'group' across the list of 5,000 sample datasets. To do this, use the function lapply() in combination with transform(), which can then be used to apply a function to a list. In this case, the transform function can be applied to the simulated list of dataframes.

```
SampleDatasets_Ch8 <- lapply(SampleDatasets_Ch8, transform, group_cf1 = group - 1)
```

A new variable called 'group_cf1' is created, where individuals in the ConquerFear group have a group value of 1, and those in the Behavioral relaxation group have a value of 0.

It is now possible to complete a Monte Carlo simulation on an analysis model. The analysis model is a latent growth curve model, conditioned on the binary grouping variable. Although this model is functionally different than the estimation model, it is mathematically a suitable approach to evaluate longitudinal data that differ across treatment conditions. The analysis model is specified below.

```
AnalysisModel_Ch8 <- "
I =~ 1*DASS_B + 1*DASS_W1 + 1*DASS_M3 + 1*DASS_M6          #intercept
S =~ 0*DASS_B + 0.25*DASS_W1 + 3*DASS_M3 + 6*DASS_M6       #slope
Q =~ 0*DASS_B + 0.0625*DASS_W1 + 9*DASS_M3 + 36*DASS_M6    #quadratic
I ~ 1          #mean of the intercept factor
S ~ 1          #mean of the slope factor
Q ~ 1          #mean of the quadratic factor
I ~~ I         #variance of the intercept factor
S ~~ S         #variance of the slope factor
Q ~~ Q         #variance of the quadratic factor

#covariances allowed among all growth factors
I ~~ S
I ~~ Q
S ~~ Q

I ~ group_cf1        #intercept conditional on group
S ~ group_cf1        #slope conditional on group
Q ~ group_cf1        #quadratic conditional on group

DASS_B ~~ DASS_B
DASS_W1 ~~ DASS_W1
DASS_M3 ~~ var1*DASS_M3 #constraining variances equal to avoid negative var estimates
DASS_M6 ~~ var1*DASS_M6
"
```

The latent growth analysis model includes intercept (I), slope (S), and quadratic (Q) change over time. Each growth factor is defined in its own line of syntax. The intercept factor loadings are fixed to 1, the slope factor loadings are fixed to 0, 0.25, 3, and 6—which reflect the months between each assessment—and the quadratic factor loadings are fixed to the squared value of the slope factor loadings. By constraining factor loadings according to observed time differences, the factor means can be interpreted as the expected DASS-21 score change per month.

Although not inherently necessary to identify the model, the lavaan AnalysisModel_Ch8 syntax shows that the intercept, slope, and quadratic factors each have an estimated mean value (~ 1), as well as estimated variances (I ~~ I, S ~~ S, Q ~~ Q) and covariances (I ~~ S, I ~~ Q, S ~~ Q) among the growth factors. Furthermore, each latent growth factor is regressed on the group variable that was created earlier, shown in the lines I ~ group_cf1, S ~ group_cf1, Q ~ group_cf1.

Observed variables have estimated residual variances, though residual variances at the 3- and 6-month follow-ups are set equal to avoid negative variance estimation. As noted earlier, some may find this a questionable practice, yet it was necessary to avoid negative variance estimation due to the pilot sample data estimates. Again as noted earlier, this practice underscores the necessity for a transparent write-up of any power analysis. If statistical power analyses are judged on plausibility and reproducibility, then a wholly transparent write-up detailing the exact description of the model is needed.

Now that the analysis model has been appropriately specified, the Monte Carlo simulation power analysis can be completed by using the previously simulated sample datasets in combination with the expected analysis model.

```
output_Ch8 <-  sim(model = AnalysisModel_Ch8,
               rawData = SampleDatasets_Ch8,
               silent = TRUE,
               lavaanfun = "growth",
               outfun = cov_coverage)
```

In this simulation, the simulated list of 5,000 population datasets are included as raw data, seen by the rawData = SampleDatasets_Ch8 line of code. This is because the data were simulated on a population model that differed from the analysis model. Note that because missingness was imposed in the simulated SampleDatasets_Ch8 object, missingness should not be included in the analysis; missingness can be imposed at either the data-generation stage or analysis stage but will be overcalculated if it is included in both stages.

An overall summary of the simulation can be evaluated.

summary(output_Ch8)

	Estimate Average	Estimate SD	Average SE	Power (Not equal 0)	Std Est	Std Est SD	Std Ave SE
I~group_cf1	-3.632	1.803	1.778	0.536	-0.193	0.093	0.092
S~group_cf1	-2.560	0.972	0.906	0.790	-0.414	0.645	26.840
Q~group_cf1	0.368	0.171	0.158	0.634	0.316	0.367	5.556

In the results, the power to detect the S~group_cf1 regression coefficient is just under .80. Mplus and R programs can lead to slightly different results, due to different starting values. To ensure transparency of analysis and replication, all information about the analysis should be provided to the audience, including the program, package, and version number of the software or other tool used to conduct the simulation analysis. In this analysis, statistical power is very close to the .80 threshold commonly used for statistical power analysis decisions about sample size. If desired, some may wish to recompute the analysis using a slightly higher sample size.

Longitudinal RCT Pilot Model Simulation Power Analysis Write-Up

"The power analysis question involved the smallest sample size needed to achieve power ≥ .80 to detect significantly greater decreases over time in Depression and Anxiety Stress Scale (DASS-21) scores for patients randomly assigned to the ConquerFear versus a Behavioral relaxation control condition in a longitudinal design that replicates the Tauber et al., (2021) study of fear of cancer recurrence. A Monte Carlo simulation power analysis was conducted using Mplus (version 8.6) assuming: (1) the means, standard deviations, and correlations for both the ConquerFear and Behavioral relaxation groups supplied by Tauber et al., constitute the best available pilot data estimates for power analysis purposes; (2) participants will be assessed at baseline, 1 week post-intervention, and at 3-month and 6-month follow-up assessments, and these assessment time points will be used to specify longitudinal growth curve analytic specifics; (3) quadratic trend would best capture DASS-21 changes over time, but the effect of randomization on linear change was the statistical power estimate of interest; (4) missing data will increase from 4% at week 1 to 10% at month 6 (MCAR), and will further increase from 5% at week 1 to 15% at month 6 per unit increases in DASS-21 scores at the previous time point; and (5) the residual variances at month 3 and month 6 were constrained to equality to avoid a negative residual variance estimate that would produce an inadmissible power analysis solution. This power analysis therefore further assumes a parsimonious modeling of residual variances prior to treatment effect testing in subsequent data analysis. Monte Carlo simulation power analysis results aggregated over 5,000 dataset replications showed power ≥ .80 to detect an unstandardized slope estimate (b) of $b \geq -2.58$ for randomization predicting linear change in DASS-21 scores over time if proper missing data handling makes $N = 142$ ($n = 71$ per group) available for analysis."

But, What If . . . ?

The previous example, which assumed a replication of Tauber et al. (2021), illustrated many key concepts in longitudinal power analysis methodology, but it is a rare occasion when a researcher's focus involves a replication study. Researchers at this point might well be wondering, and rightfully so, not only, "What if my study is not a replication?" but also, "What if my study is a novel one with little, if any, previous empirical research, and with nowhere near the amount of information available for a replication study?" These are important questions for several reasons, to be sure, not the least of which is that power analyses are most often needed for research grant funding application submissions, but another one of the criteria upon which applications are evaluated is novelty of the proposed study, and to be a truly novel study by definition means researching a subject for which published information is lacking. If this is the case, researchers' next question is often along the lines of, "So, how can I possibly begin to conduct a Monte Carlo simulation power analysis?" For many researchers and research teams, this situation constitutes the proverbial "brick wall" beyond which they find themselves unable to advance. The good news is that based on information presented in previous chapters, with the information a researcher likely knows already (or could reasonably approximate), and a little logic, a longitudinal conditional Monte Carlo simulation power analysis is well within reach.

In Chapter 7, three different unconditional models, based on published work by Bauer and Curran (2004) in which linear trend explained 50, 60, or 70% of response variable variance over time, were specified and model-reproduced correlation computations showed each to be an admissible model. Conducting a novel, conditional longitudinal Monte Carlo simulation, in which a binary indicator of treatment randomization (1 = treatment, 0 = control) is the only time-invariant covariate included, begins when a researcher assumes a linear trend will best capture response variable change over time, and a researcher needs to decide whether linear trend will explain 50, 60, or 70% of response variable variance. Two important points warrant clarification. First, with multiple assessment time points in a longitudinal research study, several trends beyond linear (e.g., quadratic, cubic, etc.) may also best capture response variable changes, but assuming linear trend for a randomized control trial (RCT) is a *reasonable* starting point. Second, deciding on how much response variable variation is explained by linear trend (50, 60, or 70%) may not have a straightforward solution, but Monte Carlo simulation power analyses can be performed at all three values of variance explained and the results can be presented in a conditional "if/then" format that demonstrates a reasonable amount of thought and consideration given to multiple possible outcomes. For demonstration purposes, it is assumed that linear trend will explain 60% of the response variable variance, and the unconditional longitudinal analysis model figure, R syntax matrices, and model-reproduced correlation matrix are all shown in Figure 8.2.

```
Lambda <- matrix(c(.7746, 0, .6527, .265, .5352, .422, .4498, .51, .3917, .561),
ncol = 2, byrow = TRUE)
Phi <- matrix(c(1, .30, .30, 1), nrow = 2, byrow = TRUE)
Psi <- matrix(c(0.40, 0, 0, 0, 0, 0, 0.40, 0, 0, 0, 0, 0, .40, 0, 0, 0, 0, 0, .40, 0, 0, 0, 0, 0, 0.40),
      nrow = 5, byrow = TRUE)
corr_matrix <- (Lambda %*% Phi %*% t(Lambda)) + Psi
corr_matrix
```

The correlation matrix once solved is as follows:

	Response Variable 1	Response Variable 2	Response Variable 3	Response Variable 4	Response Variable 5
Response Variable 1	1	0.5672	0.5126	0.4669	0.4338
Response Variable 2	0.5672	1	0.5863	0.5644	0.5453
Response Variable 3	0.5126	0.5863	1	0.5948	0.586
Response Variable 4	0.4669	0.5644	0.5948	1	0.5979
Response Variable 5	0.4338	0.5453	0.586	0.5979	1

The analysis model shown in Figure 8.3 would change to incorporate a binary treatment predictor variable as shown here.

Notice in this conditional latent growth curve model that the binary indicator of treatment randomization is specified as a predictor of latent linear slope variance only.

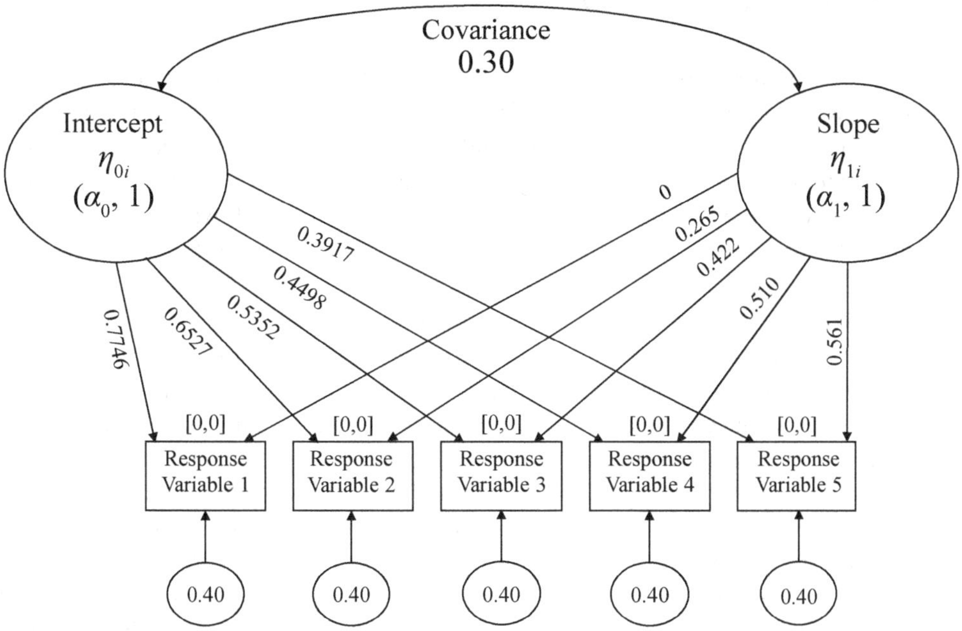

FIGURE 8.2. Longitudinal growth curve model that explains 60% of response variable variance.

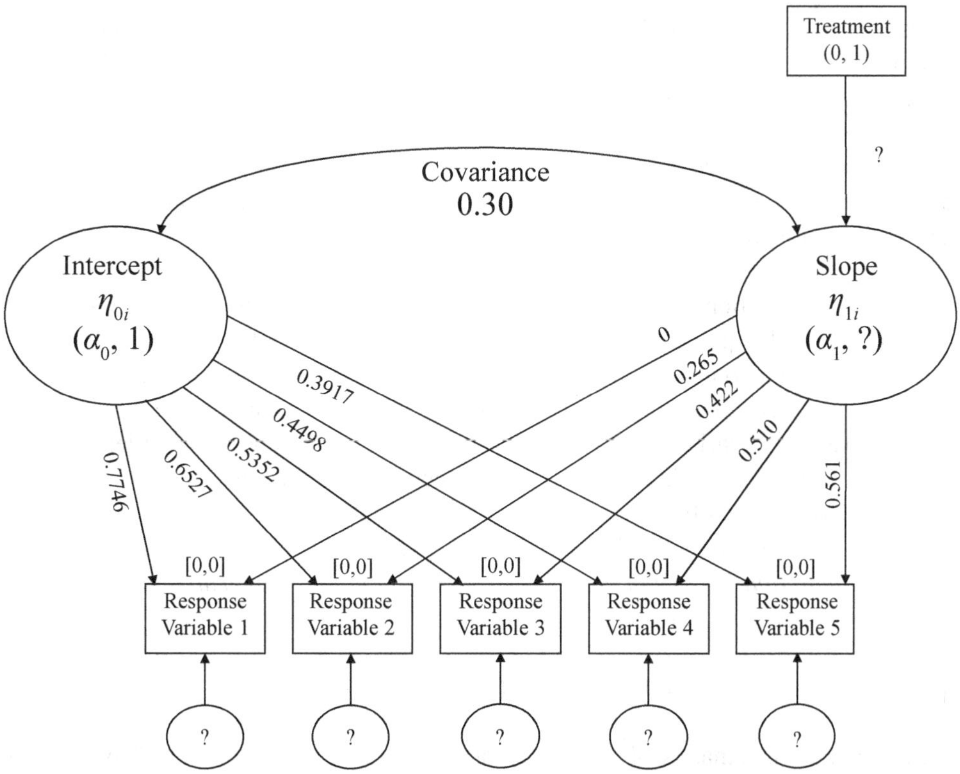

FIGURE 8.3. Main effect of treatment model; data from Corona et al. (2020).

Assuming successful random assignment to either the treatment or the control condition, a researcher would have no reason, by definition, to expect any significant response variable group differences at the outset of the study. Stated differently, if random assignment were truly random, specifying the binary treatment indicator as a predictor of intercept variance would essentially be predicting a value at or near 0, which would waste a degree of freedom. Furthermore, notice also that a number of question marks ('?') now appear in the model where specific values were previously found. The first question mark can be found next to the arrow that specifies treatment randomization as a predictor of latent linear slope variance. The second question mark can be found in the (α_1, ?) specification for latent linear slope, which indicates that treatment randomization is expected to explain a portion of slope variance that results in a value less than 1. Finally, all residual response variable variances now show question marks because of a fundamental structural equation modeling principle: "upstream" predictors will always impact "downstream" residual variances. So the two questions facing a researcher at this point involve (1) both the magnitude of the effect to be specified for the impact of treatment randomization on latent linear slope variance and the subsequent "downstream" effect on residual variances and (2) how the model-reproduced correlation matrix equation from Chapter 7 ($\mathbf{\Sigma\theta} = \mathbf{\Lambda\Phi\Lambda}^T + \mathbf{\Psi}$) needs to expand to accommodate the inclusion of time-invariant covariates into the longitudinal growth model.

As stated in previous chapters, a standardized slope estimate that explains (R^2 = 0.01) 1% of response variable variance is considered a "small" effect, and a standardized slope estimate that explains (R^2 = 0.09) 9% of response variable variance is considered a "medium" effect. Knowing that, all else being equal, binary predictor variables, such as treatment randomization, will typically explain less variance compared to continuous predictor variables, let's assume a researcher is willing to assert that treatment randomization will explain a conservative (R^2 = 0.05) 5% of response variable linear slope variance, which means a researcher is also willing to specify a standardized (β) estimate of ($\sqrt{0.05}$) β = 0.225, which results in the following analysis model (see Figure 8.4).

Notice how, in the updated analysis model in Figure 8.4, the residual variance estimates still show question marks. Readers that recall the path tracing rules from previous chapters might at this point, understandably, find the prospect of again using those rules and their subsequent computations an unappealing prospect. Plus, the question of how the model-reproduced correlation matrix formula from Chapter 7 should expand to accommodate time-invariant covariates has yet to be answered. Fortunately, a convenient answer to both scenarios can be found in the model-reproduced correlation equation for time-invariant covariate inclusion given by Grimm, Ram, and Estabrook (2017, p. 103; see also Biesanz et al., 2004, p. 32, Equation 3b) shown in Equation (8.1). (*Side Note: The equation below is correct. The equation in Grimm et al., 2017, p. 103, contains typographical errors by the authors' own admission . . .*).

$$\mathbf{\Sigma\theta} = [\mathbf{\Lambda\Phi\Lambda}^T + (\mathbf{\Lambda B\Phi\Lambda B}^T)\mathbf{\Lambda}^T] + \mathbf{\Theta} \tag{8.1}$$

where lambda ($\mathbf{\Lambda}$) is a matrix of latent variable loadings with the number of rows equal to the number of response variables and the number of columns equal to the number of latent variables, as shown in Equation (8.2).

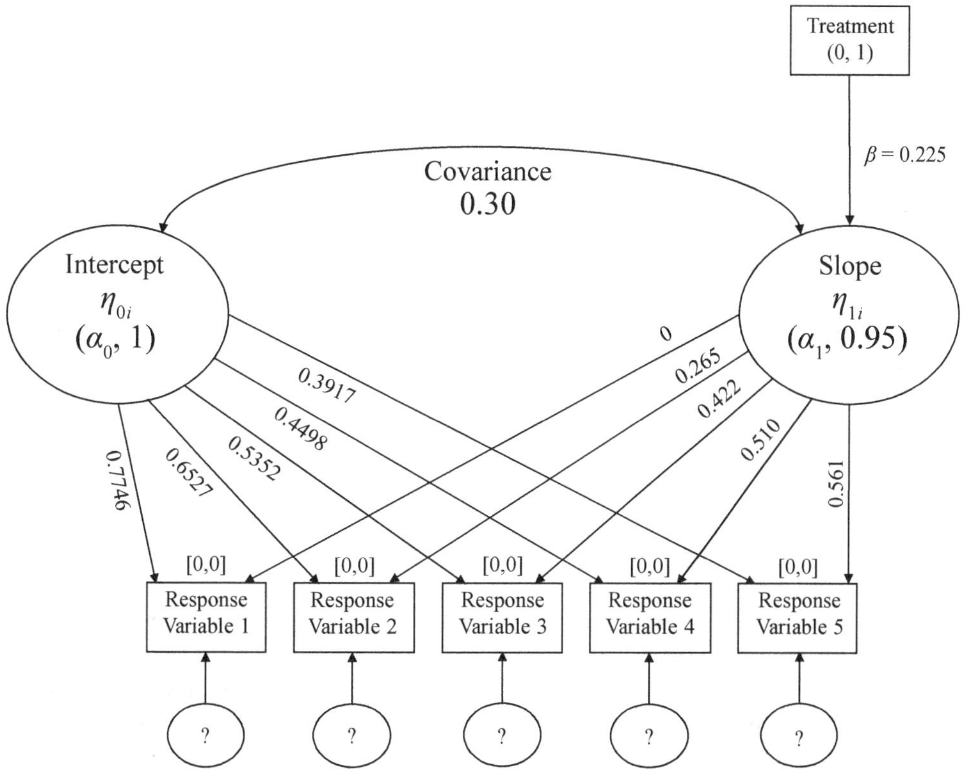

FIGURE 8.4. Partially specified main effect for treatment model.

$$\boldsymbol{\Lambda} = \begin{array}{cc|l} \text{Intercept} & \text{Slope} & \\ 0.7746 & 0 & \text{Response Variable 1} \\ 0.6527 & 0.265 & \text{Response Variable 2} \\ 0.5352 & 0.422 & \text{Response Variable 3} \\ 0.4497 & 0.510 & \text{Response Variable 4} \\ 0.3917 & 0.561 & \text{Response Variable 5} \end{array} \tag{8.2}$$

The psi ($\boldsymbol{\Psi}$) matrix is a latent variable variances (main diagonal) and covariances/correlations (off-diagonal) matrix where the number of rows and columns are equal to the number of latent variables, as shown in Equation (8.3)

$$\boldsymbol{\Psi} = \begin{array}{cc|l} \text{Intercept} & \text{Slope} & \\ 1 & 0.30 & \text{Intercept} \\ 0.30 & 0.95 & \text{Slope} \end{array} \tag{8.3}$$

Beta (**B**) is a matrix that contains regression coefficients that specify the relationships between time-invariant covariates and the latent growth variables. In the Beta matrix, the number of rows is equal to the number of latent variables and the number of columns is equal to the number of time-invariant covariates, as shown in Equation (8.4)

$$\mathbf{B} = \begin{array}{c} \text{Intercept} \\ \left| \begin{array}{c} 1 \\ 0.225 \end{array} \right| \end{array} \begin{array}{l} \\ \text{Intercept} \\ \text{Slope} \end{array} \tag{8.4}$$

The phi ($\mathbf{\Phi}$) matrix has both the number of rows and columns equal to the number of time-invariant covariates, and contains variances and correlations/covariances, as shown in Equation (8.5)

$$\mathbf{\Phi} = \begin{array}{c} \text{Treatment} \\ \left| \begin{array}{c} 1.00 \end{array} \right| \end{array} \tag{8.5}$$

As shown in Chapter 5, unit variance for a binary variable is consistent with the area under a unit normal distributional curve.

Notice in the model-reproduced correlation matrix equation from Grimm et al. (2017), we now have all the matrices enclosed in brackets []; all that remains are values for the theta ($\mathbf{\Theta}$) matrix, where the number of rows and columns are equal to the number of observed response variables, and contains residual variance values on the main diagonal. These are the values that remain unknown at this point. Notice how the model-reproduced correlation matrix ($\mathbf{\Sigma\theta}$) is the sum of the computations in brackets *plus* the theta matrix elements, the residual variances. This means that after solving the matrix computations enclosed in brackets using R, computing one minus each element on the main diagonal of the result should yield the residual variances needed for the theta matrix [shown in Equations (8.6) and (8.7)], as follows:

```
Lambda <- matrix(c(0.7746, 0, 0.6527, 0.265, 0.5352, 0.422, 0.4498, 0.51, 0.3917, 0.561),
     ncol = 2, byrow = TRUE)
Psi <- matrix(c(1, 0.30, 0.30, 0.95), nrow = 2, byrow = TRUE)
Beta <- matrix(c(0, 0.225), nrow = 2, byrow = TRUE)
Phi <- matrix(c(1), nrow = 1, byrow = TRUE)
corr_matrix <- (Lambda %*% Psi %*% t(Lambda)) + (Lambda %*% Beta %*% Phi %*%
     t(Beta) %*% t(Lambda))
corr_matrix
```

		Response Variable 1	Response Variable 2	Response Variable 3	Response Variable 4	Response Variable 5
	Response Variable 1	**0.6000**	0.5672	0.5126	0.4669	0.4338
$\mathbf{\Sigma\theta} =$	Response Variable 2	0.5672	**0.6001**	0.5684	0.5644	0.5454
	Response Variable 3	0.5126	0.5864	**0.6001**	0.5949	0.5862
	Response Variable 4	0.4669	0.5644	0.5949	**0.6002**	0.5981
	Response Variable 5	0.4338	0.5454	0.5862	0.5941	**0.6002**

(8.6)

So,

$$\theta_{\text{ResponseVariable1}} = 1 - 0.6000 = \mathbf{0.4000}$$
$$\theta_{\text{ResponseVariable2}} = 1 - 0.6001 = \mathbf{0.3999}$$

$$\theta_{\text{ResponseVariable3}} = 1 - 0.6001 = \mathbf{0.3999}$$
$$\theta_{\text{ResponseVariable4}} = 1 - 0.6002 = \mathbf{0.3998}$$
$$\theta_{\text{ResponseVariable5}} = 1 - 0.6002 = 0.3998$$

or

	Response Variable 1	Response Variable 2	Response Variable 3	Response Variable 4	Response Variable 5	
	0.4000	0	0	0	0	Response Variable 1
$\boldsymbol{\theta}$ =	0	**0.3999**	0	0	0	Response Variable 2
	0	0	**0.3999**	0	0	Response Variable 3
	0	0	0	**0.3998**	0	Response Variable 4
	0	0	0	0	**0.3998**	Response Variable 5 (8.7)

These computations can easily be checked in R by solving the complete equation given in Grimm et al. (2017) and the results shown in Equation (8.8):

```
Lambda <- matrix(c(0.7746, 0, 0.6527, 0.265, 0.5352, 0.422, 0.4498, 0.51, 0.3917, 0.561),
     ncol = 2, byrow = TRUE)
Phi <- matrix(c(1), nrow = 1, byrow = TRUE)
Beta <- matrix(c(0, 0.225), nrow = 2, byrow = TRUE)
Psi <- matrix(c(1, 0.30, 0.30, 0.95), nrow = 2, byrow = TRUE)
Theta<- matrix(c(0.4000, 0, 0, 0, 0,
     0, 0.3999, 0, 0, 0,
     0, 0, 0.3999, 0, 0,
     0, 0, 0, 0.3998, 0,
     0, 0, 0, 0, 0.3998), nrow = 5, byrow = TRUE)
corr_matrix <- (Lambda %*% Psi %*% t(Lambda)) + (Lambda %*% Beta %*% Phi %*%
     t(Beta) %*% t(Lambda)) + Theta
corr_matrix
```

		Response Variable 1	Response Variable 2	Response Variable 3	Response Variable 4	Response Variable 5	
	Response Variable 1	1	0.5672	0.5126	0.4669	0.4338	
$\boldsymbol{\Sigma\theta}$ =	Response Variable 2	0.5672	1	0.5864	0.5644	0.5454	
	Response Variable 3	0.5126	0.5864	1	0.5949	0.5862	
	Response Variable 4	0.4669	0.5644	0.5949	1	0.5981	
	Rcsponsc Variable 5	0.4338	0.5454	0.5862	0.5981	1	(8.8)

The resulting model-reproduced correlation matrix shows not only that the calculations for the observed response variable residual variances were correct, but also that the specified longitudinal growth curve model with a binary treatment randomization variable included as a time-invariant covariate is an admissible model. This result can be further verified by using the model-reproduced correlation matrix equation from Bollen and Curran (2006) shown in Chapter 7 [Equation (7.5) shown again here].

$$\boldsymbol{\Sigma\theta} = \mathbf{P}(\mathbf{I} - \mathbf{B})^{-1}\boldsymbol{\Psi}(\mathbf{I} - \mathbf{B})^{-1\mathrm{T}}\mathbf{P}^{\mathrm{T}}$$

Recall that, in the Bollen and Curran equation, the psi ($\boldsymbol{\Psi}$) matrix has a number of rows and columns equal to the total number of response (response variable is abbreviated RV below), predictor, and latent variables (in that order), and the matrix cells contain variances (main diagonal elements) and covariances/correlations among those variables (off-diagonal elements), as shown in Equation (8.9).

$\boldsymbol{\Psi}$ =

	RV1	RV2	RV3	RV4	RV5	Treatment	Intercept	Slope
RV1	0.4000	0	0	0	0	0	0	0
RV2	0	0.3999	0	0	0	0	0	0
RV3	0	0	0.3999	0	0	0	0	0
RV4	0	0	0	0.3998	0	0	0	0
RV5	0	0	0	0	0.3998	0	0	0
Treatment	0	0	0	0	0	1	0	0
Intercept	0	0	0	0	0	0	1	0.30
Slope	0	0	0	0	0	0	0.30	0.95

(8.9)

In the beta (**B**) matrix, the number of rows and columns are also equal to the total number of response, predictor, and latent variables (in that order), and the matrix cells contain regression/prediction coefficients (intercept and slope loadings, and treatment predicting slope variance), as shown in Equation (8.10).

B =

RV1	RV2	RV3	RV4	RV5	Treatment	Intercept	Slope	
0	0	0	0	0	0	0.7746	0	RV1
0	0	0	0	0	0	0.6527	0.265	RV2
0	0	0	0	0	0	0.5352	0.422	RV3
0	0	0	0	0	0	0.4498	0.51	RV4
0	0	0	0	0	0	0.3917	0.561	RV5
0	0	0	0	0	0	0	0	Treatment
0	0	0	0	0	0	0	0	Intercept
0	0	0	0	0	0.225	0	0	Slope

(8.10)

In the identity (**I**) matrix, the number of rows and columns are equal to the total number of response, predictor, and latent variables, and the matrix has values of 1 on the main diagonal, as shown in Equation (8.11).

I =

RV1	RV2	RV3	RV4	RV5	Treatment	Intercept	Slope	
1	0	0	0	0	0	0	0	RV1
0	1	0	0	0	0	0	0	RV2
0	0	1	0	0	0	0	0	RV3
0	0	0	1	0	0	0	0	RV4
0	0	0	0	1	0	0	0	RV5
0	0	0	0	0	1	0	0	Treatment
0	0	0	0	0	0	1	0	Intercept
0	0	0	0	0	0	0	1	Slope

(8.11)

Finally, recall that the (**P**) matrix can be described as a "pick" matrix where the number of columns are equal to the total number of response, predictor, and latent variables, but with a number of the rows equal to the total number of observed response and predictor variables and values of 1 on the main diagonal, as shown in Equation (8.12).

$$\mathbf{P} = \begin{array}{cccccccc|l} RV1 & RV2 & RV3 & RV4 & RV5 & Treatment & Intercept & Slope & \\ 1 & 0 & 0 & 0 & 0 & 0 & 0 & 0 & RV1 \\ 0 & 1 & 0 & 0 & 0 & 0 & 0 & 0 & RV2 \\ 0 & 0 & 1 & 0 & 0 & 0 & 0 & 0 & RV3 \\ 0 & 0 & 0 & 1 & 0 & 0 & 0 & 0 & RV4 \\ 0 & 0 & 0 & 0 & 1 & 0 & 0 & 0 & RV5 \\ 0 & 0 & 0 & 0 & 0 & 1 & 0 & 0 & Treatment \end{array} \quad (8.12)$$

Since the (**P**) matrix has an unequal number of rows and columns, the final two columns contain values of zero only. This effectively "picks" only the observed variables and drops the latent variables, resulting in a model-reproduced correlation matrix for only the observed variables, which can be shown using R syntax and results in Equation (8.13).

```
Psi <- matrix(c(
0.4000,  0,       0,       0,       0,       0,    0,     0,
0,       0.3999,  0,       0,       0,       0,    0,     0,
0,       0,       0.3999,  0,       0,       0,    0,     0,
0,       0,       0,       0.3998,  0,       0,    0,     0,
0,       0,       0,       0,       0.3998,  0,    0,     0,
0,       0,       0,       0,       0,       1,    0,     0,
0,       0,       0,       0,       0,       0,    1,     0.30,
0,       0,       0,       0,       0,       0,    0.30,  0.95
), ncol = 8, byrow = TRUE)

Beta <- matrix(c(
0,  0,  0,  0,  0,  0,      0.7746,  0,
0,  0,  0,  0,  0,  0,      0.6527,  0.265,
0,  0,  0,  0,  0,  0,      0.5352,  0.422,
0,  0,  0,  0,  0,  0,      0.4498,  0.51,
0,  0,  0,  0,  0,  0,      0.3917,  0.561,
0,  0,  0,  0,  0,  0,      0,       0,
0,  0,  0,  0,  0,  0,      0,       0,
0,  0,  0,  0,  0,  0.225,  0,       0
), ncol = 8, byrow = TRUE)

I <- matrix(c(
1,  0,  0,  0,  0,  0,  0,  0,
0,  1,  0,  0,  0,  0,  0,  0,
0,  0,  1,  0,  0,  0,  0,  0,
0,  0,  0,  1,  0,  0,  0,  0,
0,  0,  0,  0,  1,  0,  0,  0,
0,  0,  0,  0,  0,  1,  0,  0,
0,  0,  0,  0,  0,  0,  1,  0,
0,  0,  0,  0,  0,  0,  0,  1
), ncol = 8, byrow = TRUE)
```

```
P <- matrix(c(
1,   0,   0,   0,   0,   0,   0,   0,
0,   1,   0,   0,   0,   0,   0,   0,
0,   0,   1,   0,   0,   0,   0,   0,
0,   0,   0,   1,   0,   0,   0,   0,
0,   0,   0,   0,   1,   0,   0,   0,
0,   0,   0,   0,   0,   1,   0,   0
), ncol = 8, byrow = TRUE)
corr_matrix <- P %*% (solve(I-Beta)) %*% Psi %*%t(solve(I-Beta)) %*%t (P)
corr_matrix
```

$\Sigma\theta =$

	RV1	RV2	RV3	RV4	RV5	Treatment
RV1	1	0.5672	0.5126	0.4669	0.4338	0.0000
RV2	0.5672	1	0.5864	0.5644	0.5454	0.0596
RV3	0.5126	0.5864	1	0.5949	0.5862	0.0950
RV4	0.4669	0.5644	0.5949	1	0.5981	0.1148
RV5	0.4338	0.5454	0.5862	0.5981	1	0.126225
Treatment	0	0.059625	0.09495	0.11475	0.126225	1

(8.13)

Verification of the admissibility of the conditional longitudinal growth curve model using equations from both Grimm et al. (2017) and Bollen and Curran (2006) might seem to some as an exercise in redundancy. But again, the advantage of having a working knowledge of both matrix equations will be shown in the next chapter.

Mplus Monte Carlo Power Analysis: Longitudinal Treatment Effect

For now, the final step involves converting the matrix values above into Mplus syntax for a Monte Carlo simulation power analysis computation.

```
TITLE: MPLUS 8.3 Longitudinal Treatment Effect

MONTECARLO:
NAMES ARE
RV_1-RV_5 TREAT;
NOBSERVATIONS = 653;
NREPS = 5000;
MISSING = RV_2 RV_3 RV_4 RV_5;
CUTPOINTS = TREAT(0);
```

The 'NAMES ARE RV_1-RV_5 TREAT;' specification is Mplus syntax "shorthand" for specifying sequential response variables. The 'NOBSERVATIONS = 653;' allows testing of sample size $N = 653$ (treatment: $n = 327$; control: $n = 326$) for adequate statistical power. The 'MISSING' command indicates missing data will be specified for all postbaseline assessments. Recall from Chapter 5 that 'CUTPOINTS' allows the specification of a binary treatment randomization (TREAT) predictor variable. The value in parentheses after the variable(s) specified by the 'CUTPOINTS' option determines the proportion of zero and one values to be allocated to the 'TREAT' variable. Specifically, the value in parentheses is taken from the unit normal, or *z*-score, distribution that has a mean of zero and a standard deviation of one. Placing a value of zero in parentheses specifies that 50% of the values for 'TREAT' should be zeros and 50% should be values of one consistent with random assignment.

```
MODEL POPULATION:
I BY RV_1@.7746 RV_2@.6527 RV_3@.5352 RV_4@.4498 RV_5@.3917;
S BY RV_1@0 RV_2@.265 RV_3@.422 RV_4@.51 RV_5@.561;
[RV_1-RV_5@0];
```

The first two lines of syntax following the 'MODEL POPULATION:' command use the information in the lambda (**Λ**, if Grimm et al.'s [2017 equation is used, or **B** if Bollen & Curran's [2006] equation is used) matrix to specify latent intercept and latent slope loadings. The 'BY' specification is needed because standardized loadings, not traditional integer value loadings, are being used. Also, because the 'BY' specification is being used for a longitudinal growth curve model, the response variable intercepts that would typically be fixed at zero by default must be fixed at zero manually.

```
I*1;
S*0.95;
I WITH S*.30;
```

The next three lines of syntax use the information in the psi (**Ψ**) matrix to specify variances and the correlation between the latent intercept and the latent linear slope.

```
RV_1*.4;
RV_2*.3999;
RV_3*.3999;
RV_4*.3998;
RV_5*.3998;
```

The next four lines of syntax use the information from the theta (**Θ**, or psi [**Ψ**] if Bollen & Curran's [2006] equation is used) matrix to specify response variable residual variance values.

```
TREAT*1;
S ON TREAT*0.225;
```

The final two lines of code use information from the phi (**Φ**) matrix (or psi [**Ψ**] if Bollen and Curran's [2006] equation is used) and the beta (**B**) matrix to specify predictor variable variance and slope variance prediction, respectively.

```
MODEL MISSING:
[RV_2*-2.9444]; !5% MCAR;
[RV_3*-2.1972]; !10% MCAR;
[RV_4*-1.7346]; !15% MCAR;
[RV_5*-1.3862]; !20% MCAR;
```

The first four lines of syntax following the '`MODEL MISSING:`' command specify MCAR missing data using logit intercepts that indicate monotonic missing data from (exp (–2.9444) / 1 + exp (–2.9444) = 0.05) 5% missing at the first postbaseline assessment to (exp (–1.3862) / 1 + exp (–1.3862) = 0.20) 20% missing at the final time point.

```
RV_2 ON RV_1*0.0953;
RV_3 ON RV_2*0.0953 RV_1*0.0953;
RV_4 ON RV_3*0.0953 RV_2*0.0953 RV_1*0.0953;
RV_5 ON RV_4*0.0953 RV_3*0.0953 RV_2*0.0953 RV_1*0.0953;
```

The first four lines of syntax following the '`MODEL MISSING:`' command specify MAR missing data using logit slopes that indicate the odds of missing data increases ($exp^{0.0953}$ = 1.10) 10% per unit increase in response variable scores at any previous time point.

```
MODEL:
I BY RV_1@.7746 RV_2@.6527 RV_3@.5352 RV_4@.4498 RV_5@.3917;
S BY RV_1@0 RV_2@.265 RV_3@.422 RV_4@.51 RV_5@.561;

[RV_1-RV_5@0];

S ON TREAT*0.225;
```

Finally, the syntax following the '`MODEL:`' command that dictates how the generated data are to be analyzed need only contain the syntax needed to properly specify a growth model using the '`BY`' keyword as well as a line specifying the binary treatment randomization variable as a predictor of linear slope variance. The combined Mplus Monte Carlo simulation power analysis syntax is presented below followed by annotated output results from (Mplus 8.3).

```
TITLE: MPLUS 8.3 Longitudinal Treatment Effect

MONTECARLO:
NAMES ARE RV_1-RV_5 TREAT;
NOBSERVATIONS = 653;
NREPS = 5000;
MISSING = RV_2 RV_3 RV_4 RV_5;
CUTPOINTS = TREAT(0);

MODEL POPULATION:
I BY RV_1@.7746 RV_2@.6527 RV_3@.5352 RV_4@.4498 RV_5@.3917;
S BY RV_1@0 RV_2@.265 RV_3@.422 RV_4@.51 RV_5@.561;
[RV_1-RV_5@0];

I*1;
S*0.95;
I WITH S*.30;

RV_1*.4;
RV_2*.3999;
```

```
RV_3*.3999;
RV_4*.3998;
RV_5*.3998;

TREAT*1;
S ON TREAT*0.225;

MODEL MISSING:
[RV_2*-2.9444]; !5% MCAR;
[RV_3*-2.1972]; !10% MCAR;
[RV_4*-1.7346]; !15% MCAR;
[RV_5*-1.3862]; !20% MCAR;

RV_2 ON RV_1*0.0953;
RV_3 ON RV_2*0.0953 RV_1*0.0953;
RV_4 ON RV_3*0.0953 RV_2*0.0953 RV_1*0.0953;
RV_5 ON RV_4*0.0953 RV_3*0.0953 RV_2*0.0953 RV_1*0.0953;

MODEL:

I BY RV_1@.7746 RV_2@.6527 RV_3@.5352 RV_4@.4498 RV_5@.3917;
S BY RV_1@0 RV_2@.265 RV_3@.422 RV_4@.51 RV_5@.561;

[RV_1-RV_5@0];

S ON TREAT*0.225;
```

	Population	ESTIMATES Average	Std. Dev.	S. E. Average	M. S. E.	95% Cover	% Sig Coeff
S ON							
TREAT	**0.225**	0.2242	0.0804	0.0801	0.0065	0.947	**0.800**

R Monte Carlo Power Analysis: Longitudinal Treatment Effect

Unlike the straightforward extension in Mplus, inclusion of a binary covariate treatment variable was not possible in the lavaan syntax presented earlier in this chapter. Instead, we reconfigured the model using matrix notation to include a binary predictor variable. To create a matrix notation model, different aspects of each matrix should be identified: (1) whether the parameter is fixed to a specific value or freely estimated, (2) whether to impose misspecification on the value of the population parameter, and (3) whether the matrix is symmetric. Below, LYfix is used to determine which factor loading values will be fixed to a specific value; since there are specific values for each component, all factor loadings will be fixed to that value. LYpop is created to identify the population factor loadings. No misspecification matrix is created because power analyses typically do not involve model misspecification, and since the matrix is not symmetric, no symmetric component of the matrix is necessary. All components of the factor loading matrix are bound, using the 'bind' function, into a single object. Similar to the factor loading matrix, a matrix of intercepts (TY), covariances (PS), and error variances (RTE) are used to create the model.

```
LYfix <- matrix(0, nrow = 5, ncol = 2)
LYfix[1:5,1] <- c(0.7746, 0.6527, 0.5352, 0.4498, 0.3917)
LYfix[1:5,2] <- c(0, 0.265, 0.422, 0.51, 0.561)
LYpop <- matrix(0, nrow = 5, ncol = 2)
LYpop[1:5,1] <- c(0.7746, 0.6527, 0.5352, 0.4498, 0.3917)
LYpop[1:5,2] <- c(0, 0.265, 0.422, 0.51, 0.561)
LY <- bind(LYfix, LYpop)
summary(LY)
```

```
TYfix <- matrix(0, nrow = 5, ncol = 1) #for all intercepts constrained to 0
TYpop <- matrix(0, nrow = 5, ncol = 1) #intercepts set to 0
TY <- bind(TYfix, TYpop)

PSfix <- matrix(NA, nrow = 2, ncol = 2) #the covariances are all freely estimated, not
      constrained
PSpop <- matrix(.3, nrow = 2, ncol = 2)
diag(PSpop) <- c(1, .95)
PS <- binds(PSfix, PSpop) #note, binds is used when the matrix is symmetric; otherwise, bind
      is used
summary(PS)
```

```
RTEfix <- matrix(0, nrow=5, ncol = 5)
diag(RTEfix) <- NA #only the diagonals of the error variance matrix will be freely estimated; all
      other values will be constrained to 0
RTEpop <- matrix(0, nrow=5, ncol = 5)
diag(RTEpop) <- c(.4, .3999, .3999, .3998, .3998)
RTE <- binds(RTEfix, RTEpop)
```

To include a binary covariate, two additional matrices are specified: the GA and KA matrices. The GA matrix reflects the relationship between the covariate and the latent variables while the KA matrix reflects the relationship between the covariate and the manifest variables. In this example, the effect of treatment only impacts the latent slope variable.

```
GAfix <- matrix(NA, 2, 1)
GAfix[1:2] <- c(0, NA) #the tx covar only affects the slope factor, so the other is constrained to
      0
GApop <- matrix(NA, 2, 1)
GApop[1:2] <- c(0, .225)
GA <- bind(GAfix, GApop)

KA <- bind(matrix(0, 5, 1)) # the regression of the covariate on each indicator is 0
```

Similar to Chapter 5, one more model component is necessary before running the power analysis: a dataframe that reflects the configuration of the binary covariate variable. In the present case, this is the number of individuals in the treatment and control conditions.

```
treat <- data.frame(treat = rep(c(0, 1), times=c(327, 326)))
```

Because the analysis includes missing data, a missing data model is also constructed.

```
MissingModel2_Ch8 <- "
 #MCAR intercepts, which is based on known probabilities of missingness
 #MAR slopes, which is based on computed logit values from missingness at prior time
     points
 RV_2 ~ -2.9444 + .0953*RV_1
 RV_3 ~ -2.1972 + .0953*RV_2 + .0953*RV_1
 RV_4 ~ -1.7346 + .0953*RV_3 + .0953*RV_2 + .0953*RV_1
 RV_5 ~ -1.3862 + .0953*RV_4 + .0953*RV_3 + .0953*RV_2 + .0953*RV_1
"
```

Now, the power analysis can be completed.

```
Output2_Ch8 <- sim(PopulationModel2_Ch8,
             nRep = 5000,
             n = count(treat),
             covData = treat,
             miss = MissingModel2_Ch8,
             seed = 1234,
             silent = T)
```

A summary of the results is obtained and shown in Table 8.5.

As shown in Table 8.5, the statistical power to detect the effect of treatment on the slope variable was greater than .80, which suggests that a combined sample of 653, relatively equally split across treatment and control groups, is adequate to detect the expected change over time.

Longitudinal RCT Treatment Effect Model Simulation Power Analysis Write-Up

"The power analysis question involved the smallest sample size needed to achieve power ≥ .80 to detect a standardized treatment effect estimate in a longitudinal RCT. A Monte Carlo simulation power analysis was conducted using Mplus (version 8.6) assuming:

TABLE 8.5. Summary Estimates for Longitudinal Treatment Effect Power Analysis

	Estimate average	Estimate SD	Average SE	Power (not equal 0)
int~~int	1.001	0.097	0.096	1.000
int~~slope	0.298	0.088	0.088	0.916
slope~~slope	0.946	0.133	0.136	1.000
RV_1~~RV_1	0.400	0.046	0.046	1.000
RV_2~~RV_2	0.403	0.030	0.030	1.000
RV_3~~RV_3	0.407	0.031	0.030	1.000
RV_4~~RV_4	0.410	0.032	0.033	1.000
RV_5~~RV_5	0.411	0.037	0.036	1.000
slope~treat	0.224	0.079	0.080	0.802

(1) standardization of all response variables at all five assessment time points, (2) linear trend best captured response variable average changes over time and explained 60% of observed adherence response variable variance, on average, (3) random assignment results in equal sample sizes for both the treatment and control groups, (4) the magnitude of the standardized (β) effect of binary treatment randomization on linear slope variance is expected to be at least $\beta \geq 0.225$ and explain at least ($R^2 = .05$) 5% of linear slope variance, and (5) missing data are assumed to be (a) 0% at the initial assessment, (b) 5% at the first postbaseline assessment, (c) monotonically increasing in 5% increments to 20% at the final assessment, and (d) missing at random, such that unit increases in response variable values at any previous assessment time point are assumed to result in a 10% increase in the odds of missing data. Monte Carlo simulation power analysis results aggregated over 5,000 dataset replications showed power $\geq .80$ to detect a standardized "slope on binary treatment randomization" effect of $\beta \geq 0.225$ if all assumptions are met and proper missing data handling makes a total sample size of $N = 653$ available for analysis."

OK, But . . .

Even within tightly controlled randomized trials, researchers often wish to add control covariates to a longitudinal growth curve analysis model to interpret any treatment effect after having controlled for the presence of one or more potential confounding variables. Examples of common control covariates measured on a continuous scale and included in data analysis models as possible confounds include participant age, family income, IQ, and decimal years since receiving a medical or psychological diagnosis—to name only a very few. The previous power analysis, which contained only a binary treatment randomization predictor, can be expanded to include a control covariate measured on a continuous scale (cont_cov), as shown in Figure 8.5.

As indicated by the question marks shown in Figure 8.5, several new questions need to be answered, including: (1) What standardized (β) effect for the continuous covariate as a predictor of slope variance should be assumed? (2) To what extent are the binary treatment randomization predictor variable and the continuous covariate correlated? and (3) How do the answers to both questions impact linear slope variance and response variable residual variances?

Answers to the first two questions can be approached from both empirical and practical perspectives. Empirically, there is little else more useful than a complete and thorough search through the published literature on the subject matter of interest. But if a research study is truly a novel one, very little in the way of answers to the first two questions is likely to be found. However, analogous studies with similar populations and response variables can likely be found, and based on those studies, reasonable estimate bounds can be placed on the needed estimates. From a practical perspective, researchers often have accurate estimates of the number of participants they would be able to recruit, incentivize, and retain for a given research study. Assuming such a fixed a priori sample size, a researcher could then conduct multiple Monte Carlo simulation power analyses to determine the minimum

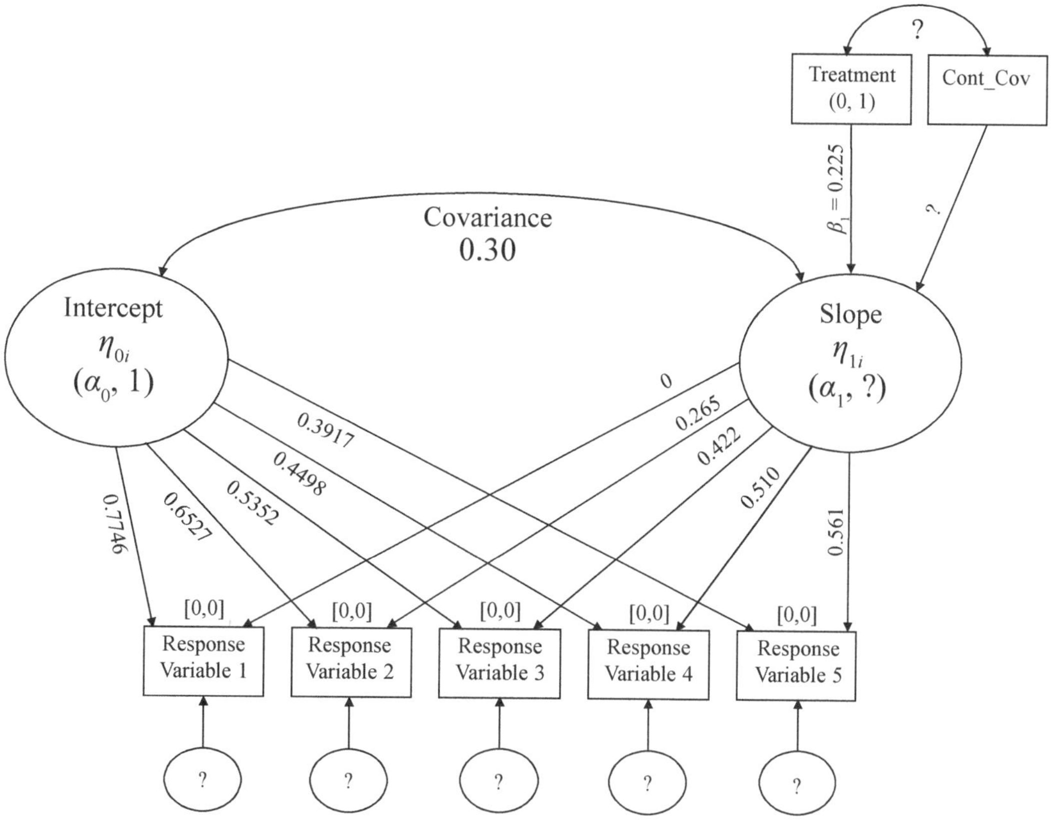

FIGURE 8.5. Longitudinal treatment with covariate model.

standardized effect detectable with power ≥ .80 to accomplish the goal of interest. For illustration purposes, let's assume, based on a literature search, multiple practical Monte Carlo simulations, or both, were found so that a researcher is willing to assume a standardized coefficient of $\beta = 0.25$ for the effect of the covariate as a predictor of linear slope variance, and is willing to specify a (point biserial) correlation of $r = .20$ between the binary treatment and continuous covariate variables, as shown in Figure 8.6.

Now that the first two questions above have been addressed, the first part of the third question can be answered using techniques discussed previously. Specifically, the path tracing rules shown previously can fill in the question mark in Figure 8.6 (α_1, ?), which refers to linear slope variance, now that a continuous covariate has been added to the model as follows. Recall that the residual linear slope variance ($\sigma^2_{\text{RESIDUAL}}$), or the variance that remains unexplained by either treatment randomization or the control covariate, is computed *assuming standardization* by ($\sigma^2_{\text{RESIDUAL}} = 1 - R^2_{\text{PREDICTORS}}$), or one minus the linear slope variance that is predicted by treatment randomization and the control covariate, or $R^2_{\text{PREDICTORS}} = R^2_{\text{SLOPE|TREATMENT}} + R^2_{\text{SLOPE|COVARIATE}}$, as shown previously. So,

$$R^2_{\text{SLOPE|TREATMENT}} = \text{Direct effect} * (\text{Direct effect} + [\text{Indirect effect product}])$$
$$R^2_{\text{SLOPE|TREATMENT}} = \beta_1 * (\beta_1 + [\text{Indirect effect product}])$$
$$R^2_{\text{SLOPE|TREATMENT}} = 0.225 * (0.225 + [\beta_2 * r])$$
$$R^2_{\text{SLOPE|TREATMENT}} = 0.225 * (0.225 + [0.25 * 0.20])$$
$$R^2_{\text{SLOPE|TREATMENT}} = \mathbf{0.061875}$$

and

$$R^2_{\text{SLOPE|COVARIATE}} = \text{Direct effect} * (\text{Direct effect} + [\text{Indirect effect product}])$$
$$R^2_{\text{SLOPE|COVARIATE}} = \beta_1 * (\beta_1 + [\text{Indirect effect product}])$$
$$R^2_{\text{SLOPE|COVARIATE}} = 0.25 * (0.25 + [\beta_1 * r])$$
$$R^2_{\text{SLOPE|COVARIATE}} = 0.25 * (0.25 + [0.225 * 0.20])$$
$$R^2_{\text{SLOPE|COVARIATE}} = \mathbf{0.07375}$$

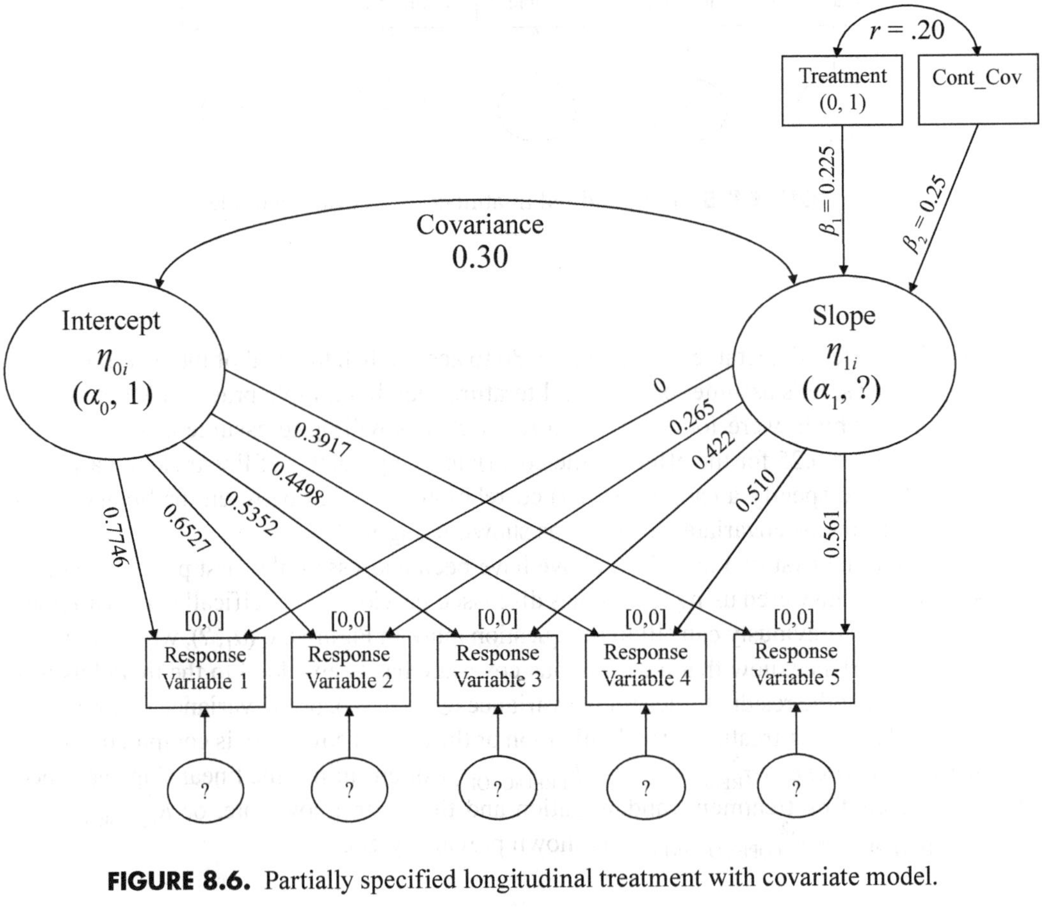

FIGURE 8.6. Partially specified longitudinal treatment with covariate model.

so

$$R^2_{\text{PREDICTORS}} = R^2_{\text{SLOPE|TREATMENT}} + R^2_{\text{SLOPE|COVARIATE}}$$

$$R^2_{\text{PREDICTORS}} = \mathbf{0.061875 + 0.07375}$$

$$R^2_{\text{PREDICTORS}} = \mathbf{0.135625}$$

And (as seen in Figure 8.7), we get

$$\sigma^2_{\text{RESIDUAL}} = 1 - R^2_{\text{PREDICTORS}}$$

$$\sigma^2_{\text{RESIDUAL}} = 1 - \mathbf{0.135625}$$

$$\sigma^2_{\text{RESIDUAL}} = \mathbf{0.864375}$$

All that now remains is an answer to the second half of the third question: specification of observed variable residual variance values. These can be computed by solving the portion of Grimm et al.'s model-reproduced equation contained in brackets

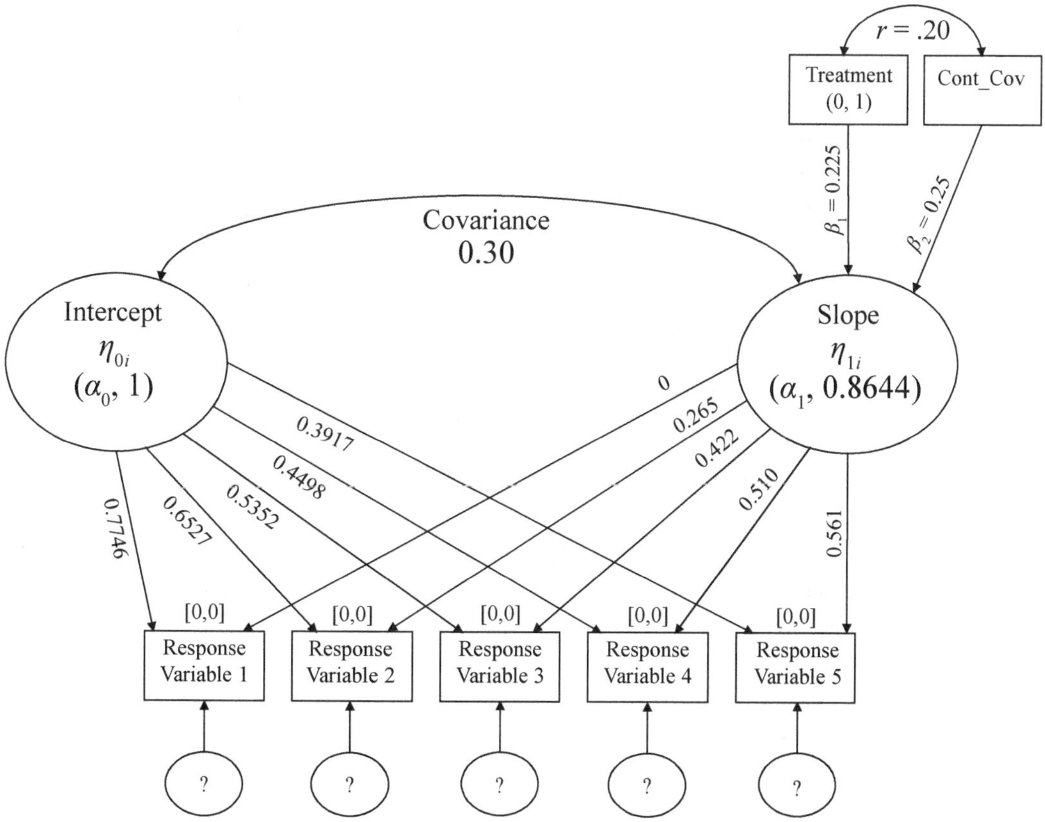

FIGURE 8.7. Slope variance specified for a longitudinal treatment with covariate model.

$$\Sigma\theta = [\Lambda\Psi\Lambda^T + (\Lambda B \Phi \Lambda B^T)\Lambda^T] + \Theta \tag{8.14}$$

and subtracting one minus the results on the main diagonal to obtain the needed theta (**Θ**) matrix values, as shown in Equation (8.15) below.

Λ =

	Intercept	Slope	
	0.7746	0	Response Variable 1
	0.6527	0.265	Response Variable 2
	0.5352	0.422	Response Variable 3
	0.4498	0.51	Response Variable 4
	0.3917	0.561	Response Variable 5

(8.15)

The lambda (**Λ**) matrix does not change from the previous power analysis, as shown in Equation (8.9).

Ψ =

	RV1	RV2	RV3	RV4	RV5	Treatment	Intercept	Slope
RV1	0.4000	0	0	0	0	0	0	0
RV2	0	0.3999	0	0	0	0	0	0
RV3	0	0	0.3999	0	0	0	0	0
RV4	0	0	0	0.3998	0	0	0	0
RV5	0	0	0	0	0.3998	0	0	0
Treatment	0	0	0	0	0	1	0	0
Intercept	0	0	0	0	0	0	1	0.30
Slope	0	0	0	0	0	0	0.30	0.95

The psi (**Ψ**) matrix changes only to reflect the additional slope variance explained by the addition of a control covariate, as shown in Equation (8.16).

B =

Treatment	Covariate	
0	0	Intercept
0.225	0.25	Slope

(8.16)

The beta (**B**) matrix expands to include both treatment and the covariate as predictors of linear slope variance with their respective standardized prediction coefficients included, as shown in Equation (8.17).

Φ =

Treatment	Covariate	
1	0.20	Treatment
0.20	1	Covariate

(8.17)

Assuming standardization, the phi (**Φ**) matrix also expands to show that both the covariate is assumed to have unit variance and the correlation between treatment and covariate is assumed to be $r = .20$. The portion of Grimm et al.'s equation enclosed in brackets can now be solved using R syntax as follows:

```
Lambda <- matrix(c(
0.7746, 0,
0.6527, 0.265,
0.5352, 0.422,
0.4498, 0.51,
0.3917, 0.561), ncol = 2, byrow = TRUE)

Phi <- matrix(c(
1, 0.20,
0.20, 1), nrow = 2, byrow = TRUE)

Beta <- matrix(c(
0, 0,
0.225, 0.25), nrow = 2, byrow = TRUE)

Psi <- matrix(c(
1, 0.30,
0.30, 0.8644 ), nrow = 2, byrow = TRUE)

corr_matrix <- (Lambda %*% Psi %*% t(Lambda)) + (Lambda %*% Beta %*% Phi %*%
    t(Beta) %*% t(Lambda))
corr_matrix
```

	Response Variable 1	Response Variable 2	Response Variable 3	Response Variable 4	Response Variable 5
Response Variable 1	**0.6000**	0.5672	0.5126	0.4669	0.4338
Response Variable 2	0.5672	**0.6000**	0.5684	0.5644	0.5453
Response Variable 3	0.5126	0.5863	**0.6000**	0.5948	0.5860
Response Variable 4	0.4669	0.5644	0.5948	**0.6001**	0.5979
Response Variable 5	0.4338	0.5453	0.5860	0.5979	**0.6000**

So as shown in Equations (8.18) and (8.19),

$$\theta_{\text{ResponseVariable1}} = 1 - 0.6000 = \mathbf{0.4000}$$
$$\theta_{\text{ResponseVariable2}} = 1 - 0.6000 = \mathbf{0.4000}$$
$$\theta_{\text{ResponseVariable3}} = 1 - 0.6000 = \mathbf{0.4000}$$
$$\theta_{\text{ResponseVariable4}} = 1 - 0.6001 = \mathbf{0.3999}$$
$$\theta_{\text{ResponseVariables5}} = 1 - 0.6000 = \mathbf{0.4000}$$

or

	Response Variable 1	Response Variable 2	Response Variable 3	Response Variable 4	Response Variable 5	
	0.4000	0	0	0	0	Response Variable 1
θ =	0	**0.4000**	0	0	0	Response Variable 2
	0	0	**0.4000**	0	0	Response Variable 3
	0	0	0	**0.3999**	0	Response Variable 4
	0	0	0	0	**0.4000**	Response Variable 5

(8.18)

Then,

```
Lambda <- matrix(c(
0.7746, 0,
0.6527, 0.265,
0.5352, 0.422,
0.4498, 0.51,
0.3917, 0.561), ncol = 2, byrow = TRUE)

Phi <- matrix(c(
1, 0.20,
0.20, 1), nrow = 2, byrow = TRUE)

Beta <- matrix(c(
0, 0,
0.225, 0.25), nrow = 2, byrow = TRUE)

Psi <- matrix(c(
1, 0.30,
0.30, 0.8644 ), nrow = 2, byrow = TRUE)

Theta<-matrix(c(

0.4000, 0, 0, 0, 0,
0, 0.4000, 0, 0, 0,
0, 0, 0.4000, 0, 0,
0, 0, 0, 0.3999, 0,
0, 0, 0, 0, 0.4000), nrow = 5, byrow = TRUE)

corr_matrix <- (Lambda %*% Psi %*% t(Lambda)) + (Lambda %*% Beta %*% Phi %*%
      t(Beta) %*% t(Lambda)) + Theta

corr_matrix
```

		Response Variable 1	Response Variable 2	Response Variable 3	Response Variable 4	Response Variable 5
	Response Variable 1	1	0.5672	0.5126	0.4669	0.4338
$\Sigma\theta =$	Response Variable 2	0.5672	1	0.5863	0.5644	0.5453
	Response Variable 3	0.5126	0.5863	1	0.5948	0.5860
	Response Variable 4	0.4669	0.5644	0.5948	1	0.5979
	Response Variable 5	0.4338	0.5453	0.5860	0.5979	1

(8.19)

Mplus Monte Carlo Power Analysis: Longitudinal RCT Covariate

Finally, the Mplus syntax from the previous Monte Carlo simulation needs only minor edits to include the control covariate and the updated matrices values. Annotated power analysis results are shown following the Mplus (8.4) syntax.

```
TITLE: MPLUS 8.4 Longitudinal RCT Covariate
```

```
MONTECARLO:
NAMES ARE
RV_1-RV_5 TREAT CONT_COV;NOBSERVATIONS = 656;
NREPS = 5000;
MISSING = RV_2 RV_3 RV_4 RV_5;
CUTPOINTS = TREAT(0);

MODEL POPULATION:
!Lambda Matrix;
I BY RV_1@.7746 RV_2@.6527 RV_3@.5352 RV_4@.4498 RV_5@.3917;
S BY RV_1@0 RV_2@.265 RV_3@.422 RV_4@.51 RV_5@.561;
[RV_1-RV_5@0];

!Psi Matrix;
I*1;
S*0.8644;
I WITH S*.30;

!Theta Matrix;
RV_1*.4;
RV_2*.4;
RV_3*.4;
RV_4*.3999;
RV_5*.4;

!Phi Matrix;
TREAT*1;
CONT_COV*1;
TREAT WITH CONT_COV*0.20;

!Beta Matrix;
S ON TREAT*0.225 CONT_COV*0.25;
```

Missing data specifications remain the same as in the previous power analysis.

```
MODEL MISSING:
[RV_2*-2.9444]; !5% MCAR;
[RV_3*-2.1972]; !10% MCAR;
[RV_4*-1.7346]; !15% MCAR;
[RV_5*-1.3862]; !20% MCAR;

RV_2 ON RV_1*0.0953;
RV_3 ON RV_2*0.0953 RV_1*0.0953;
RV_4 ON RV_3*0.0953 RV_2*0.0953 RV_1*0.0953;
RV_5 ON RV_4*0.0953 RV_3*0.0953 RV_2*0.0953 RV_1*0.0953;
```

The `MODEL:` statement changes only to include the control covariate as a predictor of linear slope variance.

```
MODEL:
[RV_1-RV_5@0];
```

```
!Lambda Matrix;
I BY RV_1@.7746 RV_2@.6527 RV_3@.5352 RV_4@.4498 RV_5@.3917;
S BY RV_1@0 RV_2@.265 RV_3@.422 RV_4@.51 RV_5@.561;

!Beta Matrix;
S ON TREAT*0.225 CONT_COV*0.25;
```

```
                          ESTIMATES              S. E.     M. S. E.  95%   % Sig
              Population  Average   Std. Dev.   Average              Cover Coeff
S        ON
 TREAT          0.225     0.2219     0.0804     0.0793     0.0065 0.943 0.804
 CONT_COV       0.250     0.2493     0.0566     0.0561     0.0032 0.949 0.992
```

R Monte Carlo Power Analysis: Longitudinal RCT Covariate Issues

In this example, a problem emerged in the R simulation, as a result of the correlation between treatment and the continuous covariate. Although it is possible to simulate correlated predictor variables, it was not possible to set a population correlation value between the binary treatment and continuous covariate in the context of the more complex SEM model, and it was not possible to allow the binary treatment and continuous covariate covary in the sample models. The analysis and results differed from those found in Mplus, and are not included in the text of this chapter; instead, they are included in the online supplemental materials at *www.guilford.com/peugh-materials.*

Longitudinal RCT Covariate Model Simulation Power Analysis Write-Up

"The power analysis question involved the smallest sample size needed to achieve power ≥ .80 to detect a standardized treatment effect estimate, with a control covariate measured on a continuous scale included, in a longitudinal RCT. A Monte Carlo simulation power analysis was conducted using Mplus (version 8.6) assuming: (1) standardization of all response variables at all five assessment time points, (2) linear trend best-captured response variable average changes over time and explained 60% of observed adherence response variable variance, on average, (3) random assignment results in equal sample sizes for both the treatment and control groups, (4) the magnitude of the standardized (β) effect of binary treatment randomization on linear slope variance is expected to be at least $\beta \geq 0.225$ and explain at least ($R^2 = .05$) 5% of linear slope variance, (5) the inclusion of a control covariate measured on a continuous scale will explain an additional ($R^2 = .085$) 8.5% of linear slope variance, and (6) missing data are assumed to be (a) 0% at the initial assessment, (b) 5% at the first postbaseline assessment, (c) monotonically increasing in 5% increments to 20% at the final assessment, and (d) missing at random, such that unit increases in response variable values at any previous assessment time point are assumed to result in a 10% increase in the odds of missing data. Monte Carlo simulation power analysis results aggregated over 5,000 dataset replications showed power ≥ .80 to detect a standardized "slope on binary treatment randomization" effect of $\beta \geq 0.225$ if all assumptions are met and proper missing data handling makes a sample size of $N = 656$ ($n = 328$ for both treatment and control groups) available for analysis."

Just One More Thing . . .

Some researchers at this point might be wondering, "What if the research question depends on whether the treatment effect is *moderated* by a continuous variable that is of theoretical interest instead of just a covariate whose potential confounding influence needs to be controlled?" Such an analysis would require the inclusion of a "treatment * covariate" interaction term in the model, as shown in Figure 8.8.

Assume that the continuous covariate is grand mean centered (i.e., the sample mean of the covariate has been subtracted from all the continuous covariate values in the dataset). Mplus then generates standardized [*z*-score] data that are essentially grand mean centered by default. The correlation between the interaction term and the binary treatment variable will likely be very low ($r_2 = .05$), while the correlation between the interaction term and the continuous covariate variable will likely be very high ($r_3 = .50$). Furthermore, the standardized effect for the interaction term as a predictor of linear slope variance ($\beta_3 = 0.175$) specifies that the effect of treatment increases by 0.175 units, on average, for those treatment participants with continuous covariate scores one standard deviation above the mean. Again, this value could come from a thorough search of published literature, multiple power analysis runs to determine the minimal effect detect able with power $\geq .80$, or both. Additionally, the answer to the question of the amount of linear slope variance left unexplained ($\sigma^2_{\text{RESIDUAL}} = 1 - R^2_{\text{PREDICTORS}}$) by the treatment or covariate main effects, or by the "treatment * covariate" interaction term, can again be computed using path tracing.

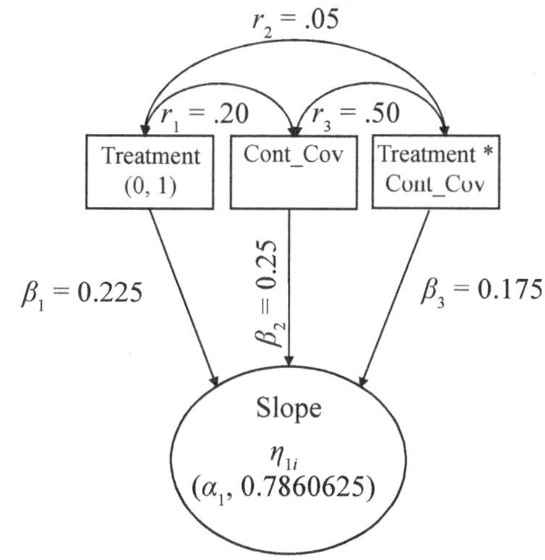

FIGURE 8.8. Moderated treatment effect longitudinal growth curve model.

$$R^2_{\text{PREDICTORS}} = R^2_{\text{SLOPE|TREATMENT}} + R^2_{\text{SLOPE|COVARIATE}} + R^2_{\text{SLOPE|INTERACTION}}$$

$$R^2_{\text{SLOPE|TREATMENT}} = \text{Direct effect} * (\text{Direct effect} + [\text{Sum of indirect effect products}])$$

$$R^2_{\text{SLOPE|TREATMENT}} = \beta_1 * (\beta_1 + [\text{Sum of indirect effect products}])$$

$$R^2_{\text{SLOPE|TREATMENT}} = 0.225 * (0.225 + [\beta_2 * r_1] + [\beta_2 * r_2])$$

$$R^2_{\text{SLOPE|TREATMENT}} = 0.225 * (0.225 + [0.25 * 0.20] + [0.175 * 0.05])$$

$$R^2_{\text{SLOPE|TREATMENT}} = 0.225 * (0.225 + [0.05] + [0.00875])$$

$$R^2_{\text{SLOPE|TREATMENT}} = 0.225 * (0.28375)$$

$$R^2_{\text{SLOPE|TREATMENT}} = \mathbf{0.06384375}$$

and

$$R^2_{\text{SLOPE|COVARIATE}} = \text{Direct effect} * (\text{Direct effect} + [\text{Sum of indirect effect products}])$$

$$R^2_{\text{SLOPE|COVARIATE}} = \beta_2 * (\beta_2 + [\text{Sum of indirect effect products}])$$

$$R^2_{\text{SLOPE|COVARIATE}} = 0.25 * (0.25 + [\beta_1 * r_1] + [\beta_3 * r_3])$$

$$R^2_{\text{SLOPE|COVARIATE}} = 0.25 * (0.25 + [0.225 * 0.20] + [0.175 * 0.50])$$

$$R^2_{\text{SLOPE|COVARIATE}} = 0.25 * (0.25 + [0.045] + [0.0875])$$

$$R^2_{\text{SLOPE|COVARIATE}} = 0.25 * (0.3825)$$

$$R^2_{\text{SLOPE|COVARIATE}} = \mathbf{0.095625}$$

and

$$R^2_{\text{SLOPE|INTERACTION}} = \text{Direct effect} * (\text{Direct effect} + [\text{Sum of indirect effect products}])$$

$$R^2_{\text{SLOPE|INTERACTION}} = \beta_3 * (\beta_3 + [\text{Sum of indirect effect products}])$$

$$R^2_{\text{SLOPE|INTERACTION}} = 0.175 * (0.175 + [\beta_1 * r_2] + [\beta_2 * r_3])$$

$$R^2_{\text{SLOPE|INTERACTION}} = 0.175 * (0.175 + [0.225 * 0.05] + [0.25 * 0.50])$$

$$R^2_{\text{SLOPE|INTERACTION}} = 0.175 * (0.175 + [0.01125] + [0.125])$$

$$R^2_{\text{SLOPE|INTERACTION}} = 0.175 * (0.31125)$$

$$R^2_{\text{SLOPE|INTERACTION}} = \mathbf{0.05446875}$$

So,

$$R^2_{\text{PREDICTORS}} = R^2_{\text{SLOPE|TREATMENT}} + R^2_{\text{SLOPE|COVARIATE}} + R^2_{\text{SLOPE|INTERACTION}}$$

$$R^2_{\text{PREDICTORS}} = \mathbf{0.06384375} + \mathbf{0.095625} + \mathbf{0.05446875}$$

$$R^2_{\text{PREDICTORS}} = \mathbf{0.2139375}$$

and

$$\sigma^2_{\text{RESIDUAL}} = 1 - R^2_{\text{PREDICTORS}}$$
$$\sigma^2_{\text{RESIDUAL}} = 1 - \mathbf{0.2139375} = \mathbf{0.7860625}$$

See Figure 8.9.

Again, the residual variance values can be computed by solving the portion of Grimm et al.'s model-reproduced equation contained in brackets in Equation (8.14) repeated here.

$$\boldsymbol{\Sigma\theta} = [\boldsymbol{\Lambda\Psi\Lambda}^T + (\boldsymbol{\Lambda B\Phi\Lambda B}^T)\boldsymbol{\Lambda}^T] + \boldsymbol{\Theta}$$

and subtracting one minus each of the main diagonal elements as follows as in Equation (8.15) repeated again here.

$\boldsymbol{\Lambda}$ =

	Intercept	Slope	
	0.7746	0	Response Variable 1
	0.6527	0.265	Response Variable 2
$\boldsymbol{\Lambda}$ =	0.5352	0.422	Response Variable 3
	0.4498	0.51	Response Variable 4
	0.3917	0.561	Response Variable 5

Again, the lambda ($\boldsymbol{\Lambda}$) matrix does not change from the previous power analysis.

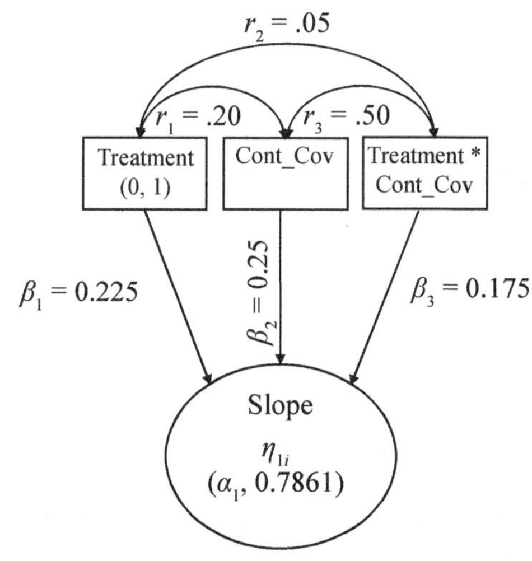

FIGURE 8.9. Specified moderated treatment effect longitudinal growth curve model.

$$\mathbf{\Psi} = \left|\begin{array}{cc} \text{Intercept} & \text{Slope} \\ 1 & 0.30 \\ 0.30 & 0.7861 \end{array}\right| \begin{array}{l} \\ \text{Intercept} \\ \text{Slope} \end{array} \quad (8.20)$$

The psi ($\mathbf{\Psi}$) matrix in Equation (8.20) changes only to reflect the additional slope variance that is explained by adding the treatment by covariate interaction term.

$$\mathbf{B} = \left|\begin{array}{ccc} \text{Treatment} & \text{Covariate} & \text{Interaction} \\ 0 & 0 & 0 \\ 0.226 & 0.25 & 0.175 \end{array}\right| \begin{array}{l} \\ \text{Intercept} \\ \text{Slope} \end{array} \quad (8.21)$$

The beta (**B**) matrix in Equation (8.21) expands to include treatment, the covariate, and the interaction as predictors of linear slope variance with all standardized coefficients for linear slope variance prediction included.

$$\mathbf{\Phi} = \left|\begin{array}{ccc} \text{Treatment} & \text{Covariate} & \text{Interaction} \\ 1 & 0.20 & 0.05 \\ 0.20 & 1 & 0.50 \\ 0.05 & 0.50 & 1 \end{array}\right| \begin{array}{l} \\ \text{Treatment} \\ \text{Covariate} \\ \text{Interaction} \end{array} \quad (8.22)$$

The phi ($\mathbf{\Phi}$) matrix in Equation (8.22) also expands to include the variances and correlations among all three predictors. Solving Grimm et al.'s equation in brackets using R:

```
Lambda <- matrix(c(
0.7746, 0,
0.6527, 0.265,
0.5352, 0.422,
0.4498, 0.51,
0.3917, 0.561), ncol = 2, byrow = TRUE)

Psi <- matrix(c(
1, 0.30,
0.30, 0.7861 ), nrow = 2, byrow = TRUE)

Beta <- matrix(c(
0, 0, 0,
0.225, 0.25, 0.175), nrow = 2, byrow = TRUE)

Phi <- matrix(c(
1, 0.20, 0.05,
0.20, 1, 0.50,
0.05, 0.50, 1), nrow = 3, byrow = TRUE)

corr_matrix <- (Lambda %*% Psi %*% t(Lambda)) + (Lambda %*% Beta %*% Phi %*%
    t(Beta) %*% t(Lambda))
corr_matrix
```

		Response Variable 1	Response Variable 2	Response Variable 3	Response Variable 4	Response Variable 5
	Response Variable 1	**0.6000**	0.5672	0.5126	0.4669	0.4338
$\Sigma\theta =$	Response Variable 2	0.5672	**0.6000**	0.5683	0.5644	0.5453
	Response Variable 3	0.5126	0.5863	**0.6000**	0.5948	0.5861
	Response Variable 4	0.4669	0.5644	0.5948	**0.6001**	0.5979
	Response Variable 5	0.4338	0.5453	0.5861	0.5979	**0.6000**

So in Equations (8.23) and (8.24),

$$\theta_{\text{ResponseVariable1}} = 1 - 0.6000 = \mathbf{0.4000}$$
$$\theta_{\text{ResponseVariable2}} = 1 - 0.6000 = \mathbf{0.4000}$$
$$\theta_{\text{ResponseVariable3}} = 1 - 0.6000 = \mathbf{0.4000}$$
$$\theta_{\text{ResponseVariable4}} = 1 - 0.6001 = \mathbf{0.3999}$$
$$\theta_{\text{ResponseVariable5}} = 1 - 0.6000 = \mathbf{0.4000}$$

or

	Response Variable 1	Response Variable 2	Response Variable 3	Response Variable 4	Response Variable 5		
	0.4000	0	0	0	0	Response Variable 1	
$\theta =$	0	**0.4000**	0	0	0	Response Variable 2	
	0	0	**0.4000**	0	0	Response Variable 3	
	0	0	0	**0.3999**	0	Response Variable 4	
	0	0	0	0	**0.4000**	Response Variable 5	(8.23)

Solving Grimm et al.'s full equation using R:

```
Lambda <- matrix(c(
0.7746, 0,
0.6527, 0.265,
0.5352, 0.422,
0.4498, 0.51,
0.3917, 0.561), ncol = 2, byrow = TRUE)

Psi <- matrix(c(
1, 0.30,
0.30, 0.7861 ), nrow = 2, byrow = TRUE)

Beta <- matrix(c(
0, 0, 0,
0.225, 0.25, 0.175), nrow = 2, byrow = TRUE)

Phi <- matrix(c(
1, 0.20, 0.05,
0.20, 1, 0.50,
0.05, 0.50, 1), nrow = 3, byrow = TRUE)

Theta<-matrix(c(
0.4000, 0, 0, 0, 0,
0, 0. 4000, 0, 0, 0,
```

```
0, 0, 0. 4000, 0, 0,
0, 0, 0, 0.3999, 0,
0, 0, 0, 0, 0.4000), nrow = 5, byrow = TRUE)

corr_matrix <- (Lambda %*% Psi %*% t(Lambda)) + (Lambda %*% Beta %*% Phi %*%
      t(Beta) %*% t(Lambda)) + Theta

corr_matrix
```

		Response Variable 1	Response Variable 2	Response Variable 3	Response Variable 4	Response Variable 5	
	Response Variable 1	1	0.5672	0.5126	0.4669	0.4338	
$\Sigma\theta =$	Response Variable 2	0.5672	1	0.5683	0.5644	0.5453	
	Response Variable 3	0.5126	0.5863	1	0.5948	0.5861	
	Response Variable 4	0.4669	0.5644	0.5948	1	0.5979	
	Response Variable 5	0.4338	0.5453	0.5861	0.5979	1	(8.24)

Mplus Monte Carlo Power Analysis: Longitudinal RCT Moderation Model

When all of the numeric information contained in all above matrices is converted into Mplus syntax, the results (MPlus 8.5) are shown here.

```
TITLE: MPLUS 8.5 Longitudinal RCT Interaction

MONTECARLO:
NAMES ARE
RV_1-RV_5 TREAT CONT_COV INT;
NOBSERVATIONS = 668;
NREPS = 5000;
MISSING = RV_2 RV_3 RV_4 RV_5;
CUTPOINTS = TREAT(0);

MODEL POPULATION:
!Lambda Matrix;
I BY RV_1@.7746 RV_2@.6527 RV_3@.5352 RV_4@.4498 RV_5@.3917;
S BY RV_1@0 RV_2@.265 RV_3@.422 RV_4@.51 RV_5@.561;
[RV_1-RV_5@0];

!Psi Matrix;
I*1;
S*0.7861;
I WITH S*.30;

!Theta Matrix;
RV_1*.4;
RV_2*.4;
RV_3*.4;
RV_4*.3999;
RV_5*.4;
```

```
!Phi Matrix;
TREAT*1;
CONT_COV*1;
INT*1;
TREAT WITH CONT_COV*0.20 INT*0.05;
CONT_COV WITH INT*0.50;

!Beta Matrix;
S ON TREAT*0.225 CONT_COV*0.25 INT*0.175;
```

Missing data specifications remain the same as in all previous power analyses.

```
MODEL MISSING:
[RV_2*-2.9444]; !5% MCAR;
[RV_3*-2.1972]; !10% MCAR;
[RV_4*-1.7346]; !15% MCAR;
[RV_5*-1.3862]; !20% MCAR;

RV_2 ON RV_1*0.0953;
RV_3 ON RV_2*0.0953 RV_1*0.0953;
RV_4 ON RV_3*0.0953 RV_2*0.0953 RV_1*0.0953;
RV_5 ON RV_4*0.0953 RV_3*0.0953 RV_2*0.0953 RV_1*0.0953;
```

The `MODEL:` statement changes only to include the interaction term as a predictor of linear slope variance.

```
MODEL:
[RV_1-RV_5@0];

!Lambda Matrix;
I BY RV_1@.7746 RV_2@.6527 RV_3@.5352 RV_4@.4498 RV_5@.3917;
S BY RV_1@0 RV_2@.265 RV_3@.422 RV_4@.51 RV_5@.561;

!Beta Matrix;
S ON TREAT*0.225 CONT_COV*0.25 INT*0.175;
```

	ESTIMATES			S. E.	M. S. E.	95%	% Sig
	Population	Average	Std. Dev.	Average		Cover	Coeff
TREAT	0.225	0.2202	0.0783	0.0769	0.0062	0.941	0.810
CONT_COV	0.250	0.2501	0.0625	0.0628	0.0039	0.949	0.977
INT	**0.175**	0.1749	0.0627	0.0624	0.0039	0.948	**0.800**

R Monte Carlo Power Analysis: Longitudinal RCT Moderation Model Issues

Similar to the model presented earlier with two correlated covariates, it was not possible to run this model clearly in R using either lavaan or simsem. The online supplemental materials (at *www.guilford.com/peugh-materials*) contain what was accomplished in R with respect to this model.

Longitudinal RCT Moderation Model Simulation Power Analysis Write-Up

"The power analysis question involved the smallest sample size needed to achieve power ≥.80 to detect a standardized 'treatment effect by control covariate' interaction in a longitudinal RCT. A Monte Carlo simulation power analysis was conducted using Mplus (version 8.6) assuming: (1) standardization of all response variables at all five assessment time points, (2) linear trend best-captured response variable average changes over time and explained 60% of observed adherence response variable variance, on average, (3) random assignment results in equal sample sizes for both the treatment and control groups, (4) the magnitude of the standardized (β) effect of binary treatment randomization on linear slope variance is expected to be at least $\beta \geq$ 0.225 and explain at least (R^2 = .05) 5% of linear slope variance, (5) the inclusion of a control covariate measured on a continuous scale will explain an additional (R^2 = .085) 8.5% of linear slope variance ($\beta \geq 0.25$), (6), including the 'treatment effect by control covariate' interaction ($\beta \geq 0.175$) will explain an additional (R^2 = .079) 7.9% of linear slope variance, and (7) missing data are assumed to be (a) 0% at the initial assessment, (b) 5% at the first postbaseline assessment, (c) monotonically increasing in 5% increments to 20% at the final assessment, and (d) missing at random, such that unit increases in response variable values at any previous assessment time point are assumed to result in a 10% increase in the odds of missing data. Monte Carlo simulation power analysis results aggregated over 5,000 dataset replications showed power ≥ .80 to detect a standardized "binary treatment randomization by continuous covariate" interaction effect of $\beta \geq 0.175$ if all assumptions are met and proper missing data handling makes a sample size of $N = 668$ ($n = 334$ for both treatment and control groups) available for analysis."

A Final Note

Notice how, in all power analyses, the intercept and slope means (α_0 and α_1, respectively) were not given specific values. Treatment group differences, with the inclusion of a continuous control covariate and an interaction term, were specified and modeled by essentially relying upon variance and covariance matrix information while ignoring the mean structure of the observed response variables that would normally be estimated as latent intercept and latent linear slope means. This is considered by many to be an advantage that SEM analyses have over mean structure models, such as a mixed factorial (between by within) ANOVA model. However, for interested readers, it is possible to obtain a Monte Carlo simulation power estimate with a reasonable amount of missing data included for a mean structure model such as a mixed factorial ANOVA, which is discussed in this chapter's appendix.

SUGGESTED READINGS

- Candel, M. J. J. M., & van Breukelen, G. J. P. (2025). Efficient design of cluster randomized trials and individually randomized group treatment trials. *Psychological Methods*. Advance online publication.
- Corona, R., Dvorsky, M. R., Romo, S., Parks, A. M., Bourchtein, E., & Smith, Z. R., et al. (2020). Integrating tobacco prevention skills into an evidence-based intervention for adolescents with ADHD: Results from a pilot efficacy randomized controlled trial. *Journal of Abnormal Child Psychology, 48,* 1439–1453.
- Feingold, A. (2021). Effect of parameterization on statistical power and effect size estimation in latent growth modeling. *Structural Equation Modeling: A Multidisciplinary Journal, 28,* 609–621.
- Goldsmith, K. A., MacKinnon, D. P., Chalder, T., White, P. D., Sharpe, M., & Pickles, A. (2018). Tutorial: The practical application of longitudinal structural equation mediation models in clinical trials. *Psychological Methods, 23,* 191–207.
- Könen, T., & Karbach, J. (2021). Analyzing individual differences in intervention-related changes. *Advances in Methods and Practices in Psychological Science, 4,* 1–19.
- Langenberg, B., Helm, J. L., & Mayer, A. (2020). Repeated measures ANOVA with latent variables to analyze interindividual differences in contrasts. *Multivariate Behavioral Research, 57,* 2–19.
- Rovine, M. J., & Molenaar, P. C. M. (2001). A structural equations modeling approach to the general linear mixed model. In L. M. Collins & A. G. Sayer (Eds.), *New methods for the analysis of change* (pp. 65–96). American Psychological Association.
- Stull, D. E. (2008). Analyzing growth and change: latent variable growth curve modeling with an application to clinical trials. *Quality of Life Research, 17,* 47–59.
- Tauber, N. M., Zachariae, R., Jensen, A. B., Thewes, B., Skyt, I., Elkjær, E., et al. (2021). ConquerFear-group: Feasibility study with pilot results of a psychological intervention for fear of cancer recurrence delivered in groups. *Psycho-Oncology, 31,* 30–38.

Appendix 8.1

"Old School" Power Analyses Using "Old School" Methods

Researchers in a number of different content areas conduct tightly controlled randomized investigations that more closely resemble traditional experiments. Often, the research question centers not only on differences in change over time between randomly assigned groups of participants, but also involves specific post hoc pairwise follow-up comparisons. Such experimental designs seek answers to research questions that address specific changes at specific points in time. Mixed factorial analysis of variance (ANOVA) designs, such as between- (i.e., treatment group versus a control group) by within- (i.e., repeated response variable assessments collected over time) subject ANOVAs are often still the data analysis of choice for tightly controlled randomized clinical trials of various sorts. But even classic ANOVA models, when viewed from a structural equation modeling perspective, have at least two notable drawbacks.

First, as shown in this chapter and in Chapter 7, longitudinal growth curve power analyses typically involve the modeling of both the response variable mean structure and covariance matrix, a task well-suited to most structural equation modeling statistical analysis software packages. ANOVA models typically focus far more on the modeling of the response variable mean structure while very strong assumptions, such as compound symmetry or sphericity, are imposed on the covariance matrix and crude adjustment factors (e.g., Greenhouse-Geisser, Hyun-Feldt, lower bound, etc.) are applied when such assumptions are often violated. Second, experimental protocol deviations, research equipment failures, participant refusal, or human error are only a few of the possible causes for missing data even in tightly controlled randomized experiments. To make matters worse, most statistical analysis software packages have made ANOVA models available with a minimum of computer mouse clicks or lines of computer code, but most also have listwise or pairwise deletion of missing data as the default handling option. For power analysis purposes, researchers conducting tightly controlled randomized studies may wonder, "Can a factorial (between-subjects by within-subjects) ANOVA Monte Carlo simulation power analysis, incorporating a reasonable amount of missing response variable data, be performed in a structural equation modeling framework?"

Research by Rovine and Molenaar (1998, 2001) has shown that factorial ANOVA models can be estimated using structural equation modeling principles that allow for modeling both the mean structure and covariance matrix, as well as easy handling of missing data. Additional work by Rovine and McDermott (2018) has shown how the model-reproduced mean structures from both factorial ANOVA models and longitudinal growth models can be shown to be equivalent, and the circumstances under which a factorial ANOVA could be a more parsimonious and statistically more powerful model than a longitudinal growth curve model. We will show how to conduct a mixed-factorial ANOVA Monte Carlo simulation power analysis within a structural equation modeling framework, incorporating reasonable expectations of missing data, using results from a published longitudinal pilot RCT by Corona et al. (2020).

The longitudinal pilot RCT by Corona et al. (2020) sought to determine the feasibility, acceptability, and effectiveness of adding tobacco prevention skills (TPS) from the Strengthening Families Program (Spoth et al., 2006, 2015) into a behavioral treatment program geared toward improving the academic performance of adolescents with ADHD (Supporting Teens' Academic Needs Daily [STAND-G]; Sibley et al., 2013, 2014). Corona et al. (2020) conducted a pilot randomized trial comparing STAND-G to STAND-G + TPS. Results from a sample ($N = 63$) of adolescents diagnosed with ADHD and assessed at baseline (B), posttreatment (P), 3-month (3M), and 6-month (6M) follow-ups showed a statistically insignificant "group by time" interaction for substance use refusal intentions ($F[2,53]$, $p = .06$) despite what appears to be a clear "group-by-time" interaction shown in the error bar plot in Figure 8A.1.

Descriptive statistics and correlation matrices for the substance use refusal intention (SURI, adolescent report [A]) response variables at all assessment time points, for both the STAND-G + TPS and STAND-G groups, respectively, are also shown in Table 8A.1.

Just as in the Tauber et al. (2021) example shown previously, covariance matrices for both groups can be computed using the descriptive information for both groups from the Table 8A.1, combined with the correlation matrices below as shown in Table 8A.2.

Now that the mean structures and covariance matrices for both independent variable groups are available, syntax very similar to that used to generate data based on Tauber et al. (2021) can be used to generate data, assuming a researcher wishes to replicate the Corona et al. (2020) study and assuming the power analysis question involves the needed sample size to reject the null hypothesis for a "group * time" interaction with power ≥ .80.

```
[TITLE: MPLUS 8S1 Old School

MONTECARLO:
NAMES ARE
SURI_B SURI_P SURI_3M SURI_6M;
NGROUPS = 2;
NOBSERVATIONS = 54 54;
NREPS = 5000;
SEED = 80351;
MISSING = SURI_P SURI_3M SURI_6M;
```

The variable names listed after the "`NAMES ARE`" syntax remain the same, data will be generated for two groups (STAND-G + TPS & STAND-G; `NGROUPS = 2`), a sample size of $N = 108$ ($n = 54$ per group) will be tested for adequate statistical power, and the

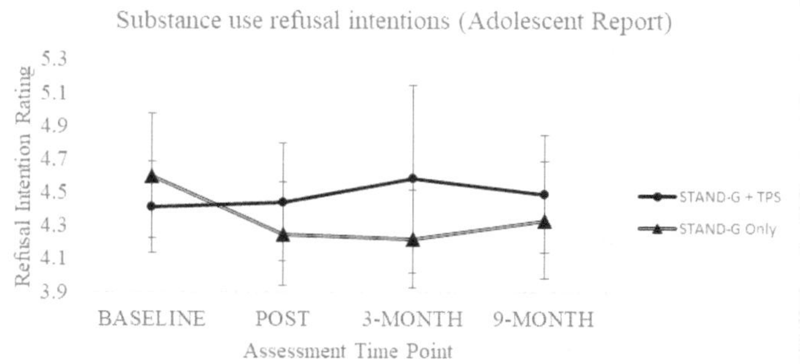

FIGURE 8A.1. Error bar graph; data from Corona et al. (2020).

"`MISSING =`" specification allows missing data to be specified for the three postbaseline assessment time points.

```
MODEL POPULATION:

[SURI_B*4.41];
[SURI_P*4.44];
[SURI_3M*4.58];
[SURI_6M*4.49];

SURI_B*.792;
SURI_P*1.300;
SURI_3M*3.349;
SURI_6M*1.300;

SURI_B WITH SURI_P*.678 SURI_3M*1.36 SURI_6M*.465;
SURI_P WITH SURI_3M*1.763 SURI_6M*.473;
SURI_3M WITH SURI_6M*1.316;
```

The "`MODEL POPULATION`" statement above specifies how data for the STAND-G + TPS group (i.e., treatment) can be generated and it has three distinct sections. The first section specifies the mean structure for the four response variables consistent with Table A8.2.

TABLE 8A.1. Response Variables to Assessment Time Points

	STAND-G + TPS		STAND-G	
	Mean	SD	Mean	SD
Baseline	4.41	0.89	4.60	0.91
Post	4.44	1.14	4.25	0.77
3 Month	4.58	1.83	4.22	0.72
6 Month	4.49	1.14	4.33	0.86

	STAND-G + TPS			
	SURI_B(A)	SURI_P(A)	SURI_3M(A)	SURI_6M(A)
SURI_B(A)	1			
SURI_P(A)	0.668	1		
SURI_3M(A)	0.835	0.845	1	
SURI_6M(A)	0.458	0.365	0.631	1

	STAND-G			
	SURI_B(A)	SURI_P(A)	SURI_3M(A)	SURI_6M(A)
SURI_B(A)	1			
SURI_P(A)	0.664	1		
SURI_3M(A)	0.568	0.780	1	
SURI_6M(A)	0.391	0.700	0.658	1

TABLE 8A.2. Corona et al. (2020) Data by Group

	STAND-G + TPS			
	SURI_B(A)	SURI_P(A)	SURI_3M(A)	SURI_6M(A)
SURI_B(A)	$(0.89)^2$			
SURI_P(A)	(0.89)(1.14)0.668	$(1.14)^2$		
SURI_3M(A)	(0.89)(1.83)0.835	(1.14)(1.83)0.845	$(1.83)^2$	
SURI_6M(A)	(0.89)(1.14)0.458	(1.14)(1.14)0.364	(1.83)(1.14)0.631	$(1.14)^2$
	STAND-G + TPS			
	SURI_B(A)	SURI_P(A)	SURI_3M(A)	SURI_6M(A)
SURI_B(A)	0.792			
SURI_P(A)	0.678	1.300		
SURI_3M(A)	1.360	1.763	3.349	
SURI_6M(A)	0.465	0.473	1.316	1.300
	STAND-G			
	SURI_B(A)	SURI_P(A)	SURI_3M(A)	SURI_6M(A)
SURI_P(A)	$(0.91)^2$			
SURI_3M(A)	(0.91)(0.77)0.664	$(0.77)^2$		
SURI_6M(A)	(0.91)(0.72)0.538	(0.77)(0.72)0.780	$(0.72)^2$	
SURI_6M(A)	(0.91)(0.86)0.391	(0.77)(0.86)0.700	(0.72)(0.86)0.658	$(0.86)^2$
	STAND-G			
	SURI_B(A)	SURI_P(A)	SURI_3M(A)	SURI_6M(A)
SURI_B(A)	0.828			
SURI_P(A)	0.465	0.593		
SURI_3M(A)	0.352	0.432	0.518	
SURI_6M(A)	0.306	0.464	0.407	0.740

The next two sections specify the variances and covariances among the response variables based on the values from the computed covariance matrix above.

```
MODEL POPULATION-G2:
[SURI_B*4.6];
[SURI_P*4.25];
[SURI_3M*4.22];
[SURI_6M*4.33];

SURI_B*.828;
SURI_P*.593;
SURI_3M*.518;
SURI_6M*.74;
SURI_B WITH SURI_P*.465 SURI_3M*.352 SURI_6M*.306;
```

```
SURI_P WITH SURI_3M*.432 SURI_6M*.464;
SURI_3M WITH SURI_6M*.407;
```

The "MODEL POPULATION-G2" statement above specifies how data for the STAND-G group (i.e., active control) is to be generated based on the mean structure and covariance matrix values in similar fashion.

```
MODEL MISSING:
[SURI_P*-3.17805]; !4% missing MCAR;
[SURI_3M*-1.81528];!14% missing MCAR;
[SURI_6M*-1.0986]; !25% missing MCAR;

!10% increase in odds of missing data per unit decrease;
SURI_P ON SURI_B*-0.09531;
SURI_3M ON SURI_P*-0.09531;
SURI_6M ON SURI_3M*-0.09531;
```

The "MODEL MISSING:" statement contains two distinct sections of syntax. The first three lines indicate missing completely at random (MCAR) missing data for all postbaseline response variable assessment time points. The logit intercept values contained in brackets specify MCAR missing data rates of ($\exp^{-3.17805}/1 + [\exp^{-3.17805}] = 0.04$) 4% at the posttreatment assessment, ($\exp^{-1.81528}/1 + [\exp^{-1.81528}] = 0.14$) 14% at the 3-month follow-up assessment, and ($\exp^{-1.0986}/1 + [\exp^{-1.0986}] = 0.25$) 25% at the 6-month follow-up assessment. The next three lines of syntax (the "ON" statements) change the missing data assumption from MCAR to missing at random (MAR) by relating missing data at a subsequent assessment time point to substance use refusal intentions (SURI) values at the previous assessment time point. The logit slope values specified in the "ON" statements specify a ($\exp^{-0.09531} = 0.9091$, $1/0.9091 = 1.10$) 10% increase in the odds of missing data at a subsequent assessment time point per unit decrease in SURI scores at any previous time point. Now that syntax specifications have been provided for how both observed and missing response variable data are to be generated, all that remains to be done in order to obtain a Monte Carlo simulation power estimate is to specify how the data are to be analyzed.

Mixed-Factorial ANOVA Design Matrices

One way to define and describe a *design matrix* is by presenting a design matrix that readers, at this point, are familiar with already, as shown in Equation (8A.1).

$$\Lambda = \begin{vmatrix} 1 & 0 \\ 1 & 1 \\ 1 & 2 \\ 1 & 3 \end{vmatrix} \tag{8A.1}$$

where lambda (Λ) indicates this design matrix contains values that mathematically define the relationship between four observed variables (because there are four rows) and two latent variables (because there are two columns). This particular lambda design matrix specifies loadings that define a linear latent growth curve with slope loadings (second column) centered to define the intercept mean as the expected response variable score at the first measurement occasion (second column, first row). For the purposes of specifying a mixed factorial ANOVA power analysis, the point to keep in mind is that a lambda design matrix will mathematically specify relationships between observed response variables and latent variables.

Rovine and Molenaar (1998, 2001) have shown that, to perform a mixed factorial ANOVA power analysis, two lambda design matrices are needed to represent the two independent variable groups (STAND-G + TPS & STAND-G), as shown in Equations (8A.2) and (8A.3).

$\Lambda_{\text{STAND-G+TPS}} =$

	Intercept η_1	Between (Group) η_2	Within (SURI_P) η_3	Within (SURI_3M) η_4	Within (SURI_6M) η_5	Between*Within (Group*SURI_P) η_6	Between*Within (Group*SURI_3M) η_7	Between*Within (Group*SURI_6M) η_8
SURI_B(A)	1	1	0	0	0	0	0	0
SURI_P(A)	1	1	1	0	0	1	0	0
SURI_3M(A)	1	1	0	1	0	0	1	0
SURI_6M(A)	1	1	0	0	1	0	0	1

(8A.2)

$\Lambda_{\text{STAND-G}} =$

	Intercept η_1	Between (Group) η_2	Within (SURI_P) η_3	Within (SURI_3M) η_4	Within (SURI_6M) η_5	Between*Within (Group*SURI_P) η_6	Between*Within (Group*SURI_3M) η_7	Between*Within (Group*SURI_6M) η_8
SURI_B(A)	1	0	0	0	0	0	0	0
SURI_P(A)	1	0	1	0	0	0	0	0
SURI_3M(A)	1	0	0	1	0	0	0	0
SURI_6M(A)	1	0	0	0	1	0	0	0

(8A.3)

As shown in the lambda design matrices for the two independent variable groups in Equations (8A.2) and (8A.3), the rows of both matrices contain the names of the response variables assessed over time, the eight columns (labeled η_1–η_8) correspond to latent variables that capture between-subjects, within-subjects, and the between-subjects * within-subjects interaction effects estimated in a mixed factorial ANOVA. The first column, η_1 (Intercept), shows values of one across all SURI variables in both design matrices. This intercept specification is the same as the intercept specification that assumes a linear growth curve model shown previously. The second column, η_2 (Group), shows values of one across all SURI variables in the STAND-G + TPS design matrix, but also shows values of zero across all SURI variables in the STAND-G design matrix. The values of zero in the STAND-G design matrix establish a baseline against which the average incremental change in the SURI intercept score that result from random assignment to the STAND-G + TPS group (i.e., the between-subject effect) can be estimated. The next three columns, labeled η_3–η_5,, show values of zero in the first row of both design matrices. This both defines the intercept estimate as the expected SURI score at baseline (SURI_B) but also establishes the baseline assessment as the reference class. The values of one for SURI_P, SURI_3M, and SURI_6M in columns η_3–η_5 specify orthogonal polynomial contrast coefficients at each assessment time point and, taken together, comprise the within-subjects effect, or average change in SURI scores over time. Similar to the way the between-subjects, or group, effect was specified in the second (η_2) column, the last three columns labeled η_6–η_8, show values of zero in the STAND-G design matrix, but show values of one for SURI_P, SURI_3M and SURI_6M across columns η_6–η_8, respectively, for the STAND-G + TPS design matrix. The values of zero in the STAND-G design matrix establish a baseline against which the average difference in SURI score changes over time resulting from random assignment to the STAND-G + TPS condition can be estimated. Taken together, columns η_6–η_8 enable the estimation of the between-subject * within-subject (or, group * time) interaction effect.

To convert the information in the two design matrices above into Mplus syntax to analyze the generated Monte Caro simulation data specified above, three `MODEL:` statements will be needed: `MODEL:`, `MODEL G1:`, and `MODEL G2:`.

```
MODEL:
[SURI_B-SURI_6M@0];
ETA1-ETA8@0;
ETA1-ETA8 WITH ETA1-ETA8@0;
```

The first line of syntax in the `MODEL:` command in Mplus is shorthand for constraining the observed SURI response variable means at all assessment time points to zero. The next two lines of syntax constrain the latent variable (`ETA1-ETA8`) variances and covariances, respectively, to zero. These commands have the effect of estimating SURI response variable means at the latent variable (`ETA1-ETA8`) level to obtain the between-subject and within- subject main effect estimates, and the between-subject * within-subject interaction effect estimate, for a mixed factorial ANOVA. These commands also have the effect of emphasizing the modeling of the mean structure while minimizing the number of estimated parameters.

```
SURI_B-SURI_6M (1);
SURI_B-SURI_6M WITH SURI_B-SURI_6M (2);
```

The next two lines of Mplus syntax constrain the observed SURI response variable variances to equality using (1) and constrains all possible SURI response variable covariance/correlations separately to equality using (2). Constraining observed variable residual variances and covariances separately to equality is the definition of *compound symmetry*, a common assumption in mixed factorial ANOVA.

```
ETA1 | SURI_B@1 SURI_P@1 SURI_3M@1 SURI_6M@1;
ETA2 | SURI_B@1 SURI_P@1 SURI_3M@1 SURI_6M@1;
ETA3 | SURI_P@1;
ETA4 | SURI_3M@1;
ETA5 | SURI_6M@1;
ETA6 | SURI_P@1;
ETA7 | SURI_3M@1;
ETA8 | SURI_6M@1;
```

Notice how, in the final Mplus syntax lines for the first MODEL: command, each of the latent variables (ETA1–ETA8) is measured by (|) each of the observed SURI variables as specified by the design matrices above, but loadings are fixed (@, rather than allowed to vary, *) at values taken from the STAND-G + TPS design matrix. These syntax specifications can be thought of as an "overall" model that includes all needed parameter estimates. The necessary group-specific (STAND-G + TPS & STAND-G) deviations from this "overall" model are specified in the MODEL G1: and MODEL G2: statements, respectively, as shown.

```
MODEL G1:

[ETA1](3);
[ETA2];
[ETA3](4);
[ETA4](4);
[ETA5](4);
[ETA6](5);
[ETA7](5);
[ETA8](5);

MODEL G2:
ETA2|SURI_B@0SURI_P@0SURI_3M@0SURI_6M@0;
ETA6|SURI_B@0;
ETA7|SURI_P@0;
ETA8|SURI_3M@0;

[ETA1](3);
[ETA2@0];
[ETA3](4);
[ETA4](4);
[ETA5](4);
[ETA6@0];
[ETA7@0];
[ETA8@0];
```

The MODEL G2: statement allows deviations from the "overall" model specific to the design matrix specifications for the STAND-G group. Notice how, in the first line of syntax under MODEL G2:, the latent variable ETA2 is measured by (|) SURI variables whose values have been fixed at zero (@0). This is to establish a baseline against which the between-subjects effect (group) will be estimated. The next three lines of syntax show that the latent variables ETA6–ETA8 are measured by (|) specific SURI variables with values again fixed at zero (@0). This is to establish a baseline against which the between-subjects * within-subjects (or, group*time) interaction effect can be estimated. Further, the eight lines of code containing brackets ([]) common to both the MODEL G1: and MODEL G2: statements show how the between-subjects and within-subjects main effects, and the between-subjects * within-subjects interaction effect, are estimated. First, the syntax line [ETA1] (3); allows a single intercept estimate, or expected SURI_B value for the STAND-G group, by constraining the estimated latent variable mean to equality between the two groups. The latent variable mean [ETA2] estimate, the between-subjects or group effect, is fixed at zero `[ETA2@0]` in the STAND-G group to establish a baseline against which the between-subjects (i.e., the group effect or treatment effect) is estimated in the STAND-G + TPS group: `[ETA2]`.

The next three lines of Mplus code are identical in both groups

```
[ETA3](4);
[ETA4](4);
[ETA5](4);
```

and are constrained to equality both over time (`ETA3`–`ETA5` represent SURI_P, SURI_3M, and SURI_6M average score changes over time) and between the two groups. This is done so that a single within-subjects main effect is estimated. Finally, notice how the last three latent variable means

```
[ETA6](5);
[ETA7](5);
[ETA8](5);
```

are estimated, but constrained to equality over time in the STAND-G + TPS group, but are fixed at zero

```
[ETA6@0];
[ETA7@0];
[ETA8@0];
```

in the STAND-G group. The zeros for the means in the STAND-G group establish a baseline against which the between-subjects * within-subjects interaction effect can be estimated in the STAND-G + TPS group. Constraining the `ETA6`–`ETA8` estimated means to equality over time in the STAND-G + TPS group is done so that a single between-subjects * within-subjects interaction effect can be estimated.

The statements in the '`MODEL POPULATION:`' Mplus syntax shown below are straightforward mean, variance, and covariance specifications, as well as MAR '`MODEL MISSING:`' statements, consistent with such statements shown in previous chapters. Far more attention will be given to the "old school" specifications shown in the '`MODEL:`' statements below. Specifically, the general '`MODEL:`' statement specification, as well as the group-specific (`MODEL: G1`' & '`MODEL: G2`') specification statements, will be illustrated in two analysis model figures (8A.2, 8A.3, and 8A.4), followed immediately by the combined Mplus Monte Carlo simulation syntax and the annotated power analysis (8A.1) estimation results.

```
TITLE: MPLUS 8S1 Old School

MONTECARLO:
NAMES ARE
SURI_B SURI_P SURI_3M SURI_6M;
NGROUPS = 2;
NOBSERVATIONS = 54 54;
NREPS = 5000;
SEED = 80351;
MISSING = SURI_P SURI_3M SURI_6M;
```

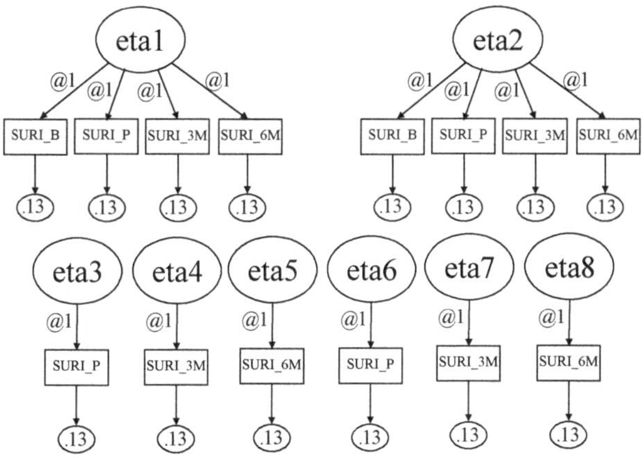

FIGURE 8A.2. General 'Model:' statement. (Note: Observed variable [SURI] variances and covariances constrained separately to equality, i.e., compound symmetry.) All other parameters fixed at zero. Residual variance values rounded (.13) for illustration.

```
MODEL POPULATION:

[SURI_B*4.41];
[SURI_P*4.44];
[SURI_3M*4.58];
[SURI_6M*4.49];

SURI_B*.792;
SURI_P*1.300;
SURI_3M*3.349;
SURI_6M*1.300;

SURI_B WITH SURI_P*.678 SURI_3M*1.36 SURI_6M*.465;
SURI_P WITH SURI_3M*1.763 SURI_6M*.473;
SURI_3M WITH SURI_6M*1.316;
```

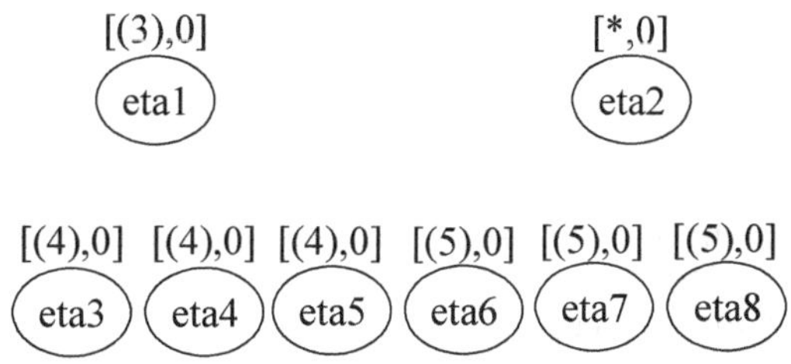

FIGURE 8A.3. 'Model G1:' statement. (Note: Integer values in parentheses indicate latent variable means constrained to equality with two exceptions. First, the '*' represents the 'between-subjects' effect estimated in the first group but fixed to zero in the second group. Second, the '(5)' represents an equality constraint to estimate a single 'between * within' interaction effect in this group. Those latent variable means will also be fixed to zero in the second group.)

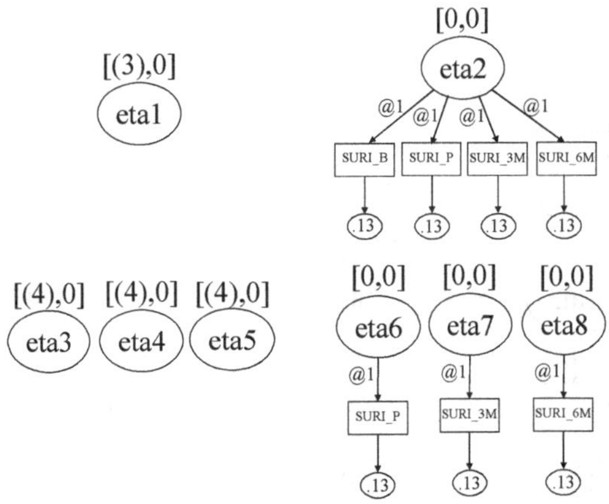

FIGURE 8A.4. 'Model G2:' statement. (Note: The latent variable mean 'eta2' is fixed at zero to establish a baseline for the 'between-subjects' effect estimated in the G1 model. The latent variable means for 'eta6-8' are also fixed at zero to establish a baseline for the 'between*within' effect also estimated in the G1 model.)

```
MODEL POPULATION-G2:
[SURI_B*4.6];
[SURI_P*4.25];
[SURI_3M*4.22];
[SURI_6M*4.33];

SURI_B*.828;
SURI_P*.593;
SURI_3M*.518;
SURI_6M*.74;

SURI_B WITH SURI_P*.465 SURI_3M*.352 SURI_6M*.306;
SURI_P WITH SURI_3M*.432 SURI_6M*.464;
SURI_3M WITH SURI_6M*.407;

MODEL MISSING:
[SURI_P*-3.17805]; !4% missing MCAR;
[SURI_3M*-1.81528];!14% missing MCAR;

[SURI_6M*-1.0986]; !25% missing MCAR;

!10% increase in odds of missing data per unit decrease;
SURI_P ON SURI_B*-0.09531;
SURI_3M ON SURI_P*-0.09531;
SURI_6M ON SURI_3M*-0.09531;

MODEL:
[SURI_B-SURI_6M@0];
ETA1-ETA8@0;
ETA1-ETA8 WITH ETA1-ETA8@0;
```

```
SURI_B-SURI_6M (1);
SURI_B-SURI_6M WITH SURI_B-SURI_6M (2);

ETA1 | SURI_B@1 SURI_P@1 SURI_3M@1 SURI_6M@1;
ETA2 | SURI_B@1 SURI_P@1 SURI_3M@1 SURI_6M@1;
ETA3 | SURI_P@1;
ETA4 | SURI_3M@1;
ETA5 | SURI_6M@1;
ETA6 | SURI_P@1;
ETA7 | SURI_3M@1;
ETA8 | SURI_6M@1;

MODEL G1:

[ETA1](3);
[ETA2];
[ETA3](4);
[ETA4](4);
[ETA5](4);
[ETA6](5);
[ETA7](5);
[ETA8](5);

MODEL G2:

ETA2|SURI_B@0SURI_P@0SURI_3M@0SURI_6M@0;
ETA6|SURI_B@0;
ETA7|SURI_P@0;
ETA8|SURI_3M@0;

[ETA1](3);
[ETA2@0];
[ETA3](4);
[ETA4](4);
[ETA5](4);
[ETA6@0];
[ETA7@0];
[ETA8@0];
```

	Population	ESTIMATES Average	Std. Dev.	S. E. Average	M. S. E.	95% Cover	% Sig Coeff
Means							
ETA1 (Intercept)	3.571	4.5984	0.1252	0.1457	1.0714	0.000	1.000
ETA2 (Between-Subjects)	0.852	-0.1869	0.1740	0.2060	1.1098	0.000	0.108
ETA3	-0.201	-0.3352	0.1025	0.1082	0.0284	0.774	0.883
ETA4 (Within-Subjects)	-0.201	-0.3352	0.1025	0.1082	0.0284	0.774	0.883
ETA5	-0.201	-0.3352	0.1025	0.1082	0.0284	0.774	0.883
ETA6	**0.277**	0.4282	0.1479	0.1529	0.0449	0.839	**0.808**
ETA7 (Between*Within)	**0.277**	0.4282	0.1479	0.1529	0.0449	0.839	**0.808**
ETA8	**0.277**	0.4282	0.1479	0.1529	0.0449	0.839	**0.808**

Before presenting an example Monte Carlo simulation power analysis write-up for a mixed factorial ANOVA using Rovine and Molenaar's (1998, 2001) design matrix specifications, it is important to note that this technique holds both potential power analytic and subsequent data analytic advantages. The first power analysis advantage is the ability to specify and incorporate a reasonable amount of anticipated missing data into the power estimate. The second potential power analysis advantage, assuming compound symmetry is reasonable, is that the mixed factorial ANOVA model for Corona et al.'s (2020) data estimates only six parameters. A comparable standard linear latent growth curve model would estimate 10 parameters, meaning a mixed factorial ANOVA model could be the statistically more powerful option under certain conditions. Analytically, the first advantage of Rovine and Molenaar's design matrix mixed factorial ANOVA model would be the ability to handle missing data by default using maximum likelihood estimation. The second data analysis advantage, assuming a significant between-subjects * within-subjects interaction effect, is that post hoc pairwise follow-up comparisons can be estimated by simply removing the equality constraints for the interaction effect(5) in the STAND-G + TPS group. Finally, if an assumption is made that compound symmetry is not reasonable, the design matrix approach affords the ability to test several different combinations of fixed and freely estimated residual variance and covariance combinations to determine the best fitting residual variance/ covariance matrix based on model fit. Making this flexibility available to researchers is a far more appealing option than the traditional mixed factorial ANOVA route of assuming sphericity and applying coarse adjustments to significance tests prior to interpretation if sphericity is violated (e.g., Greenhouse-Geisser, Hyun-Feldt, Lower Bound, etc.).

A Mixed-Factorial ANOVA Model Simulation Power Analysis Write-Up

> "The power analysis question under consideration regards the minimal sample size needed to replicate Corona, et al's. (2020) study and reject the null hypothesis for a "group*time" (or, between-subjects*within-subjects) interaction with power $\geq$ .80 in a 2 (between: STAND-G + TPS vs. STAND-G) by 4 (baseline, postintervention, 3-month follow-up, and 6-month follow-up) mixed factorial ANOVA using Rovine and Molenaar's (1998, 2001) design matrix model specifications. A Monte Carlo simulation power analysis was conducted using Mplus (version 8.6) assuming: (1) descriptive statistics, including means, standard deviations, and correlations for the substance use refusal intentions (SURI) data for both the STAND-G + TPS and STAND-G groups constitute reliable and reasonable pilot data estimates for Monte Carlo data-generation purposes, (2) random assignment will produce equal STAND-G + TPS and STAND-G group sample sizes with no missing data at the baseline assessment, (3) missing data are assumed to be MAR, 4% at the first postbaseline assessment, 14% at the 3-month follow-up, 25% at the 6-month follow-up, and the odds of missing data at any postbaseline assessment increase 10% per unit decrease in SURI scores at any previous time point, and (4) compound symmetry, defined as all SURI residual variances constrained to equality, and all residual covariances constrained separately to equality. Monte Carlo simulation power analysis results aggregated over 5,000 dataset replications showed power $\geq$ .80 to detect a between-subjects*within-subjects interaction effect $\geq$ 0.227 if proper missing data handling makes N = 108 (n = 54 for both the STAND-G + TPS & STAND-G groups) available for analysis."

9

Adding Time-Varying Covariates

Chapter 8 showed how to conduct a Monte Carlo simulation power analysis for a longitudinal growth model that included time-invariant covariates to explain between-participant differences in average response variable changes over time. *Time-invariant covariates* were defined as predictor variables whose values do not change over the course of the longitudinal study, and examples included random assignment to a treatment or a control condition, or biological sex. *Time-varying covariates*, which are defined predictor variables whose values are expected to change over time and are usually collected in conjunction with response variable measures at each assessment time point, can also be added to a longitudinal growth curve model to explain within-participant variation in response variable changes over time. Examples of time-varying covariates include state anxiety, mood assessment, current stress level, urges to smoke, and symptom severity. To illustrate, a longitudinal growth curve model with only time-varying covariates (TVC) included is shown in Figure 9.1.

Several features unique to time-varying covariate additions can be contrasted with the addition of time-invariant covariates to a longitudinal model. First, as indicated by the integer values from 1–5, time-varying covariate data are collected at each assessment time point along with response variable data. Time-invariant covariate data, by definition, need only be collected once. Second, in contrast to time-invariant covariates specified to predict latent variable variance (intercept, linear slope, etc.), time-varying covariates are specified as direct predictors of response variable variances. Finally, just like time-invariant covariates, and as indicated by the curved, double-headed arrows, time-varying covariates are also correlated.

Recall in Chapter 7 that a Monte Carlo simulation power analysis was conducted on an unconditional longitudinal growth curve model to determine the sample size needed to detect a 5% decrease in adherence over time from an 80% baseline adherence rate. Recall also that results showed an $N = 297$ was needed that was conditional on proper handling of

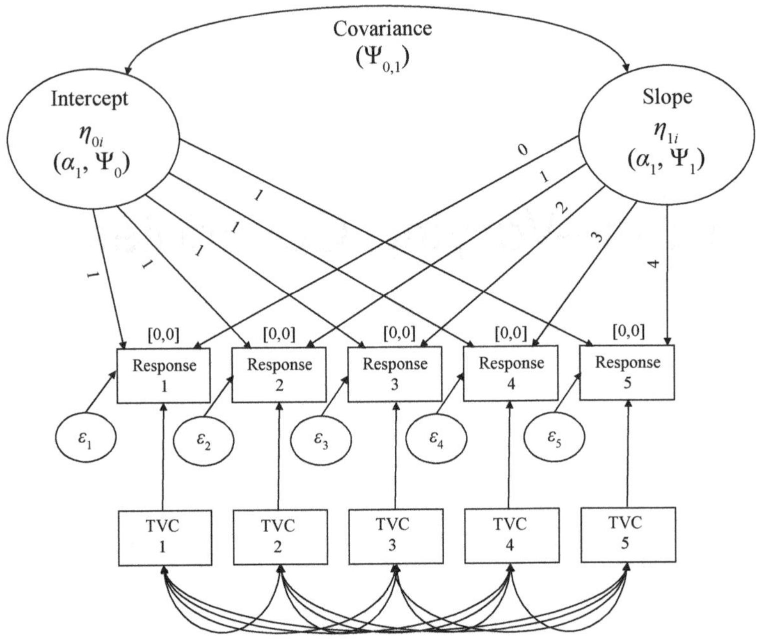

FIGURE 9.1. Adding time-varying covariates to a longitudinal growth curve model.

missing data. For illustration purposes, let's assume a researcher has decided that $N = 297$ is not feasible and wants to add a time-varying covariate such as symptom severity (SympSev) and perform a revised power analysis. Further, let's assume the researcher is willing to make stronger assumptions, such as linear trend is expected to explain 70% of the variation in adherence changes over time, while keeping the same missing data assumptions from the original Monte Carlo simulation power analysis. The revised power analysis model is shown in Figure 9.2.

The 10 question marks (?) between the rectangles representing observed adherence percentage and symptom severity scores are all related: A researcher is willing to propose that linear trend explains 70% of adherence percentage variance over time, but the magnitude of the standardized coefficient for symptom severity as a predictor of observed adherence (i.e., the five question marks on the regression arrows) will alter the amount of adherence variance left unexplained (i.e., the five question marks in the residual variance circles). The last question mark at the lower right of the analysis figure indicates that the 10 correlations among the symptom severity scores collected over time must be specified also. Let's further assume that, based on a search of published literature, pilot data, or previous experience, a researcher believes that symptom severity will explain an additional 10% of adherence percentage variance at each assessment time point and will specify a standardized coefficient (β) of ($\sqrt{0.10}$ =) $\beta = 0.3162$ for symptom severity, thus predicting adherence percentage at each longitudinal assessment. This leaves the correlations among the symptom severity scores over time to be specified. Recall from Chapter 7 that, without knowing the extent to which adherence percentages were correlated over time, a researcher was willing to assume a band diagonal correlation structure that specifies adjacent time point adherence values

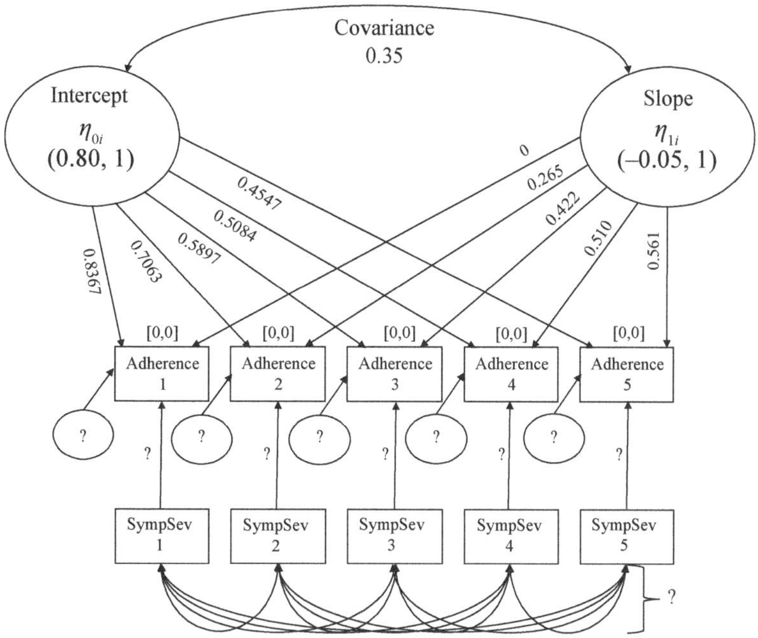

FIGURE 9.2. Correlated residuals in a longitudinal growth curve model.

that were more highly correlated (r = .50) than adherence values separated by one (r = .40) or two (r = .30) assessment time points. A researcher can assume the same band diagonal correlation structure (shown within rectangles in the following chart) for symptom severity score correlations over time if the actual correlations are not known.

	SympSev1	SympSev2	SympSev3	SympSev4	SympSev5
SympSev1	1				
SympSev2	0.50	1			
SympSev3	0.40	0.50	1		
SympSev4	0.30	0.40	0.50	1	
SympSev5	0.20	0.30	0.40	0.50	1

The updated time-varying covariate Monte Carlo simulation model is shown in Figure 9.3. Notice how the question marks within the residual variance circles remain. This is because the model-reproduced ($\mathbf{\Sigma}$) correlation matrix formula for a time-varying covariate longitudinal growth model is shown by Grimm et al. (2017, p. 183, Equation 8.12) to be

$$\mathbf{\Sigma\theta} = [\mathbf{\Lambda\Psi\Lambda}^T + \mathbf{A\Phi A}^T] + \mathbf{\Theta} \tag{9.1}$$

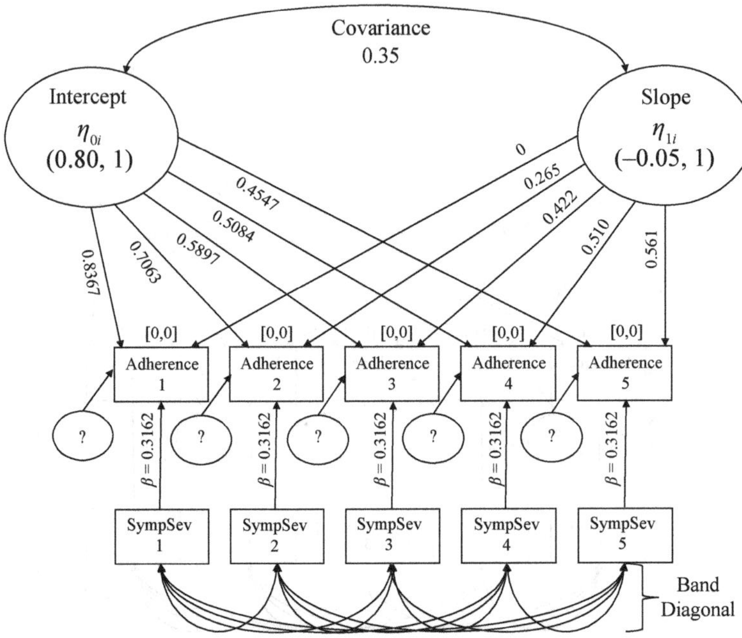

FIGURE 9.3. Band diagonal correlated residuals in a longitudinal growth curve model.

where the residual variance matrix (**Θ**) is again an additive term and the needed values can be obtained by solving the portion of the equation in brackets and subtracting as follows, as in Equation (9.2).

$$\mathbf{\Lambda} = \begin{array}{|cc|l} \text{Intercept} & \text{Slope} & \\ 0.8367 & 0 & \text{Adherence 1} \\ 0.7063 & 0.265 & \text{Adherence 2} \\ 0.5987 & 0.422 & \text{Adherence 3} \\ 0.5084 & 0.51 & \text{Adherence 4} \\ 0.4547 & 0.561 & \text{Adherence 5} \end{array} \tag{9.2}$$

where the lambda (**Λ**) matrix contains the loadings that specify the observed adherence response variable values to the latent intercept and latent linear slope, as shown in Equation (9.3).

$$\mathbf{\Psi} = \begin{array}{|cc|l} \text{Intercept} & \text{Slope} & \\ 1 & 0.35 & \text{Intercept} \\ 0.35 & 1 & \text{Slope} \end{array} \tag{9.3}$$

where the psi (**Ψ**) matrix contains the latent intercept and latent linear slope variances and correlation, as shown in Equation (9.4).

$$
\mathbf{A} = \begin{array}{|ccccc|l}
\text{SympSev1} & \text{SympSev2} & \text{SympSev3} & \text{SympSev4} & \text{SympSev5} & \\
0.3162 & 0 & 0 & 0 & 0 & \text{Adherence 1} \\
0 & 0.3162 & 0 & 0 & 0 & \text{Adherence 2} \\
0 & 0 & 0.3162 & 0 & 0 & \text{Adherence 3} \\
0 & 0 & 0 & 0.3162 & 0 & \text{Adherence 4} \\
0 & 0 & 0 & 0 & 0.3162 & \text{Adherence 5}
\end{array} \quad (9.4)
$$

where the alpha (**A**) matrix has a number of rows and columns equal to the number of response variables and time-varying covariate variables, respectively. The value on the main diagonal of the alpha matrix is the standardized regression coefficient for symptom severity, which predicts the adherence percentage scores at each assessment time point, as shown in Equation (9.5).

$$
\mathbf{\Phi} = \begin{array}{|ccccc|l}
\text{SympSev1} & \text{SympSev2} & \text{SympSev3} & \text{SympSev4} & \text{SympSev5} & \\
1 & 0.50 & 0.40 & 0.30 & 0.20 & \text{SympSev1} \\
0.50 & 1 & 0.50 & 0.40 & 0.30 & \text{SympSev2} \\
0.40 & 0.50 & 1 & 0.50 & 0.40 & \text{SympSev3} \\
0.30 & 0.40 & 0.50 & 1 & 0.50 & \text{SympSev4} \\
0.30 & 0.40 & 0.50 & 1 & & \text{SympSev5}
\end{array} \quad (9.5)
$$

where the phi (**Φ**) matrix contains the variances and the correlations for the time-varying covariates. Assuming standardization, the main diagonal elements show unit variances, and the off-diagonal elements show a band diagonal correlation structure. The portion of Grimm 's et al.(2017) equation contained in brackets can now be solved as follows, as shown in Equations (9.6) and (9.7):

```
Lambda <- matrix(c(
0.8367, 0,
0.7063, 0.265,
0.5987, 0.422,
0.5084, 0.51,
0.4547, 0.561), ncol = 2, byrow = TRUE)

Psi <- matrix(c(
1, 0.35,
0.35, 1), nrow = 2, byrow = TRUE)

Alpha <- matrix(c(
0.3162, 0, 0, 0, 0,
0, 0.3162, 0, 0, 0,
0, 0, 0.3162, 0, 0,
0, 0, 0, 0.3162, 0,
0, 0, 0, 0, 0.3162), nrow = 5, byrow = TRUE)
```

```
Phi <- matrix(c(
1, 0.50, 0.40, 0.30, 0.20,
0.50, 1, 0.50, 0.40, 0.30,
0.40, 0.50, 1, 0.50, 0.40,
0.30, 0.40, 0.50, 1, 0.50,
0.20, 0.30, 0.40, 0.50, 1), nrow = 5, byrow = TRUE)

corr_matrix <- (Lambda %*% Psi %*% t(Lambda)) + (Alpha %*% Phi %*% t(Alpha))

corr_matrix
```

	Adherence 1	Adherence 2	Adherence 3	Adherence 4	Adherence 5
Adherence 1	0.8000	0.7186	0.6645	0.6047	0.5647
Adherence 2	0.7186	0.8001	0.7445	0.7075	0.6807
Adherence 3	0.6645	0.7445	0.8134	0.7515	0.7337
Adherence 4	0.6047	0.7075	0.7515	0.8001	0.7483
Adherence 5	0.5647	0.6807	0.7337	0.7483	0.8000

So,

$$\theta_{\text{Adherence1}} = 1 - 0.8000 = \mathbf{0.2000}$$
$$\theta_{\text{Adherence2}} = 1 - 0.8001 = \mathbf{0.1999}$$
$$\theta_{\text{Adherence3}} = 1 - 0.8134 = \mathbf{0.1866}$$
$$\theta_{\text{Adherence4}} = 1 - 0.8001 = \mathbf{0.1999}$$
$$\theta_{\text{Adherence5}} = 1 - 0.8000 = \mathbf{0.2000}$$

or

$$\boldsymbol{\Theta} = \begin{array}{c} \text{Adherence 1 Adherence 2 Adherence 3 Adherence 4 Adherence 5} \\ \left|\begin{array}{ccccc} 0.2000 & 0 & 0 & 0 & 0 \\ 0 & 0.1999 & 0 & 0 & 0 \\ 0 & 0 & 0.1866 & 0 & 0 \\ 0 & 0 & 0 & 0.1999 & 0 \\ 0 & 0 & 0 & 0 & 0.2000 \end{array}\right| \begin{array}{l} \text{Adherence 1} \\ \text{Adherence 2} \\ \text{Adherence 3} \\ \text{Adherence 4} \\ \text{Adherence 5} \end{array} \end{array} \quad (9.6)$$

Solving the full equation:

```
Lambda <- matrix(c(
0.8367, 0,
0.7063, 0.265,
0.5987, 0.422,
0.5084, 0.51,
0.4547, 0.561), ncol = 2, byrow = TRUE)

Psi <- matrix(c(
1, 0.35,
0.35, 1), nrow = 2, byrow = TRUE)
```

```
Alpha <- matrix(c(
0.3162, 0, 0, 0, 0,
0, 0.3162, 0, 0, 0,
0, 0, 0.3162, 0, 0,
0, 0, 0, 0.3162, 0,
0, 0, 0, 0, 0.3162), nrow = 5, byrow = TRUE)

Phi <- matrix(c(
1, 0.50, 0.40, 0.30, 0.20,
0.50, 1, 0.50, 0.40, 0.30,
0.40, 0.50, 1, 0.50, 0.40,
0.30, 0.40, 0.50, 1, 0.50,
0.20, 0.30, 0.40, 0.50, 1), nrow = 5, byrow = TRUE)

Theta<-matrix(c(
0.2000, 0, 0, 0, 0,
0, 0.1999, 0, 0, 0,
0, 0, 0.1866, 0, 0,
0, 0, 0, 0.1999, 0,
0, 0, 0, 0, 0.2000
), nrow = 5, byrow = TRUE)

corr_matrix <- (Lambda %*% Psi %*% t(Lambda)) + (Alpha %*% Phi %*% t(Alpha)) + Theta

corr_matrix
```

$\Sigma =$

	Adherence 1	Adherence 2	Adherence 3	Adherence 4	Adherence 5
Adherence 1	1	0.7186	0.6645	0.6047	0.5647
Adherence 2	0.7186	1	0.7445	0.7075	0.6807
Adherence 3	0.6645	0.7445	1	0.7515	0.7337
Adherence 4	0.6047	0.7075	0.7515	1	0.7483
Adherence 5	0.5647	0.6807	0.7337	0.7483	1

(9.7)

Grimm et al.'s (2017) equation has confirmed an admissible model and the information in the above matrices could now be converted into Mplus power analysis syntax.

However, it is the rare case where a linear slope mean, estimated in the presence of time-varying covariates, is the parameter estimate needed to answer a research question. Far more commonplace are analyses that include time-varying covariates, in the service of controlling for their influence on the response variable, while interpreting one or more time-invariant covariate effects to answer a research question.

Recall that, at the conclusion of Chapter 8, the results from a time-invariant covariate (TIC) power analysis showed an $N = 668$ was needed for power $\geq .80$ to reject the null hypothesis for a binary treatment indicator by continuous covariate interaction for a given response variable (RV). Suppose a researcher decides that $N = 668$ is not feasible and wants to add time-varying covariates (TVC) to the model in an attempt to decrease the needed sample size. The time-varying covariate specifications shown in Figure 9.3 can be added to the time-invariant covariate model from Chapter 8 to produce the following (see Figure 9.4).

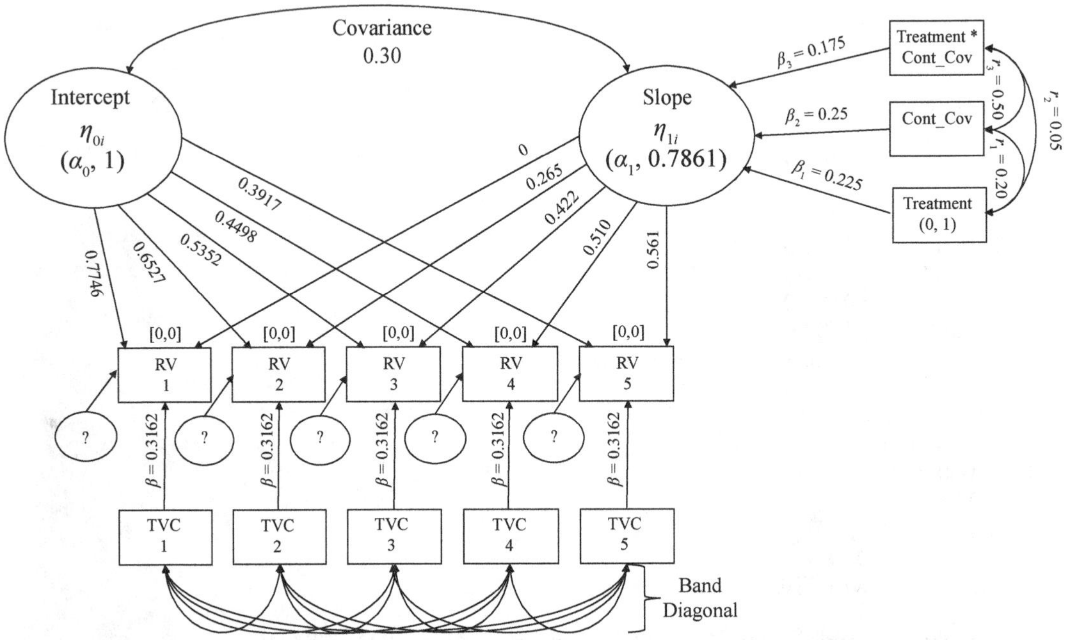

FIGURE 9.4. Adding time-invariant covariates to a longitudinal growth curve model.

Notice again the five question marks within the circles representing the observed RV residual variances, which indicates values that need to be specified. Again, the model-reproduced correlation matrix [Σ; Equation (9.8)] for a longitudinal growth curve model that contains both time-invariant and time-varying covariates[1]

$$\Sigma\theta = [\Lambda(\mathbf{B}\Phi_{TIC}\mathbf{B}^T)\Lambda^T + (\Lambda\Psi\Lambda^T) + (\Lambda\Phi_{TVC}\Lambda^T)] + \Theta \quad (9.8)$$

shows that the observed RV residual variances matrix, Θ, remains additive, which means the residual variances can again be obtained by subtraction as shown in Equation (9.9).

$$\begin{array}{cc} & \begin{array}{cc}\text{Intercept} & \text{Slope}\end{array} \\ \Lambda = & \left|\begin{array}{cc} 0.7746 & 0 \\ 0.6527 & 0.265 \\ 0.5352 & 0.422 \\ 0.4498 & 0.51 \\ 0.3917 & 0.561 \end{array}\right| \begin{array}{l} \text{RV 1} \\ \text{RV 2} \\ \text{RV 3} \\ \text{RV 4} \\ \text{RV 5} \end{array} \end{array} \quad (9.9)$$

where the lambda (Λ) matrix remains a loading matrix for the latent intercept and latent slope as they relate to the observed response variables, as shown in Equation (9.10).

[1]The authors extend their thanks and gratitude to Drs. Kevin Grimm, Nilam Ram, and Ryan Estabrook for all of their assistance with model-reproduced equations.

$$\mathbf{B} = \begin{array}{c} \\ \\ \end{array}\begin{array}{ccc|l} \text{Treatment} & \text{Covariate} & \text{Interaction} & \\ \hline 0 & 0 & 0 & \text{Intercept} \\ 0.225 & 0.25 & 0.175 & \text{Slope} \end{array} \quad (9.10)$$

where the beta (**B**) matrix specifies the relationships between the time-invariant covariates as predictors of latent linear slope variance as in Chapter 8 and as shown in Equation (9.11).

$$\boldsymbol{\Phi}_{\text{TIC}} = \begin{array}{ccc|l} \text{Treatment} & \text{Covariate} & \text{Interaction} & \\ \hline 1 & 0.20 & 0.05 & \text{Treatment} \\ 0.20 & 1 & 0.50 & \text{Covariate} \\ 0.05 & 0.50 & 1 & \text{Interaction} \end{array} \quad (9.11)$$

where the phi matrix for the time-invariant covariates ($\boldsymbol{\Phi}_{\text{TIC}}$) specifies the variances and correlations among the time-invariant covariates as in Chapter 8 and as shown in Equation (9.12).

$$\boldsymbol{\Psi} = \begin{array}{cc|l} \text{Intercept} & \text{Slope} & \\ \hline 1 & 0.30 & \text{Intercept} \\ 0.30 & 0.7861 & \text{Slope} \end{array} \quad (9.12)$$

where the psi ($\boldsymbol{\Psi}$) matrix contains variances and correlations for the latent intercept and latent slope variables. These values are also the same as in Chapter 8 and as shown in Equation (9.13).

$$\mathbf{A} = \begin{array}{ccccc|l} \text{TVC1} & \text{TVC2} & \text{TVC3} & \text{TVC4} & \text{TVC5} & \\ \hline 0.3162 & 0 & 0 & 0 & 0 & \text{RV1} \\ 0 & 0.3162 & 0 & 0 & 0 & \text{RV2} \\ 0 & 0 & 0.3162 & 0 & 0 & \text{RV3} \\ 0 & 0 & 0 & 0.3162 & 0 & \text{RV4} \\ 0 & 0 & 0 & 0 & 0.3162 & \text{RV5} \end{array} \quad (9.13)$$

As shown in the earlier example, the alpha (**A**) matrix in Equation (9.13) contains the standardized slopes for the TVC as predictors of observed RV variances.

$$\boldsymbol{\Phi}_{\text{TVC}} = \begin{array}{ccccc|l} \text{TVC1} & \text{TVC2} & \text{TVC3} & \text{TVC4} & \text{TVC5} & \\ \hline 1 & 0.50 & 0.40 & 0.30 & 0.20 & \text{TVC1} \\ 0.50 & 1 & 0.50 & 0.40 & 0.30 & \text{TVC2} \\ 0.40 & 0.50 & 1 & 0.50 & 0.40 & \text{TVC3} \\ 0.30 & 0.40 & 0.50 & 1 & 0.50 & \text{TVC4} \\ 0.20 & 0.30 & 0.40 & 0.40 & 1 & \text{TVC5} \end{array} \quad (9.14)$$

where the phi matrix for the time-varying covariates ($\mathbf{\Phi}_{TVC}$) specifies the variances and band diagonal correlations among the time-varying covariates consistent with the earlier example. Now the portion of Equation (9.14) in brackets can be solved as follows:

```
Lambda <- matrix(c(
0.7746, 0,
0.6527, 0.265,
0.5352, 0.422,
0.4498, 0.51,
0.3917, 0.561), ncol = 2, byrow = TRUE)

Beta <- matrix(c(
0, 0, 0,
0.225, 0.25, 0.175), nrow = 2, byrow = TRUE)

Phi_TIC <- matrix(c(
1, 0.20, 0.05,
0.20, 1, 0.50,
0.05, 0.50, 1), nrow = 3, byrow = TRUE)

Psi <- matrix(c(
1, 0.30,
0.30, 0.7861 ), nrow = 2, byrow = TRUE)

Alpha <- matrix(c(
0.3162, 0, 0, 0, 0,
0, 0.3162, 0, 0, 0,
0, 0, 0.3162, 0, 0,
0, 0, 0, 0.3162, 0,
0, 0, 0, 0, 0.3162), nrow = 5, byrow = TRUE)

Phi_TVC <- matrix(c(
1, 0.50, 0.40, 0.30, 0.20,
0.50, 1, 0.50, 0.40, 0.30,
0.40, 0.50, 1, 0.50, 0.40,
0.30, 0.40, 0.50, 1, 0.50,
0.20, 0.30, 0.40, 0.50, 1), nrow = 5, byrow = TRUE)
corr_matrix <- Lambda%*%(Beta%*%Phi_TIC%*%t(Beta))%*%t(Lambda)
      +Lambda%*%(Psi)%*%t(Lambda) + Alpha%*%Phi_TVC%*%t(Alpha)

corr_matrix
```

	RV 1	RV 2	RV 3	RV 4	RV 5
RV 1	0.7000	0.6172	0.5526	0.4969	0.4538
RV 2	0.6172	0.7000	0.6363	0.6044	0.5753
RV 3	0.5526	0.6363	0.7000	0.6448	0.6260
RV 4	0.4969	0.6044	0.6448	0.7001	0.6479
RV 5	0.4538	0.5753	0.6260	0.6479	0.7000

So from Equations (9.15) and (9.16),

$$\theta_{RV1} = 1 - 0.7000 = \mathbf{0.3000}$$
$$\theta_{RV2} = 1 - 0.7000 = \mathbf{0.3000}$$
$$\theta_{RV3} = 1 - 0.7000 = \mathbf{0.3000}$$
$$\theta_{RV4} = 1 - 0.7001 = \mathbf{0.2999}$$
$$\theta_{RV5} = 1 - 0.7000 = \mathbf{0.3000}$$

or

$$\boldsymbol{\Theta} = \begin{array}{c} \\ \\ \end{array}\begin{array}{ccccc} \text{RV 1} & \text{RV 2} & \text{RV 3} & \text{RV 4} & \text{RV 5} \\ \left|\begin{array}{ccccc} 0.3000 & 0 & 0 & 0 & 0 \\ 0 & 0.3000 & 0 & 0 & 0 \\ 0 & 0 & 0.3000 & 0 & 0 \\ 0 & 0 & 0 & 0.3000 & 0 \\ 0 & 0 & 0 & 0 & 0.3000 \end{array}\right| \end{array} \begin{array}{c} \\ \text{RV 1} \\ \text{RV 2} \\ \text{RV 3} \\ \text{RV 4} \\ \text{RV 5} \end{array} \quad (9.15)$$

At this point, it would appear that all the necessary information to confirm an admissible longitudinal growth model with time-invariant and time-varying covariates has been obtained. However, although not readily apparent, the above model-reproduced correlation matrix formula makes an unlikely assumption. Specifically, the ($\boldsymbol{\Phi}_{TIC}$) matrix allows correlations among the time-invariant covariates to be specified, and the ($\boldsymbol{\Phi}_{TVC}$) matrix allows a band diagonal correlation structure among the time-varying covariates to also be specified. But notice that nowhere in the above matrix formula is there an opportunity to specify correlations between the time-invariant and time-varying covariates. Both sets of covariates are predicting response variable variance(s) and are likely correlated at a magnitude that should not be assumed to be zero. As stated in previous chapters, knowledge of how to enter the information from the seven matrices for the expanded Grimm et al. (2017) equation above into the model-reproduced correlation matrix equation from Bollen and Curran (2006) can allow for correlations between the time-invariant and time-varying covariates to be specified.

$$\boldsymbol{\Sigma} = \mathbf{P}(\mathbf{I} - \mathbf{B})^{-1}\boldsymbol{\Psi}(\mathbf{I} - \mathbf{B})^{-1T}\mathbf{P}^{T} \quad (9.16)$$

Recall that in the beta (**B**) and psi (**Ψ**) matrices a number of both rows and columns are equal to the number of: response variables (RV1–RV5), time-varying covariates (TVC1–TVC5), time-invariant covariates (treatment [treat], continuous covariate [cont_cov], and the treatment by continuous covariate interaction [INT]), and number of latent variables (intercept and slope), in that order, as shown in Equation (9.17).

B =

RV1	RV2	RV3	RV4	RV5	TVC1	TVC2	TVC3	TVC4	TVC5	TREAT	CONT_COV	INT	I	S	
0	0	0	0	0	0.3162	0	0	0	0	0	0	0	0.7746	0	RV1
0	0	0	0	0	0	0.3162	0	0	0	0	0	0	0.6527	0.265	RV2
0	0	0	0	0	0	0	0.3162	0	0	0	0	0	0.5352	0.422	RV3
0	0	0	0	0	0	0	0	0.3162	0	0	0	0	0.4498	0.51	RV4
0	0	0	0	0	0	0	0	0	0.3162	0	0	0	0.3917	0.561	RV5
0	0	0	0	0	0	0	0	0	0	0	0	0	0	0	TVC1
0	0	0	0	0	0	0	0	0	0	0	0	0	0	0	TVC2
0	0	0	0	0	0	0	0	0	0	0	0	0	0	0	TVC3
0	0	0	0	0	0	0	0	0	0	0	0	0	0	0	TVC4
0	0	0	0	0	0	0	0	0	0	0	0	0	0	0	TVC5
0	0	0	0	0	0	0	0	0	0	0	0	0	0	0	TREAT
0	0	0	0	0	0	0	0	0	0	0	0	0	0	0	CONT_COV
0	0	0	0	0	0	0	0	0	0	0	0	0	0	0	INT
0	0	0	0	0	0	0	0	0	0	0	0	0	0	0	I
0	0	0	0	0	0	0	0	0	0	0.225	0.25	0.175	0	0	S

(A) (A) (B)

RV1	RV2	RV3	RV4	RV5	TVC1	TVC2	TVC3	TVC4	TVC5	TREAT	CONT_COV	INT	I	S	
0.3000	0	0	0	0	0	0	0	0	0	0	0	0	0	0	RV1
0	0.3000	0	0	0	0	0	0	0	0	0	0	0	0	0	RV2
0	0	0.3000	0	0	0	0	0	0	0	0	0	0	0	0	RV3
0	0	0	0.2999	0	0	0	0	0	0	0	0	0	0	0	RV4
0	0	0	0	0.3000	0	0	0	0	0	0	0	0	0	0	RV5
0	0	0	0	0	1	0.50	0.40	0.30	0.20	0.20	0.40	0.30	0	0	TVC1
0	0	0	0	0	0.50	1	0.50	0.40	0.30	0.20	0.40	0.30	0	0	TVC2
0	0	0	0	0	0.40	0.50	1	0.50	0.40	0.20	0.40	0.30	0	0	TVC3
0	0	0	0	0	0.30	0.40	0.50	1	0.50	0.20	0.40	0.30	0	0	TVC4
0	0	0	0	0	0.20	0.30	0.40	0.50	1	0.20	0.40	0.30	0	0	TVC5
0	0	0	0	0	0.20	0.20	0.20	0.20	0.20	1	0.20	0.05	0	0	TREAT
0	0	0	0	0	0.40	0.40	0.40	0.40	0.40	0.20	1	0.50	0	0	CONT_COV
0	0	0	0	0	0.30	0.30	0.30	0.30	0.30	0.05	0.50	1	0	0	INT
0	0	0	0	0	0	0	0	0	0	0	0	0	1	0.30	I
0	0	0	0	0	0	0	0	0	0	0	0	0	0.30	0.7861	S

(Θ) (Φ_{TVC}) (Φ_{TIC}) (Ψ) (9.17)

As shown by the dashed rectangles above, the information contained in the seven matrices that extend Grimm et al.'s (2017) model-reproduced equations can easily be incorporated into Bollen and Curran's (2006) beta (**B**) and psi (**Ψ**) matrices. However, as shown by the solid line rectangles above, Bollen and Curran's psi (**Ψ**) matrix can also allow correlations to be specified between the time-invariant and time-varying covariates (r = .20–.40). Recall also that the identity (**I**) matrix has a number of rows and columns equal to both the beta (**B**) and psi (**Ψ**) matrices, while the **P** ("pick") matrix has a number of columns equal to the number of response variables (RV1–RV5), time-varying covariates (TVC1–TVC5), time-invariant covariates (treatment [treat], continuous covariate [cont_cov], the treatment by continuous covariate interaction [INT]), and number of latent variables (intercept and slope), but it has a number of rows that excludes the latent variables (intercept and slope), as shown in Equations (9.18) and (9.19).

P =

RV1	RV2	RV3	RV4	RV5	TVC1	TVC2	TVC3	TVC4	TVC5	TREAT	CONT_COV	INT	I	S	
1	0	0	0	0	0	0	0	0	0	0	0	0	0	0	RV1
0	1	0	0	0	0	0	0	0	0	0	0	0	0	0	RV2
0	0	1	0	0	0	0	0	0	0	0	0	0	0	0	RV3
0	0	0	1	0	0	0	0	0	0	0	0	0	0	0	RV4
0	0	0	0	1	0	0	0	0	0	0	0	0	0	0	RV5
0	0	0	0	0	1	0	0	0	0	0	0	0	0	0	TVC1
0	0	0	0	0	0	1	0	0	0	0	0	0	0	0	TVC2
0	0	0	0	0	0	0	1	0	0	0	0	0	0	0	TVC3
0	0	0	0	0	0	0	0	1	0	0	0	0	0	0	TVC4
0	0	0	0	0	0	0	0	0	1	0	0	0	0	0	TVC5
0	0	0	0	0	0	0	0	0	0	1	0	0	0	0	TREAT
0	0	0	0	0	0	0	0	0	0	0	1	0	0	0	CONT_COV
0	0	0	0	0	0	0	0	0	0	0	0	1	0	0	INT

(9.18)

I =

RV1	RV2	RV3	RV4	RV5	TVC1	TVC2	TVC3	TVC4	TVC5	TREAT	CONT_COV	INT	I	S	
1	0	0	0	0	0	0	0	0	0	0	0	0	0	0	RV1
0	1	0	0	0	0	0	0	0	0	0	0	0	0	0	RV2
0	0	1	0	0	0	0	0	0	0	0	0	0	0	0	RV3
0	0	0	1	0	0	0	0	0	0	0	0	0	0	0	RV4
0	0	0	0	1	0	0	0	0	0	0	0	0	0	0	RV5
0	0	0	0	0	1	0	0	0	0	0	0	0	0	0	TVC1
0	0	0	0	0	0	1	0	0	0	0	0	0	0	0	TVC2
0	0	0	0	0	0	0	1	0	0	0	0	0	0	0	TVC3
0	0	0	0	0	0	0	0	1	0	0	0	0	0	0	TVC4
0	0	0	0	0	0	0	0	0	1	0	0	0	0	0	TVC5
0	0	0	0	0	0	0	0	0	0	1	0	0	0	0	TREAT
0	0	0	0	0	0	0	0	0	0	0	1	0	0	0	CONT_COV
0	0	0	0	0	0	0	0	0	0	0	0	1	0	0	INT
0	0	0	0	0	0	0	0	0	0	0	0	0	1	0	I
0	0	0	0	0	0	0	0	0	0	0	0	0	0	1	S

(9.19)

Now that all information has been entered into Bollen and Curran's (2006) beta (**B**) and psi (**Ψ**) matrices, their model-reproduced correlation matrix equation can be solved as follows, as shown in Equation (9.20):

```
Beta <- matrix(c(
0, 0, 0, 0, 0, 0.3162, 0, 0, 0, 0, 0, 0, 0.7746, 0,
0, 0, 0, 0, 0, 0, 0.3162, 0, 0, 0, 0, 0, 0.6527, 0.265,
0, 0, 0, 0, 0, 0, 0, 0.3162, 0, 0, 0, 0, 0.5352, 0.422,
0, 0, 0, 0, 0, 0, 0, 0, 0.3162, 0, 0, 0, 0.4498, 0.51,
0, 0, 0, 0, 0, 0, 0, 0, 0, 0.3162, 0, 0, 0, 0.3917, 0.561,
0, 0, 0, 0, 0, 0, 0, 0, 0, 0, 0, 0, 0, 0,
0, 0, 0, 0, 0, 0, 0, 0, 0, 0, 0, 0, 0, 0,
0, 0, 0, 0, 0, 0, 0, 0, 0, 0, 0, 0, 0, 0,
0, 0, 0, 0, 0, 0, 0, 0, 0, 0, 0, 0, 0, 0,
0, 0, 0, 0, 0, 0, 0, 0, 0, 0, 0, 0, 0, 0,
0, 0, 0, 0, 0, 0, 0, 0, 0, 0, 0, 0, 0, 0,
0, 0, 0, 0, 0, 0, 0, 0, 0, 0, 0, 0, 0, 0,
0, 0, 0, 0, 0, 0, 0, 0, 0, 0, 0, 0, 0, 0,
0, 0, 0, 0, 0, 0, 0, 0, 0, 0, 0, 0, 0, 0,
0, 0, 0, 0, 0, 0, 0, 0, 0, 0.225, 0.25, 0.175, 0, 0), ncol = 15, byrow = TRUE)

Psi <- matrix(c(
0.3000, 0, 0, 0, 0, 0, 0, 0, 0, 0, 0, 0, 0, 0,
0, 0.3000, 0, 0, 0, 0, 0, 0, 0, 0, 0, 0, 0, 0,
0, 0, 0.3000, 0, 0, 0, 0, 0, 0, 0, 0, 0, 0, 0,
0, 0, 0, 0.2999, 0, 0, 0, 0, 0, 0, 0, 0, 0, 0,
0, 0, 0, 0, 0.3000, 0, 0, 0, 0, 0, 0, 0, 0, 0,
0, 0, 0, 0, 0, 1, 0.50, 0.40, 0.30, 0.20, 0.20, 0.40, 0.30, 0, 0,
0, 0, 0, 0, 0, 0.50, 1, 0.50, 0.40, 0.30, 0.20, 0.40, 0.30, 0, 0,
0, 0, 0, 0, 0, 0.40, 0.50, 1, 0.50, 0.40, 0.20, 0.40, 0.30, 0, 0,
0, 0, 0, 0, 0, 0.30, 0.40, 0.50, 1, 0.50, 0.20, 0.40, 0.30, 0, 0,
0, 0, 0, 0, 0, 0.20, 0.30, 0.40, 0.50, 1, 0.20, 0.40, 0.30, 0, 0,
0, 0, 0, 0, 0, 0.20, 0.20, 0.20, 0.20, 0.20, 1, 0.20, 0.05, 0, 0,
0, 0, 0, 0, 0, 0.40, 0.40, 0.40, 0.40, 0.40, 0.20, 1, 0.50, 0, 0,
0, 0, 0, 0, 0, 0.30, 0.30, 0.30, 0.30, 0.30, 0.05, 0.50, 1, 0, 0,
0, 0, 0, 0, 0, 0, 0, 0, 0, 0, 0, 0, 1, 0.30,
0, 0, 0, 0, 0, 0, 0, 0, 0, 0, 0, 0, 0.30, 0.7861), ncol = 15, byrow = TRUE)
```

```
P <- matrix(c(
1, 0, 0, 0, 0, 0, 0, 0, 0, 0, 0, 0, 0, 0, 0,
0, 1, 0, 0, 0, 0, 0, 0, 0, 0, 0, 0, 0, 0, 0,
0, 0, 1, 0, 0, 0, 0, 0, 0, 0, 0, 0, 0, 0, 0,
0, 0, 0, 1, 0, 0, 0, 0, 0, 0, 0, 0, 0, 0, 0,
0, 0, 0, 0, 1, 0, 0, 0, 0, 0, 0, 0, 0, 0, 0,
0, 0, 0, 0, 0, 1, 0, 0, 0, 0, 0, 0, 0, 0, 0,
0, 0, 0, 0, 0, 0, 1, 0, 0, 0, 0, 0, 0, 0, 0,
0, 0, 0, 0, 0, 0, 0, 1, 0, 0, 0, 0, 0, 0, 0,
0, 0, 0, 0, 0, 0, 0, 0, 1, 0, 0, 0, 0, 0, 0,
0, 0, 0, 0, 0, 0, 0, 0, 0, 1, 0, 0, 0, 0, 0,
0, 0, 0, 0, 0, 0, 0, 0, 0, 0, 1, 0, 0, 0, 0,
0, 0, 0, 0, 0, 0, 0, 0, 0, 0, 0, 1, 0, 0, 0,
0, 0, 0, 0, 0, 0, 0, 0, 0, 0, 0, 0, 1, 0, 0), ncol = 15, byrow = TRUE)

I <- matrix(c(
1, 0, 0, 0, 0, 0, 0, 0, 0, 0, 0, 0, 0, 0, 0,
0, 1, 0, 0, 0, 0, 0, 0, 0, 0, 0, 0, 0, 0, 0,
0, 0, 1, 0, 0, 0, 0, 0, 0, 0, 0, 0, 0, 0, 0,
0, 0, 0, 1, 0, 0, 0, 0, 0, 0, 0, 0, 0, 0, 0,
0, 0, 0, 0, 1, 0, 0, 0, 0, 0, 0, 0, 0, 0, 0,
0, 0, 0, 0, 0, 1, 0, 0, 0, 0, 0, 0, 0, 0, 0,
0, 0, 0, 0, 0, 0, 1, 0, 0, 0, 0, 0, 0, 0, 0,
0, 0, 0, 0, 0, 0, 0, 1, 0, 0, 0, 0, 0, 0, 0,
0, 0, 0, 0, 0, 0, 0, 0, 1, 0, 0, 0, 0, 0, 0,
0, 0, 0, 0, 0, 0, 0, 0, 0, 1, 0, 0, 0, 0, 0,
0, 0, 0, 0, 0, 0, 0, 0, 0, 0, 1, 0, 0, 0, 0,
0, 0, 0, 0, 0, 0, 0, 0, 0, 0, 0, 1, 0, 0, 0,
0, 0, 0, 0, 0, 0, 0, 0, 0, 0, 0, 0, 1, 0, 0,
0, 0, 0, 0, 0, 0, 0, 0, 0, 0, 0, 0, 0, 1, 0,
0, 0, 0, 0, 0, 0, 0, 0, 0, 0, 0, 0, 0, 0, 1), ncol = 15, byrow = TRUE)

corr_matrix <- P %*% (solve(I-Beta)) %*% Psi %*%t(solve(I-Beta)) %*%t(P)

corr_matrix
```

Σ = (9.20)

	RV1	RV2	RV3	RV4	RV5	TVC1	TVC2	TVC3	TVC4	TVC5	TREAT	CONT_ COV	INT
RV1	1.0000	0.6337025	0.5789769	0.5287729	0.4888067	0.3162	0.1581	0.12648	0.09486	0.06324	0.06324	0.12648	0.09486
RV2	0.6337025	**1.0331**	0.6792335	0.6527531	0.6269007	0.2104375	0.3685375	0.2104375	0.1788175	0.1471975	0.1384338	0.2278425	0.1773413
RV3	0.5789769	0.6792335	**1.0527**	0.7029855	0.6874329	0.209825	0.241445	0.399545	0.241445	0.209825	0.1829825	0.287895	0.2262075
RV4	0.5287729	0.6527531	0.7029855	**1.0636**	0.7148135	0.195585	0.227205	0.258825	0.416925	0.258825	0.2079525	0.321555	0.2535975
RV5	0.4888067	0.6269007	0.6874329	0.7148135	**1.0701**	0.1740375	0.2056575	0.2372775	0.2688975	0.4269975	0.2224238	0.3410625	0.2694712
TVC1	0.3162	0.2104375	0.209825	0.195585	0.1740375	1	0.5	0.4	0.3	0.2	0.2	0.4	0.3
TVC2	0.1581	0.3685375	0.241445	0.227205	0.2056575	0.5	1	0.5	0.4	0.3	0.2	0.4	0.3
TVC3	0.12648	0.2104375	0.399545	0.258825	0.2372775	0.4	0.5	1	0.5	0.4	0.2	0.4	0.3
TVC4	0.09486	0.1788175	0.241445	0.416925	0.2688975	0.3	0.4	0.5	1	0.5	0.2	0.4	0.3
TVC5	0.06324	0.1471975	0.209825	0.258825	0.4269975	0.2	0.3	0.4	0.5	1	0.2	0.4	0.3
TREAT	0.06324	0.1384338	0.1829825	0.2079525	0.2224238	0.2	0.2	0.2	0.2	0.2	1	0.2	0.05
CONT_ COV	0.12648	0.2278425	0.287895	0.321555	0.3410625	0.4	0.4	0.4	0.4	0.4	0.2	1	0.5
INT	0.09486	0.1773413	0.2262075	0.2535975	0.2694712	0.3	0.3	0.3	0.3	0.3	0.05	0.5	1

As shown above by bold underlined terms, using values based on an expansion of Grimm et al.'s (2017) model-reproduced equations that do not take into account the likely correlations between the time-invariant and time-varying covariates have resulted in model-reproduced variances for RV2–RV5 that are larger than one. Notice how the psi (**Ψ**) matrix, which contains residual variance estimates from Grimm et al.'s theta (**Θ**) matrix, is not an additive term but a multiplier in Bollen and Curran's (2006) equation, which complicates matters. However, after a bit of trial and error, the underlined and bold values below will result in the correct correlation matrix, as shown in Equation (9.21):

```
Beta <- matrix(c(
0, 0, 0, 0, 0, 0.3162, 0, 0, 0, 0, 0, 0, 0.7746, 0,
0, 0, 0, 0, 0, 0, 0.3162, 0, 0, 0, 0, 0, 0.6527, 0.265,
0, 0, 0, 0, 0, 0, 0, 0.3162, 0, 0, 0, 0, 0.5352, 0.422,
0, 0, 0, 0, 0, 0, 0, 0, 0.3162, 0, 0, 0, 0.4498, 0.51,
0, 0, 0, 0, 0, 0, 0, 0, 0, 0.3162, 0, 0, 0, 0.3917, 0.561,
0, 0, 0, 0, 0, 0, 0, 0, 0, 0, 0, 0, 0, 0, 0,
0, 0, 0, 0, 0, 0, 0, 0, 0, 0, 0, 0, 0, 0, 0,
0, 0, 0, 0, 0, 0, 0, 0, 0, 0, 0, 0, 0, 0, 0,
0, 0, 0, 0, 0, 0, 0, 0, 0, 0, 0, 0, 0, 0, 0,
0, 0, 0, 0, 0, 0, 0, 0, 0, 0, 0, 0, 0, 0, 0,
0, 0, 0, 0, 0, 0, 0, 0, 0, 0, 0, 0, 0, 0, 0,
0, 0, 0, 0, 0, 0, 0, 0, 0, 0, 0, 0, 0, 0, 0,
0, 0, 0, 0, 0, 0, 0, 0, 0, 0, 0, 0, 0, 0, 0,
0, 0, 0, 0, 0, 0, 0, 0, 0, 0, 0, 0, 0, 0, 0,
0, 0, 0, 0, 0, 0, 0, 0, 0, 0, 0.225, 0.25, 0.175, 0, 0), ncol = 15, byrow = TRUE)

Psi <- matrix(c(
0.3000, 0, 0, 0, 0, 0, 0, 0, 0, 0, 0, 0, 0, 0, 0,
0, 0.2696, 0, 0, 0, 0, 0, 0, 0, 0, 0, 0, 0, 0, 0,
0, 0, 0.2540, 0, 0, 0, 0, 0, 0, 0, 0, 0, 0, 0, 0,
0, 0, 0, 0.2461, 0, 0, 0, 0, 0, 0, 0, 0, 0, 0, 0,
0, 0, 0, 0, 0.2419, 0, 0, 0, 0, 0, 0, 0, 0, 0, 0,
0, 0, 0, 0, 0, 1, 0.50, 0.40, 0.30, 0.20, 0.20, 0.40, 0.30, 0, 0,
0, 0, 0, 0, 0, 0.50, 1, 0.50, 0.40, 0.30, 0.20, 0.40, 0.30, 0, 0,
0, 0, 0, 0, 0, 0.40, 0.50, 1, 0.50, 0.40, 0.20, 0.40, 0.30, 0, 0,
0, 0, 0, 0, 0, 0.30, 0.40, 0.50, 1, 0.50, 0.20, 0.40, 0.30, 0, 0,
0, 0, 0, 0, 0, 0.20, 0.30, 0.40, 0.50, 1, 0.20, 0.40, 0.30, 0, 0,
0, 0, 0, 0, 0, 0.20, 0.20, 0.20, 0.20, 0.20, 0.25, 0.20, 0.05, 0, 0,
0, 0, 0, 0, 0, 0.40, 0.40, 0.40, 0.40, 0.40, 0.20, 1, 0.50, 0, 0,
0, 0, 0, 0, 0, 0.30, 0.30, 0.30, 0.30, 0.30, 0.05, 0.50, 1, 0, 0,
0, 0, 0, 0, 0, 0, 0, 0, 0, 0, 0, 0, 0, 1, 0.30,
0, 0, 0, 0, 0, 0, 0, 0, 0, 0, 0, 0, 0, 0.30, 0.7861), ncol = 15, byrow = TRUE)

P <- matrix(c(
1, 0, 0, 0, 0, 0, 0, 0, 0, 0, 0, 0, 0, 0, 0,
0, 1, 0, 0, 0, 0, 0, 0, 0, 0, 0, 0, 0, 0, 0,
0, 0, 1, 0, 0, 0, 0, 0, 0, 0, 0, 0, 0, 0, 0,
0, 0, 0, 1, 0, 0, 0, 0, 0, 0, 0, 0, 0, 0, 0,
0, 0, 0, 0, 1, 0, 0, 0, 0, 0, 0, 0, 0, 0, 0,
0, 0, 0, 0, 0, 1, 0, 0, 0, 0, 0, 0, 0, 0, 0,
0, 0, 0, 0, 0, 0, 1, 0, 0, 0, 0, 0, 0, 0, 0,
0, 0, 0, 0, 0, 0, 0, 1, 0, 0, 0, 0, 0, 0, 0,
0, 0, 0, 0, 0, 0, 0, 0, 1, 0, 0, 0, 0, 0, 0,
0, 0, 0, 0, 0, 0, 0, 0, 0, 1, 0, 0, 0, 0, 0,
0, 0, 0, 0, 0, 0, 0, 0, 0, 0, 1, 0, 0, 0, 0,
0, 0, 0, 0, 0, 0, 0, 0, 0, 0, 0, 1, 0, 0, 0,
0, 0, 0, 0, 0, 0, 0, 0, 0, 0, 0, 0, 1, 0, 0), ncol = 15, byrow = TRUE)
```

```
I <- matrix(c(
1, 0, 0, 0, 0, 0, 0, 0, 0, 0, 0, 0, 0, 0, 0,
0, 1, 0, 0, 0, 0, 0, 0, 0, 0, 0, 0, 0, 0, 0,
0, 0, 1, 0, 0, 0, 0, 0, 0, 0, 0, 0, 0, 0, 0,
0, 0, 0, 1, 0, 0, 0, 0, 0, 0, 0, 0, 0, 0, 0,
0, 0, 0, 0, 1, 0, 0, 0, 0, 0, 0, 0, 0, 0, 0,
0, 0, 0, 0, 0, 1, 0, 0, 0, 0, 0, 0, 0, 0, 0,
0, 0, 0, 0, 0, 0, 1, 0, 0, 0, 0, 0, 0, 0, 0,
0, 0, 0, 0, 0, 0, 0, 1, 0, 0, 0, 0, 0, 0, 0,
0, 0, 0, 0, 0, 0, 0, 0, 1, 0, 0, 0, 0, 0, 0,
0, 0, 0, 0, 0, 0, 0, 0, 0, 1, 0, 0, 0, 0, 0,
0, 0, 0, 0, 0, 0, 0, 0, 0, 0, 1, 0, 0, 0, 0,
0, 0, 0, 0, 0, 0, 0, 0, 0, 0, 0, 1, 0, 0, 0,
0, 0, 0, 0, 0, 0, 0, 0, 0, 0, 0, 0, 1, 0, 0,
0, 0, 0, 0, 0, 0, 0, 0, 0, 0, 0, 0, 0, 1, 0,
0, 0, 0, 0, 0, 0, 0, 0, 0, 0, 0, 0, 0, 0, 1), ncol = 15, byrow = TRUE)

corr_matrix <- P %*% (solve(I-Beta)) %*% Psi %*%t(solve(I-Beta)) %*%t(P)

corr_matrix
```

$\Sigma =$

	RV1	RV2	RV3	RV4	RV5	TVC1	TVC2	TVC3	TVC4	TVC5	TREAT	CONT_COV	INT
RV1	1	0.6337025	0.5789769	0.5287729	0.4888067	0.3162	0.1581	0.12648	0.09486	0.06324	0.06324	0.12648	0.09486
RV2	0.6337025	1	0.6749874	0.6476216	0.6212561	0.2104375	0.3685375	0.2104375	0.1788175	0.1471975	0.093715	0.2278425	0.1773413
RV3	0.5789769	0.6749874	1	0.6948138	0.6784441	0.209825	0.241445	0.399545	0.241445	0.209825	0.11177	0.287895	0.2262075
RV4	0.5287729	0.6476216	0.6948138	1	0.7039502	0.195585	0.227205	0.258825	0.416925	0.258825	0.12189	0.321555	0.2535975
RV5	0.4888067	0.6212561	0.6784441	0.7039502	1	0.1740375	0.2056575	0.2372775	0.2688975	0.4269975	0.127755	0.3410625	0.2694712
TVC1	0.3162	0.2104375	0.209825	0.195585	0.1740375	1	0.5	0.4	0.3	0.2	0.2	0.4	0.3
TVC2	0.1581	0.3685375	0.241445	0.227205	0.2056575	0.5	1	0.5	0.4	0.3	0.2	0.4	0.3
TVC3	0.12648	0.2104375	0.399545	0.258825	0.2372775	0.4	0.5	1	0.5	0.4	0.2	0.4	0.3
TVC4	0.09486	0.1788175	0.241445	0.416925	0.2688975	0.3	0.4	0.5	1	0.5	0.2	0.4	0.3
TVC5	0.06324	0.1471975	0.209825	0.258825	0.4269975	0.2	0.3	0.4	0.5	1	0.2	0.4	0.3
TREAT	0.06324	0.093715	0.11177	0.12189	0.127755	0.2	0.2	0.2	0.2	0.2	0.25	0.2	0.05
CONT_COV	0.12648	0.2278425	0.287895	0.321555	0.3410625	0.4	0.4	0.4	0.4	0.4	0.2	1	0.5
INT	0.09486	0.1773413	0.2262075	0.2535975	0.2694712	0.3	0.3	0.3	0.3	0.3	0.05	0.5	1

(9.21)

Mplus Monte Carlo Power Analysis: Adding Time-Varying Covariates

Now that the correct model-reproduced correlation matrix has been computed by confirming an admissible analysis model, all of the information contained in the matrices above can be converted into Mplus Monte Carlo simulation power analysis syntax.

```
TITLE: MPLUS 9.1 TVC

MONTECARLO:
NAMES ARE
RV_1-RV_5
TVC_1 - TVC_5
TREAT CONT_COV INT;
OBSERVATIONS = 560;
NREPS = 5000;
MISSING = RV_2 RV_3 RV_4 RV_5;
CUTPOINTS = TREAT(0);
```

The initial lines of syntax are the same as those for the final interaction model from Chapter 8 with two exceptions: the time-varying covariates (TVC_1 - TVC_5) are added to the model, and based on the inclusion of the time-varying covariates, a decrease in the sample size needed ($N = 560$) to reject the null hypothesis for the treatment by continuous covariate interaction (INT) with power ≥ .80 is expected.

```
MODEL POPULATION:

[RV_1-RV_5@0];

!Lambda Matrix;
I BY RV_1@.7746 RV_2@.6527 RV_3@.5352 RV_4@.4498 RV_5@.3917;
S BY RV_1@0 RV_2@.265 RV_3@.422 RV_4@.51 RV_5@.561;
```

Recall from previous chapters that the first line of syntax in the MODEL POPULATION: command fixes all response variable means to zero so that a linear growth model can be specified placing standardized values from the lambda (**Λ**) matrix after the BY statements in the next two lines.

```
!Alpha Matrix;
RV_1 ON TVC_1*0.3162(1);
RV_2 ON TVC_2*0.3162(1);
RV_3 ON TVC_3*0.3162(1);
RV_4 ON TVC_4*0.3162(1);
RV_5 ON TVC_5*0.3162(1);
```

The next five lines of syntax specify the time-varying covariates (TVC1 – TVC5) as predictors of response variable variances based on values taken from the alpha (**A**) matrix. The values of one in parentheses (1) constrain each time point specific prediction to equality over time in the data generation process.

```
!Beta Matrix;
S ON TREAT*0.225 CONT_COV*0.25 INT*0.175;
```

The next line of syntax specifies the binary treatment indicator (TREAT), the continuous covariate (CONT_COV), and the interaction between those two variables (INT) as predictors of linear slope variance using values taken from the beta (**B**) matrix.

```
!Psi Matrix;
I*1;
S*0.7861;
I WITH S*.30;
```

These syntax lines specify latent intercept (I) variance, latent slope (S) residual variance, and the correlation between the intercept and slope (I WITH S) using values from the psi (**Ψ**) matrix.

```
!Phi_TIC Matrix;
TREAT*1;
CONT_COV*1;
INT*1;
TREAT WITH CONT_COV*0.20 INT*0.05;
CONT_COV WITH INT*0.50;
```

The first three lines of syntax in the next section specify unit time-invariant covariate variances, and the next two lines specify correlations among the time-invariant covariates based on values from the phi_TIC ($\mathbf{\Phi}_{\text{TIC}}$) matrix.

```
!Phi_TVC;
TVC_1*1;
TVC_2*1;
TVC_3*1;
TVC_4*1;
TVC_5*1;

TVC_1 WITH TVC_2*.50 TVC_3*.40 TVC_4*.30 TVC_5*.20;
TVC_2 WITH TVC_3*.50 TVC_4*.40 TVC_5*.30;
TVC_3 WITH TVC_4*.50 TVC_5*.40;
TVC_4 WITH TVC_5*.50;
```

The next nine syntax lines specify time-varying covariate (TVC) variances (first five lines) and correlations (last four lines) based on values from the phi_TVC ($\mathbf{\Phi}_{\text{TVC}}$) matrix.

```
!TIC & TVC correlations;
TREAT WITH TVC_1 - TVC_5*.20;
CONT_COV WITH TVC_1 - TVC_5*.40;
INT WITH TVC_1 - TVC_5*.30
```

The next three lines of syntax allow band diagonal correlations between the time-invariant and time-varying covariates to be specified based on the Bollen and Curran (2006) version of the psi ($\mathbf{\Psi}$) matrix (values enclosed within Equations 9.17 and 9.18).

```
!Theta Matrix;
RV_1*.3;
RV_2*.2696;
RV_3*.2540;
RV_4*.2461;
RV_5*.2419;
```

The final five lines specify the response variable residual variances based on values from the theta ($\mathbf{\Theta}$) matrix.

```
MODEL MISSING:
[RV_2*-2.9444]; !5% MCAR;
[RV_3*-2.1972]; !10% MCAR;
[RV_4*-1.7346]; !15% MCAR;
[RV_5*-1.3862]; !20% MCAR;
```

```
!MAR
RV_2 ON RV_1*0.0953;
RV_3 ON RV_2*0.0953 RV_1*0.0953;
RV_4 ON RV_3*0.0953 RV_2*0.0953 RV_1*0.0953;
RV_5 ON RV_4*0.0953 RV_3*0.0953 RV_2*0.0953 RV_1*0.0953;
```

The missing data specifications remain the same as in the final example from Chapter 8. The first four syntax lines in brackets specify MCAR missing data that increase monotonically from 5 to 20% at all postbaseline assessments. The next four lines change the missing data specifications from MCAR to MAR. The `ON` statements specify a ($exp^{0.0953} = 1.10$) 10% increase in the odds of missing data at a given assessment time point per unit response variable increase at any previous time point.

```
MODEL:
[RV_1-RV_5@0];

!Lambda Matrix;
I BY RV_1@.7746 RV_2@.6527 RV_3@.5352 RV_4@.4498 RV_5@.3917;
S BY RV_1@0 RV_2@.265 RV_3@.422 RV_4@.51 RV_5@.561;

!Beta Matrix;
S ON TREAT*0.225 CONT_COV*0.25 INT*0.175;

!Alpha Matrix;
RV_1 ON TVC_1*0.3162(1);
RV_2 ON TVC_2*0.3162(1);
RV_3 ON TVC_3*0.3162(1);
RV_4 ON TVC_4*0.3162(1);
RV_5 ON TVC_5*0.3162(1);
```

Only the information contained in Grimm et al.'s (2017) lambda (**Λ**), beta (**B**), and alpha (**Α**) matrices, all of which can be found in Bollen and Curran's (2006) beta (**B**) matrix, needs to be specified in the `MODEL:` command. The complete Mplus syntax is shown below, followed by the syntax results and an example write-up.

```
TITLE: MPLUS 9.1 TVC

MONTECARLO:
NAMES ARE
RV_1-RV_5
TVC_1 - TVC_5
TREAT CONT_COV INT;
OBSERVATIONS = 560;
NREPS = 5000;
MISSING = RV_2 RV_3 RV_4 RV_5;
CUTPOINTS = TREAT(0);

MODEL POPULATION:

[RV_1-RV_5@0];
```

```
!Lambda Matrix;
I BY RV_1@.7746 RV_2@.6527 RV_3@.5352 RV_4@.4498 RV_5@.3917;
S BY RV_1@0 RV_2@.265 RV_3@.422 RV_4@.51 RV_5@.561;

!Alpha Matrix;
RV_1 ON TVC_1*0.3162(1);
RV_2 ON TVC_2*0.3162(1);
RV_3 ON TVC_3*0.3162(1);
RV_4 ON TVC_4*0.3162(1);
RV_5 ON TVC_5*0.3162(1);

!Beta Matrix;
S ON TREAT*0.225 CONT_COV*0.25 INT*0.175;

!Psi Matrix;
I*1;
S*0.7861;
I WITH S*.30;

!Phi_TIC Matrix;
TREAT*1;
CONT_COV*1;
INT*1;
TREAT WITH CONT_COV*0.20 INT*0.05;
CONT_COV WITH INT*0.50;

!Phi_TVC;
TVC_1*1;
TVC_2*1;
TVC_3*1;
TVC_4*1;
TVC_5*1;

TVC_1 WITH TVC_2*.50 TVC_3*.40 TVC_4*.30 TVC_5*.20;
TVC_2 WITH TVC_3*.50 TVC_4*.40 TVC_5*.30;
TVC_3 WITH TVC_4*.50 TVC_5*.40;
TVC_4 WITH TVC_5*.50;

!TIC & TVC correlations;
TREAT WITH TVC_1 - TVC_5*.20;
CONT_COV WITH TVC_1 - TVC_5*.40;
INT WITH TVC_1 - TVC_5*.30

!Theta Matrix;
RV_1*.3;
RV_2*.2696;
RV_3*.2540;
RV_4*.2461;
RV_5*.2419;
```

```
MODEL MISSING:
[RV_2*-2.9444]; !5% MCAR;
[RV_3*-2.1972]; !10% MCAR;
[RV_4*-1.7346]; !15% MCAR;
[RV_5*-1.3862]; !20% MCAR;

!MAR
RV_2 ON RV_1*0.0953;
RV_3 ON RV_2*0.0953 RV_1*0.0953;
RV_4 ON RV_3*0.0953 RV_2*0.0953 RV_1*0.0953;
RV_5 ON RV_4*0.0953 RV_3*0.0953 RV_2*0.0953 RV_1*0.0953;

MODEL:

[RV_1-RV_5@0];

!Lambda Matrix;
I BY RV_1@.7746 RV_2@.6527 RV_3@.5352 RV_4@.4498 RV_5@.3917;
S BY RV_1@0 RV_2@.265 RV_3@.422 RV_4@.51 RV_5@.561;

!Beta Matrix;
S ON TREAT*0.225 CONT_COV*0.25 INT*0.175;

!Alpha Matrix;
RV_1 ON TVC_1*0.3162(1);
RV_2 ON TVC_2*0.3162(1);
RV_3 ON TVC_3*0.3162(1);
RV_4 ON TVC_4*0.3162(1);
RV_5 ON TVC_5*0.3162(1);
```

		ESTIMATES		S. E.	M. S. E.	95%	% Sig
	Population	Average	Std. Dev.	Average		Cover	Coeff
S ON							
TREAT	0.225	0.2212	0.0775	0.0763	0.0060	0.951	0.817
CONT_COV	0.250	0.2490	0.0626	0.0625	0.0039	0.949	0.980
INT	**0.175**	0.1753	0.0624	0.0619	0.0039	0.949	**0.804**

R Monte Carlo Power Analysis: Adding Time-Varying Covariates Issues

As also happened with a similar model in Chapter 8, a problem emerged in the R simulation in this example, due to the correlation between treatment and the continuous covariate. Although possible to simulate correlated predictor variables, it was not possible to set a population correlation value between the binary treatment and continuous covariate in the context of the more complex SEM model, nor was it possible to allow the binary treatment and continuous covariate covary in the sample models. The analysis and results differed from those found in Mplus and they are not included in the text of this chapter; the online supplemental materials include more information and detail (see *www.guilford.com/peugh-materials*).

Longitudinal Time-Varying Covariates Simulation Power Analysis Write-Up

"The power analysis question involved the smallest sample size needed to achieve power ≥ .80 to detect a standardized 'treatment effect by control covariate' interaction in a longitudinal randomized control trial. A Monte Carlo simulation power analysis was conducted using Mplus (version 8.6) assuming: (1) standardization of all response variables at all five assessment time points, (2) linear trend best-captured response variable average changes over time and explained 60% of observed adherence response variable variance, on average, (3) random assignment results in equal sample sizes for both the treatment and control groups, (4) the magnitude of the standardized (β) effect of binary treatment randomization on linear slope variance is expected to be at least $\beta \geq 0.225$ and explain at least ($R^2 = .05$) 5% of linear slope variance, (5) the inclusion of a control covariate measured on a continuous scale will explain an additional ($R^2 = .085$) 8.5% of linear slope variance ($\beta \geq 0.25$), (6) inclusion of the 'treatment effect by control covariate' interaction ($\beta \geq 0.175$) will explain an additional ($R^2 = .079$) 7.9% of linear slope variance, (7) inclusion of time-varying covariates will explain an additional ($R^2 = .10$) 10% of response variable variance, (8) correlations among the time-varying covariates follows a band diagonal structure where adjacent time-varying covariate values are more highly correlated ($r = .50$) than time-varying covariate values separated by one ($r = .40$) or two ($r = .30$) assessment time points, (9) correlations between the time-varying and time-invariant covariates ranged between ($r = .20$–$.40$), and (10) missing data are assumed to be (a) 0% at the initial assessment, (b) 5% at the first postbaseline assessment, (c) monotonically increasing in 5% increments to 20% at the final assessment, and (d) missing at random, such that unit increases in response variable values at any previous assessment time point are assumed to result in a 10% increase in the odds of missing data. Monte Carlo simulation power analysis results aggregated over 5,000 dataset replications showed power ≥ .80 to detect a standardized 'binary treatment randomization by continuous covariate' interaction effect of $\beta \geq 0.175$ if all assumptions are met and proper missing data handling makes a sample size of $N = 560$ ($n = 280$ for both treatment and control groups) available for analysis."

Mplus Monte Carlo Power Analysis: A Random Effect Model

A useful feature available in Mplus is the ability to allow parameter estimates to vary randomly across participants, to estimate the amount of variation, and to allow the variation to be predicted by other analysis variable in the model. For example, suppose a researcher wanted to allow the effect of the time-varying covariates as predictors of response variable variance (i.e., $\beta = 0.3162$) to vary randomly across participants (*Side Note: For those familiar with multilevel or hierarchical linear modeling, this is conceptually the same as allowing the effect of a level 1 predictor to vary randomly across level 2 units*). Such an extension of the previous time-invariant and time-varying covariates model is shown in Figure 9.5.

Notice how the effect for the time-varying covariates (i.e., $\beta = 0.3162$) has been removed from each of the arrows specifying the time-varying covariates as predictors of response

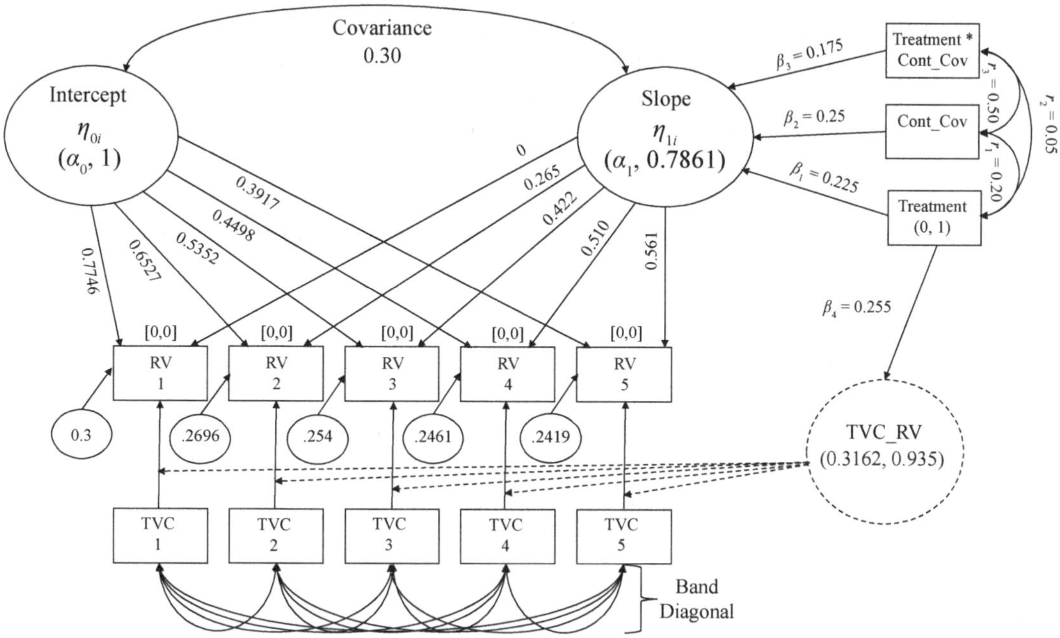

FIGURE 9.5. A random effects longitudinal growth curve model.

variable variances. Time-varying covariate effect random variation (TVC_RV) across participants is now estimated, as indicated by both the dashed circle and dashed arrows pointing to the time-varying covariate prediction arrows. Notice also how the standardized coefficient for the effect of the time-varying covariates as predictors of response variable variation (i.e., $\beta = 0.3162$) is now included in the dashed circle as the mean or average effect, as was specified in the previous power analysis example. But now that effect is allowed to vary randomly across participants. Under standardization, a researcher would assume unit variance for the time-varying covariate effect. However, notice also how a researcher has specified a standardized effect of ($\beta_4 = 0.255$) for the binary treatment indicator as a predictor of time-varying covariate effect variance. As the only predictor, a standardized effect estimate of ($\beta_4 = 0.255$) means a researcher expects treatment to explain $R^2 =$ 6.5% (i.e., $\sqrt{0.065} = 0.255$) of time-varying covariate effect variance, leaving ($1 - 0.065 = 0.935$) 0.935 residual variance. That value is also included in the dashed circle. Taken together, the values contained in the dashed circle (0.3162, 0.935) specify the mean and the residual variance of the time-varying covariate effect. A model such as this one would answer research questions such as whether there is a further incremental effect of treatment for participants with higher time-varying covariate scores.

Typically, the next step in the power analysis process would be to verify the admissibility of the proposed model using model-reproduced correlation matrix equations, but there is no model-reproduced equation for the proposed model. Allowing the effect of the time-varying covariates to vary randomly across participants raises the possibility of several model-reproduced matrix possibilities. However, this is not a concern for the present example for two reasons. First, as shown in the previous chapters, all aspects of the model other than the random variation in the time-varying covariate effect have been verified as admissible. Second, assuming unit variance for the effect of the time-varying covariates and a reasonable standardized effect for treatment as a predictor, correctly computing residual variance for the random effect (TVC_RV) is straightforward. Stated differently, a researcher at this point would have no reason to suspect an inadmissible model.

Furthermore, as shown below, only a few alterations to the previous Mplus syntax for the time-invariant and time-varying covariate model are needed to specify a random effect model.

```
ANALYSIS:
TYPE = RANDOM;
```

None of the previous power analysis examples required specifications to the `ANALYSIS:` command. For this model example, the `TYPE = RANDOM;` specification is needed to allow random variation in the effects for the time-varying covariates.

```
!Alpha Matrix;
TVC_RV | RV_1 ON TVC_1(1);
TVC_RV | RV_2 ON TVC_2(1);
TVC_RV | RV_3 ON TVC_3(1);
TVC_RV | RV_4 ON TVC_4(1);
TVC_RV | RV_5 ON TVC_5(1);

[TVC_RV*0.3162];
TVC_RV*0.935;

TVC_RV ON TREAT*0.255;
```

The five lines of Mplus syntax that specified each time-varying covariate as a predictor of its respective response variable based on values from the alpha matrix in the previous analysis example (i.e., `RV_1 ON TVC_1*0.3162(1);`, ... `RV_5 ON TVC_5*0.3162(1);`) are now replaced by the eight lines above in both the `MODEL POPULATION:` and the `MODEL:` commands. The first five lines of Mplus syntax above state that random variation in the effects of the time-varying covariates (TVC_RV) is measured by (|) the effects of the time-varying covariates as predictors of response variable variances constrained to equality over time (`RV_1 ON TVC_1*0.3162(1);`, ... `RV_5 ON TVC_5*0.3162(1);`). The final three lines state that the average effect for the time-varying covariates as predictors of response variable variances is 0.3162 (`[TVC_RV*0.3162];`), but instead of specifying unit variance, the residual variance for `TVC_RV` is specified to be 0.935 (`TVC_RV*0.935;`) because the expected standardized effect for the binary treatment variable as a predictor of `TVC_RV` variation is $\beta_4 = 0.255$, which is expected to explain $R^2 = 6.5\%$ of `TVC_RV` variance, as described above. The complete Mplus syntax for a random effects model, followed by syntax results and an example write-up is shown here.

```
MONTECARLO:
NAMES ARE
RV_1-RV_5
```

```
TVC_1 - TVC_5
TREAT CONT_COV INT;
OBSERVATIONS = 560;
NREPS = 5000;
MISSING = RV_2 RV_3 RV_4 RV_5;
CUTPOINTS = TREAT(0);

MODEL POPULATION:

[RV_1-RV_5@0];

!Lambda Matrix;
I BY RV_1@.7746 RV_2@.6527 RV_3@.5352 RV_4@.4498 RV_5@.3917;
S BY RV_1@0 RV_2@.265 RV_3@.422 RV_4@.51 RV_5@.561;

!Alpha Matrix;
TVC_RV | RV_1 ON TVC_1(1);
TVC_RV | RV_2 ON TVC_2(1);
TVC_RV | RV_3 ON TVC_3(1);
TVC_RV | RV_4 ON TVC_4(1);
TVC_RV | RV_5 ON TVC_5(1);

[TVC_RV*0.3162];
TVC_RV*0.935;

TVC_RV ON TREAT*0.255;

!Beta Matrix;
S ON TREAT*0.225 CONT_COV*0.25 INT*0.175;

!Psi Matrix;
I*1;
S*0.7861;
I WITH S*.30;

!Phi_TIC Matrix;
TREAT*1;
CONT_COV*1;
INT*1;
TREAT WITH CONT_COV*0.20 INT*0.05;
CONT_COV WITH INT*0.50;

!Phi_TVC;
TVC_1*1;
TVC_2*1;
TVC_3*1;
TVC_4*1;
TVC_5*1;

TVC_1 WITH TVC_2*.50 TVC_3*.40 TVC_4*.30 TVC_5*.20;
TVC_2 WITH TVC_3*.50 TVC_4*.40 TVC_5*.30;
TVC_3 WITH TVC_4*.50 TVC_5*.40;
TVC_4 WITH TVC_5*.50;
```

```
!TIC & TVC correlations;
TREAT WITH TVC_1 - TVC_5*.20;
CONT_COV WITH TVC_1 - TVC_5*.40;
INT WITH TVC_1 - TVC_5*.30

!Theta Matrix;
RV_1*.3;
RV_2*.2696;
RV_3*.2540;
RV_4*.2461;
RV_5*.2419;

MODEL MISSING:
[RV_2*-2.9444]; !5% MCAR;
[RV_3*-2.1972]; !10% MCAR;
[RV_4*-1.7346]; !15% MCAR;
[RV_5*-1.3862]; !20% MCAR;

!MAR
RV_2 ON RV_1*0.0953;
RV_3 ON RV_2*0.0953 RV_1*0.0953;
RV_4 ON RV_3*0.0953 RV_2*0.0953 RV_1*0.0953;
RV_5 ON RV_4*0.0953 RV_3*0.0953 RV_2*0.0953 RV_1*0.0953;

MODEL:

[RV_1-RV_5@0];

!Lambda Matrix;
I BY RV_1@.7746 RV_2@.6527 RV_3@.5352 RV_4@.4498 RV_5@.3917;
S BY RV_1@0 RV_2@.265 RV_3@.422 RV_4@.51 RV_5@.561;

!Beta Matrix;
S ON TREAT*0.225 CONT_COV*0.25 INT*0.175;

!Alpha Matrix;
TVC_RV | RV_1 ON TVC_1(1);
TVC_RV | RV_2 ON TVC_2(1);
TVC_RV | RV_3 ON TVC_3(1);
TVC_RV | RV_4 ON TVC_4(1);
TVC_RV | RV_5 ON TVC_5(1);

[TVC_RV*0.3162];

TVC_RV*0.935;
TVC_RV ON TREAT*0.255;
```

	Population	ESTIMATES Average	Std. Dev.	S. E. Average	M. S. E.	95% Cover	% Sig Coeff
TVC_RV ON							
TREAT	**0.255**	0.2582	0.0903	0.0903	0.0082	0.949	**0.807**

R Monte Carlo Power Analysis: Random Effect Model Issues

Just as in the earlier example, a problem emerged in the R simulation in this example, due primarily to the correlation between treatment and the continuous covariate. Although it was possible to simulate correlated predictor variables, it was not possible to set a population correlation value between the binary treatment and continuous covariate in the context of the more complex SEM model, nor was it possible to allow the binary treatment and continuous covariate covary in the sample models.

Longitudinal Random Effect Model Simulation Power Analysis Write-Up

> "The power analysis question involved the smallest sample size needed to achieve power ≥ .80 to detect a standardized effect of $\beta \geq 0.255$ for the effect of a binary treatment group indicator as a predictor of random variation in the effects of time-varying covariates in a longitudinal randomized control trial. A Monte Carlo simulation power analysis was conducted using Mplus (version 8.6) assuming: (1) standardization of all response variables at all five assessment time points, (2) linear trend best-captured response variable average changes over time and explained 60% of observed adherence response variable variance, on average, (3) random assignment results in equal sample sizes for both the treatment and control groups, (4) the magnitude of the standardized (β) effect of binary treatment randomization on linear slope variance is expected to be at least $\beta \geq 0.225$ and explain at least ($R^2 = 0.05$) 5% of linear slope variance, (5) the inclusion of a control covariate measured on a continuous scale will explain an additional ($R^2 = 0.085$) 8.5% of linear slope variance ($\beta \geq 0.25$), (6) including the 'treatment effect by control covariate' interaction ($\beta \geq 0.175$) will explain an additional ($R^2 = 0.079$) 7.9% of linear slope variance, (7) inclusion of time-varying covariates will explain an additional ($R^2 = 0.10$) 10% of response variable variance, (8) correlations among the time-varying covariates follows a band diagonal structure where adjacent time-varying covariate values are more highly correlated ($r = .50$) than time-varying covariate values separated by one ($r = .40$) or two ($r = .30$) assessment time points, (9) correlations between the time-varying and time-invariant covariates ranged between ($r = .20$–$.40$), (10) assumption of unit variance for the random effect of the time-varying covariates, a standardized slope of ($\beta = 0.255$) for treatment as a predictor will explain ($R^2 = 0.065$) 6.5% of time-varying covariate variance, and (11) missing data are assumed to be (a) 0% at the initial assessment, (b) 5% at the first postbaseline assessment, (c) monotonically increasing in 5% increments to 20% at the final assessment, and (d) missing at random, such that unit increases in response variable values at any previous assessment time point are assumed to result in a 10% increase in the odds of missing data. Monte Carlo simulation power analysis results aggregated over 5,000 dataset replications showed power ≥ .80 to detect a standardized effect of $\beta \geq 0.255$ for treatment as a predictor of time-varying covariate effect variance if all assumptions are met and proper missing data handling makes a sample size of $N = 560$ ($n = 280$ for both treatment and control groups) available for analysis."

SUGGESTED READINGS

- Baird, R., & Maxwell, S. E. (2016). Performance of time-varying predictors in multilevel models under an assumption of fixed or random effects. *Psychological Methods, 21,* 175–188.
- Bauer, D. J., Gottfredson, N. C., Dean, D., & Zucker, R. A. (2013). Analyzing repeated measures data on individuals nested within groups: Accounting for dynamic group effects. *Psychological Methods, 18,* 1–14.
- Bianconcini, S., & Bollen, K. A. (2018). The latent variable-autoregressive latent trajectory model: A general framework for longitudinal data analysis. *Structural Equation Modeling: A Multidisciplinary Journal, 25,* 791–808.
- Dziak, J. J., Li, R., Tan, X., Shiffman, S., & Shiyko, M. P. (2015). Modeling intensive longitudinal data with mixtures of nonparametric trajectories and time-varying effects. *Psychological Methods, 20,* 444–469.
- Feingold, A. (2009). Effect sizes for growth-modeling analysis for controlled clinical trials in the same metric as for classical analysis. *Psychological Methods, 14,* 43–53.
- Feingold, A. (2019). Time-varying effect sizes for quadratic growth models in multilevel and latent growth modeling. *Structural Equation Modeling: A Multidisciplinary Journal, 26,* 418–429.
- Koch, T., Holtmann, J., Bohn, J., & Eid, M. (2018). Explaining general and specific factors in longitudinal, multimethod, and bifactor models: Some caveats and recommendations. *Psychological Methods, 23,* 505–523.
- McNeish, D., & Kelley, K. (2019). Fixed effects models versus mixed effects models for clustered data: Reviewing the approaches, disentangling the differences, and making recommendations. *Psychological Methods, 24,* 20–35.
- McNeish, D., & Matta, T. H. (2020). Flexible treatment of time-varying covariates with time unstructured data. *Structural Equation Modeling: A Multidisciplinary Journal, 27,* 298–317.
- Tan, X., Shiyko, M. P., Li, R., Li, Y., & Dierker, L. (2012). A time-varying effect model for intensive longitudinal data. *Psychological Methods, 17,* 61–77.
- Wu, W., West, S. G., & Taylor, A. B. (2009). Evaluating model fit for growth curve models: Integration of fit indices from SEM and MLM frameworks. *Psychological Methods, 14,* s183–s201.

10

Parallel-Process Mediation

Chapter 9 showed how the inclusion of time-varying covariates to a longitudinal growth model that tests the effects of one or more time-invariant covariates allows for control of the influence of potential confounding variables. This affords researchers the advantages of both estimating a more accurate picture of response variable change over time and also allows the interpretation of the effects of time-invariant covariates after having controlled for such time-varying confounds. Correlations among the time-varying covariates were specified as having a band diagonal structure in the alpha (**A**) matrix from Grimm et al. (2017). But as also shown in Chapter 9, likely correlations between the time-invariant and time-varying covariates could also be within the psi ($\boldsymbol{\Psi}$) matrix from Bollen and Curran (2006). The two key points of emphasis from Chapter 9 were: (1) knowledge that the model-reproduced matrix equations from both Grimm et al. (2017) and Bollen and Curran (2006) were shown to be both advantageous and necessary, and (2) adjustments made to the response variable residual variance estimates using simple subtraction resulted in an admissible model and enabled power for a longitudinal model that included both time-invariant and time-varying covariates to be estimated.

Recall that Chapter 2 showed how to estimate statistical power for comparing changes between two groups (e.g., treatment and control) across multiple correlated response variables: a multivariate two-group comparison power analysis model. The thinking behind that model was predicated on the idea that researchers are often interested in how treatment impacts two or more correlated response variables that occur simultaneously. Applying this cross-sectional line of thought to a longitudinal growth model could involve estimating a second growth model for what would have been time-varying covariates and allowing the growth curve models for both the response variable and the time-varying covariates to correlate, which is known as a *parallel-process growth model* (also called *multivariate latent curve models*, see Bollen & Curran, 2006, pp. 198–207). Time-invariant covariates could predict trajectory variation for both the response variable and time-varying covariate. But parallel-process growth models also allow predictions between growth trajectory components, such as allowing the intercept of one growth process to predict the linear slope of the other growth process for example. Such analyses can answer research questions such as whether a participant's initial status on one variable predicts their rate of change on a second variable. Parallel-process growth models can also be expanded to answer research questions such as whether the effects of initial status on one variable and its effect on change over time on a second variable is mediated by one or more intervening predictor variables.

To illustrate, let's assume a researcher wants to start from the assumption that linear change will explain 60% of the variance in their response variable (RV1) of interest, as shown in Figure 10.1.

Let's further assume that a researcher wants to estimate a second longitudinal growth model (RV2) for a second response variable rather than include the second variable as time-varying covariates (TVC). Because the researcher has less a priori information about change over time, let's assume a researcher takes a conservative approach and assumes linear change will explain 50% of variance in the second variable, as shown in Figure 10.2.

Recall from Chapter 7 that both models shown here have already been verified *separately* as admissible growth models through model-reproduced correlation matrix equations. Focusing only on the trajectory components of both growth models, an unconditional parallel-process growth model would estimate both growth curves simultaneously as well as all possible trajectory component correlations between the two growth processes, as shown in see Figure 10.3.

An important first step, even though the separate RV1 and RV2 models shown above have been verified as admissible in Chapter 7, is to verify the admissibility of combining the two models into an unconditional parallel-process growth model. As will be shown, the model-reproduced matrix equation from Bollen and Curran (2006) will be needed to combine the longitudinal growth curve parameter estimate specifications from both the RV1 and RV2 models. Recall from previous chapters that Bollen and Curran's beta (**B**) matrix specifies predictive relationships between observed and latent trajectory variables,

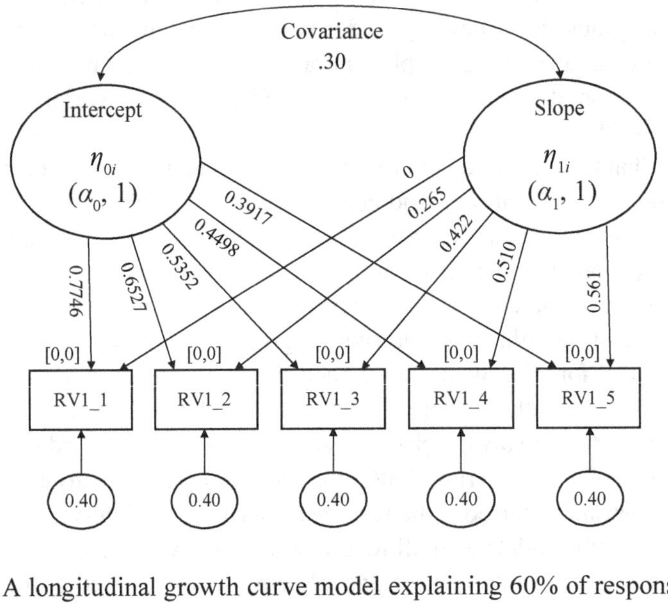

FIGURE 10.1. A longitudinal growth curve model explaining 60% of response variable variance.

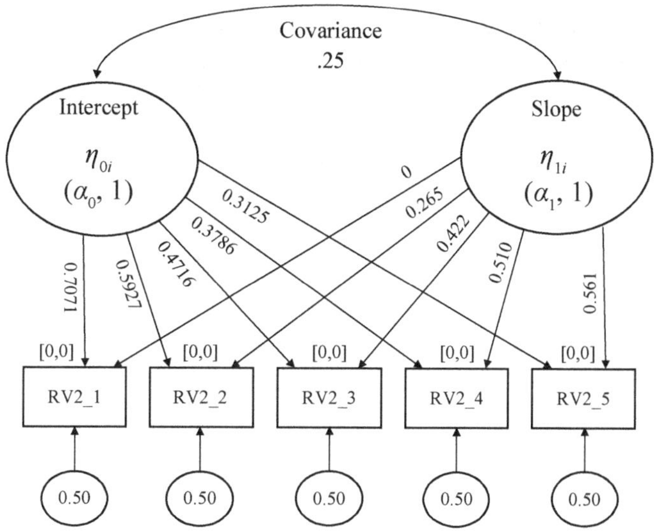

FIGURE 10.2. A longitudinal growth curve model explaining 50% of response variable variance.

while the psi (**Ψ**) matrix specifies covariances/correlations and residual variances. It is important to remember the order of variable entry into both of Bollen and Curran's beta (**B**) and psi (**Ψ**) matrices: all observed response variables, all time-varying covariates, all time-invariant covariates, all intercepts, all slopes, and then all additional latent trajectory components (quadratic, cubic, etc.) as needed. Let's assume that RV1 represents depression scores (DEP), and RV2 represents sluggish cognitive tempo (SCT; now referred to as *cognitive disengagement syndrome*) both collected over time and modeled as separate but parallel

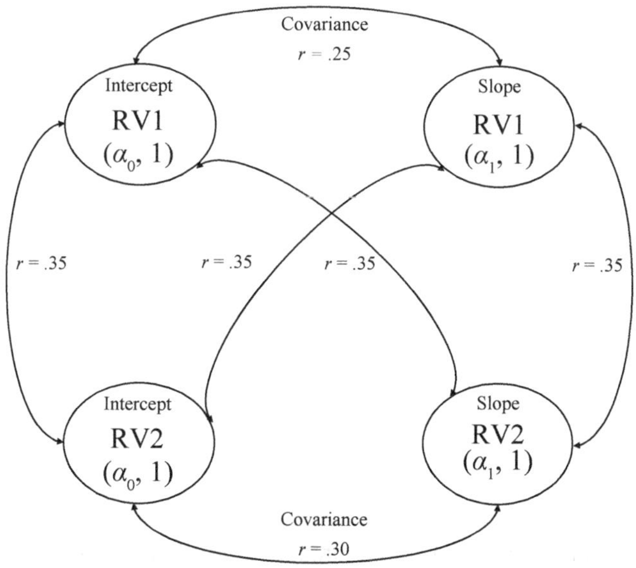

FIGURE 10.3. A conceptual parallel-process trajectory correlations model.

growth curve processes. Verifying the admissibility of the unconditional parallel-process growth model shown here involves dealing only with observed response variables, latent intercepts (INT), and latent slopes (SLOPE) as shown in Equations (10.1–10.4).

$\Lambda_{SCT} + \Lambda_{DEP}$

B =

	SCT1	SCT2	SCT3	SCT4	SCT5	DEP1	DEP2	DEP3	DEP4	DEP5	INT_{SCT}	INT_{DEP}	$SLOPE_{SCT}$	$SLOPE_{DEP}$
SCT1	0	0	0	0	0	0	0	0	0	0	0.7071	0	0	0
SCT2	0	0	0	0	0	0	0	0	0	0	0.5927	0	0.265	0
SCT3	0	0	0	0	0	0	0	0	0	0	0.4716	0	0.422	0
SCT4	0	0	0	0	0	0	0	0	0	0	0.3786	0	0.510	0
SCT5	0	0	0	0	0	0	0	0	0	0	0.3125	0	0.561	0
DEP1	0	0	0	0	0	0	0	0	0	0	0	0.7746	0	0
DEP2	0	0	0	0	0	0	0	0	0	0	0	0.6527	0	0.265
DEP3	0	0	0	0	0	0	0	0	0	0	0	0.5352	0	0.422
DEP4	0	0	0	0	0	0	0	0	0	0	0	0.4498	0	0.510
DEP5	0	0	0	0	0	0	0	0	0	0	0	0.3917	0	0.561
INT_{SCT}	0	0	0	0	0	0	0	0	0	0	0	0	0	0
INT_{DEP}	0	0	0	0	0	0	0	0	0	0	0	0	0	0
$SLOPE_{SCT}$	0	0	0	0	0	0	0	0	0	0	0	0	0	0
$SLOPE_{DEP}$	0	0	0	0	0	0	0	0	0	0	0	0	0	0

(10.1)

$\theta_{SCT} + \theta_{DEP}$

ψ =

	SCT1	SCT2	SCT3	SCT4	SCT5	DEP1	DEP2	DEP3	DEP4	DEP5	INT_{SCT}	INT_{DEP}	$SLOPE_{SCT}$	$SLOPE_{DEP}$
SCT1	0.50	0	0	0	0	0	0	0	0	0	0	0	0	0
SCT2	0	0.50	0	0	0	0	0	0	0	0	0	0	0	0
SCT3	0	0	0.50	0	0	0	0	0	0	0	0	0	0	0
SCT4	0	0	0	0.50	0	0	0	0	0	0	0	0	0	0
SCT5	0	0	0	0	0.50	0	0	0	0	0	0	0	0	0
DEP1	0	0	0	0	0	0.40	0	0	0	0	0	0	0	0
DEP2	0	0	0	0	0	0	0.40	0	0	0	0	0	0	0
DEP3	0	0	0	0	0	0	0	0.40	0	0	0	0	0	0
DEP4	0	0	0	0	0	0	0	0	0.40	0	0	0	0	0
DEP5	0	0	0	0	0	0	0	0	0	0.40	0	0	0	0
INT_{SCT}	0	0	0	0	0	0	0	0	0	0	1	0.35	0.25	0.35
INT_{DEP}	0	0	0	0	0	0	0	0	0	0	0.35	1	0.35	0.30
$SLOPE_{SCT}$	0	0	0	0	0	0	0	0	0	0	0.25	0.35	1	0.35
$SLOPE_{DEP}$	0	0	0	0	0	0	0	0	0	0	0.35	0.30	0.35	1

$\Phi_{SCT} + \Phi_{DEP}$

(10.2)

I =

	SCT1	SCT2	SCT3	SCT4	SCT5	DEP1	DEP2	DEP3	DEP4	DEP5	INT_{SCT}	INT_{DEP}	$SLOPE_{SCT}$	$SLOPE_{DEP}$
SCT1	1	0	0	0	0	0	0	0	0	0	0	0	0	0
SCT2	0	1	0	0	0	0	0	0	0	0	0	0	0	0
SCT3	0	0	1	0	0	0	0	0	0	0	0	0	0	0
SCT4	0	0	0	1	0	0	0	0	0	0	0	0	0	0
SCT5	0	0	0	0	1	0	0	0	0	0	0	0	0	0
DEP1	0	0	0	0	0	1	0	0	0	0	0	0	0	0
DEP2	0	0	0	0	0	0	1	0	0	0	0	0	0	0
DEP3	0	0	0	0	0	0	0	1	0	0	0	0	0	0
DEP4	0	0	0	0	0	0	0	0	1	0	0	0	0	0
DEP5	0	0	0	0	0	0	0	0	0	1	0	0	0	0
INT_{SCT}	0	0	0	0	0	0	0	0	0	0	1	0	0	0
INT_{DEP}	0	0	0	0	0	0	0	0	0	0	0	1	0	0
$SLOPE_{SCT}$	0	0	0	0	0	0	0	0	0	0	0	0	1	0
$SLOPE_{DEP}$	0	0	0	0	0	0	0	0	0	0	0	0	0	1

(10.3)

P =

	SCT1	SCT2	SCT3	SCT4	SCT5	DEP1	DEP2	DEP3	DEP4	DEP5	INT_{SCT}	INT_{DEP}	$SLOPE_{SCT}$	$SLOPE_{DEP}$
SCT1	1	0	0	0	0	0	0	0	0	0	0	0	0	0
SCT2	0	1	0	0	0	0	0	0	0	0	0	0	0	0
SCT3	0	0	1	0	0	0	0	0	0	0	0	0	0	0
SCT4	0	0	0	1	0	0	0	0	0	0	0	0	0	0
SCT5	0	0	0	0	1	0	0	0	0	0	0	0	0	0
DEP1	0	0	0	0	0	1	0	0	0	0	0	0	0	0
DEP2	0	0	0	0	0	0	1	0	0	0	0	0	0	0
DEP3	0	0	0	0	0	0	0	1	0	0	0	0	0	0
DEP4	0	0	0	0	0	0	0	0	1	0	0	0	0	0
DEP5	0	0	0	0	0	0	0	0	0	1	0	0	0	0

(10.4)

As shown in these equations, a key advantage to Bollen and Curran's (2006) model-reproduced matrix equation is the ease with which what would be separate lambda (**Λ**), theta (**Θ**), and phi (**Φ**) matrices for SCT and depression using Grimm et al.'s (2017) equations can be combined and integrated into the flexible beta (**B**) and psi (**Ψ**) matrices. Also shown in Equation (10.3) is the identity (**I**) matrix, which has the same number of rows and columns as the beta (**B**) and psi (**Ψ**) matrices with values of one on the main diagonal, while the "pick" (**P**) matrix in Equation (10.4) has the same number of columns as beta (**B**) and psi (**Ψ**), but the number of rows are equal only to the number of observed variables, and having values of one on the main diagonal similar to the (**I**) matrix.

As shown in previous chapters, Bollen and Curran's (2006) model-reproduced (**Σθ**) matrix Equation (7.5), which is shown again here; [see also Equation (10.5)].

$$\mathbf{\Sigma\theta} = \mathbf{P}(\mathbf{I} - \mathbf{B})^{-1}\mathbf{\Psi}(\mathbf{I} - \mathbf{B})^{-1\mathrm{T}}\mathbf{P}^{\mathrm{T}}$$

can be solved using the information in the above matrices together with the following R code:

```
Beta <- matrix(c(
0, 0, 0, 0, 0, 0, 0, 0, 0, 0, 0.7071, 0, 0, 0,
0, 0, 0, 0, 0, 0, 0, 0, 0, 0, 0.5927, 0, 0.265, 0,
0, 0, 0, 0, 0, 0, 0, 0, 0, 0, 0.4716, 0, 0.422, 0,
0, 0, 0, 0, 0, 0, 0, 0, 0, 0, 0.3786, 0, 0.510, 0,
0, 0, 0, 0, 0, 0, 0, 0, 0, 0, 0.3125, 0, 0.561, 0,
0, 0, 0, 0, 0, 0, 0, 0, 0, 0, 0, 0.7746, 0, 0,
0, 0, 0, 0, 0, 0, 0, 0, 0, 0, 0, 0.6527, 0, 0.265,
0, 0, 0, 0, 0, 0, 0, 0, 0, 0, 0, 0.5352, 0, 0.422,
0, 0, 0, 0, 0, 0, 0, 0, 0, 0, 0, 0.4498, 0, 0.510,
0, 0, 0, 0, 0, 0, 0, 0, 0, 0, 0, 0.3917, 0, 0.561,
0, 0, 0, 0, 0, 0, 0, 0, 0, 0, 0, 0, 0, 0,
0, 0, 0, 0, 0, 0, 0, 0, 0, 0, 0, 0, 0, 0,
0, 0, 0, 0, 0, 0, 0, 0, 0, 0, 0, 0, 0, 0,
0, 0, 0, 0, 0, 0, 0, 0, 0, 0, 0, 0, 0, 0), ncol = 14, byrow = TRUE)

Psi <- matrix(c(
0.50, 0, 0, 0, 0, 0, 0, 0, 0, 0, 0, 0, 0, 0,
0, 0.50, 0, 0, 0, 0, 0, 0, 0, 0, 0, 0, 0, 0,
0, 0, 0.50, 0, 0, 0, 0, 0, 0, 0, 0, 0, 0, 0,
0, 0, 0, 0.50, 0, 0, 0, 0, 0, 0, 0, 0, 0, 0,
0, 0, 0, 0, 0.50, 0, 0, 0, 0, 0, 0, 0, 0, 0,
0, 0, 0, 0, 0, 0.40, 0, 0, 0, 0, 0, 0, 0, 0,
0, 0, 0, 0, 0, 0, 0.40, 0, 0, 0, 0, 0, 0, 0,
0, 0, 0, 0, 0, 0, 0, 0.40, 0, 0, 0, 0, 0, 0,
0, 0, 0, 0, 0, 0, 0, 0, 0.40, 0, 0, 0, 0, 0,
0, 0, 0, 0, 0, 0, 0, 0, 0, 0.40, 0, 0, 0, 0,
0, 0, 0, 0, 0, 0, 0, 0, 0, 0, 1, 0.35, 0.25, 0.35,
0, 0, 0, 0, 0, 0, 0, 0, 0, 0, 0.35, 1, 0.35, 0.30,
0, 0, 0, 0, 0, 0, 0, 0, 0, 0, 0.25, 0.35, 1, 0.35,
0, 0, 0, 0, 0, 0, 0, 0, 0, 0, 0.35, 0.30, 0.35, 1), ncol = 14, byrow = TRUE)

P <- matrix(c(
1, 0, 0, 0, 0, 0, 0, 0, 0, 0, 0, 0, 0, 0,
0, 1, 0, 0, 0, 0, 0, 0, 0, 0, 0, 0, 0, 0,
0, 0, 1, 0, 0, 0, 0, 0, 0, 0, 0, 0, 0, 0,
0, 0, 0, 1, 0, 0, 0, 0, 0, 0, 0, 0, 0, 0,
```

```
0, 0, 0, 0, 1, 0, 0, 0, 0, 0, 0, 0, 0, 0,
0, 0, 0, 0, 0, 1, 0, 0, 0, 0, 0, 0, 0, 0,
0, 0, 0, 0, 0, 0, 1, 0, 0, 0, 0, 0, 0, 0,
0, 0, 0, 0, 0, 0, 0, 1, 0, 0, 0, 0, 0, 0,
0, 0, 0, 0, 0, 0, 0, 0, 1, 0, 0, 0, 0, 0,
0, 0, 0, 0, 0, 0, 0, 0, 0, 1, 0, 0, 0, 0), ncol = 14, byrow = TRUE)

I <- matrix(c(
1, 0, 0, 0, 0, 0, 0, 0, 0, 0, 0, 0, 0, 0,
0, 1, 0, 0, 0, 0, 0, 0, 0, 0, 0, 0, 0, 0,
0, 0, 1, 0, 0, 0, 0, 0, 0, 0, 0, 0, 0, 0,
0, 0, 0, 1, 0, 0, 0, 0, 0, 0, 0, 0, 0, 0,
0, 0, 0, 0, 1, 0, 0, 0, 0, 0, 0, 0, 0, 0,
0, 0, 0, 0, 0, 1, 0, 0, 0, 0, 0, 0, 0, 0,
0, 0, 0, 0, 0, 0, 1, 0, 0, 0, 0, 0, 0, 0,
0, 0, 0, 0, 0, 0, 0, 1, 0, 0, 0, 0, 0, 0,
0, 0, 0, 0, 0, 0, 0, 0, 1, 0, 0, 0, 0, 0,
0, 0, 0, 0, 0, 0, 0, 0, 0, 1, 0, 0, 0, 0,
0, 0, 0, 0, 0, 0, 0, 0, 0, 0, 1, 0, 0, 0,
0, 0, 0, 0, 0, 0, 0, 0, 0, 0, 0, 1, 0, 0,
0, 0, 0, 0, 0, 0, 0, 0, 0, 0, 0, 0, 1, 0,
0, 0, 0, 0, 0, 0, 0, 0, 0, 0, 0, 0, 0, 1), ncol = 14, byrow = TRUE)

corr_matrix <- P %*% (solve(I-Beta)) %*% Psi %*%t(solve(I-Beta)) %*%t(P)

corr_matrix
```

$\Sigma\Theta =$

	SCT1	SCT2	SCT3	SCT4	SCT5	DEP1	DEP2	DEP3	DEP4	DEP5
SCT1	1	0.4659	0.4081	0.3579	0.3201	0.1917	0.2271	0.2369	0.2375	0.2358
SCT2	0.4659	1	0.4851	0.4602	0.4377	0.2325	0.2755	0.2873	0.2881	0.2860
SCT3	0.4081	0.4851	1	0.4938	0.4832	0.2423	0.2870	0.2994	0.3002	0.2980
SCT4	0.3579	0.4602	0.4938	1	0.4974	0.2409	0.2854	0.2977	0.2985	0.2963
SCT5	0.3201	0.4377	0.4832	0.4974	1	02368	0.2806	0.2926	0.2934	0.2913
DEP1	0.1917	0.2325	0.2423	0.2409	0.2368	1	0.5672	0.5126	0.4669	0.4338
DEP2	0.2271	0.2755	0.2870	0.2854	0.2806	0.5672	1	0.5863	0.5644	0.5453
DEP3	0.2369	0.2873	0.2994	0.2977	0.2926	0.5126	0.5863	1	0.5948	0.55860
DEP4	0.2375	0.2881	0.3002	0.2985	0.2934	0.4669	0.5644	0.5948	1	0.5979
DEP5	0.2358	0.2860	0.2980	0.2963	0.2913	0.4338	0.5453	0.55860	0.5979	1

(10.5)

As shown here, the results from solving Bollen and Curran's (2006) model-reproduced correlation matrix equation for an unconditional parallel-process model confirms that the model is admissible. These unconditional parallel-process growth curve model could be modified to allow the intercepts of the two processes to predict the slopes of the opposite process as shown. Such parallel-process models answer research questions about whether a participant's initial status on one variable impacts the change over time on another (see Figure 10.4).

But for illustration purposes, the parallel-process power analysis shown below will expand further on the trajectory prediction model shown above to determine the sample size needed for power ≥ .80 to reject the null hypothesis that the influence of the intercept for the first variable (RV1; depression [DEP]) on the slope of the second variable (RV2; slug-

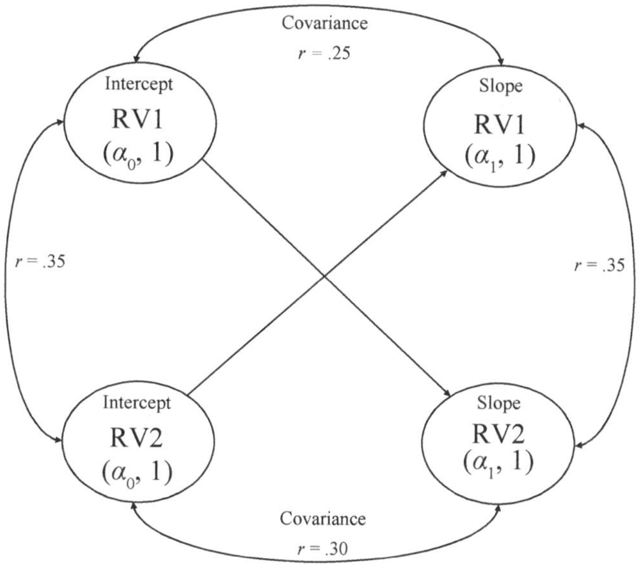

FIGURE 10.4. A conceptual parallel-process trajectory prediction model.

gish cognitive tempo [SCT]) is mediated by two observed covariates based on research by Becker et al. (2016).

A Parallel-Process Power Analysis Based on Becker et al. (2016)

Using a meta-analysis, Becker and colleagues (2016) sought to establish the psychometric validity and diagnostic viability of a construct called *sluggish cognitive tempo* (SCT; now referred to as *cognitive disengagement syndrome*). Through a systematic review of the published research, the authors sought to both identify symptomatology unique to SCT, and to further clarify the relationship between SCT and the diagnosis of ADHD—Inattentive Type as well as internalizing psychological symptoms such as depression. The authors found 13 symptoms associated with SCT, ranging from tendencies to daydream and underachievement to difficulties following directions and slow task completion. Among the many additional conclusions resulting from the meta-analysis, two were of particular interest for further research. First, as stated by Becker and colleagues (2016, p. 173, *italics added*): "It would be interesting to know whether the *developmental progression* of SCT *parallels* the progression of depressive symptoms . . . ." This statement suggests that depression scores should not be considered as time-varying covariates in a longitudinal growth model that examines changes over time in SCT, but rather changes over time in both SCT and depression scores should be estimated simultaneously to enable predictive relationships among the trajectory components of both to be estimated. Second, as also stated by the authors (p. 174): "There is some indication that SCT is linked to social withdrawal specifically, but this needs to be further evaluated. . . ."

Pursuant to the meta-analysis conclusions, Becker[1] and colleagues proposed a parallel-process model to answer research questions on whether social withdrawal (WithDr) and self-reported loneliness (LoneLin) mediate the relationship between SCT initial status and changes in depression scores over time. Assuming linear trend explains 60% of the variance in depression scores and 50% of the variance in SCT scores collected over time, the analysis model proposed to answer the research question is shown in (see Figures 10.5 to 10.7). Figure 10.5 shows the sluggish cognitive tempo growth curve model, Figure 10.6 shows the depression growth curve model, and Figure 10.7 shows the mediated parallel-process growth curve model.

Several aspects of the parallel-process mediation model shown in Figure 10.7 warrant clarification. First, notice how large effect size correlations (r = .50) are specified for correlation between the intercepts and slopes for SCT and depression scores. These inferences are a direct result from the conclusions drawn from Becker et al. (2016). Second, the alpha (α_1 and α_2) and beta (β_1 and β_2) paths are needed to form the mediated pathways for withdrawal ($\alpha_1 * \beta_1$) and loneliness ($\alpha_2 * \beta_2$). The symbol tau prime (τ') refers to the effect of SCT initial status as a predictor of depression score changes over time in the presence of one or more mediating variables. Finally, notice the question mark (?) that indicates that depression score residual slope variance will need to be calculated using Wright's path tracing rules.

However, before applying path tracing rules, a researcher must specify standardized relationships for the alpha, beta, and tau prime predictions, as well as the correlation between social withdrawal and loneliness. Let's assume, based on meta-analysis results, pilot data analyses, a published literature search, or limits testing on feasible participant

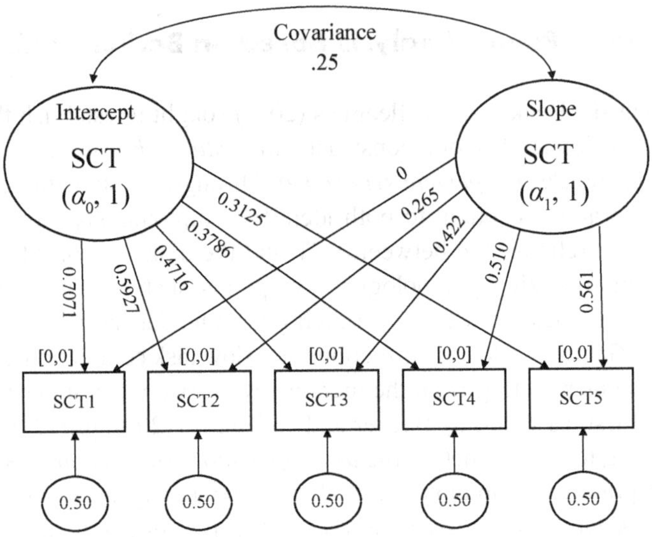

FIGURE 10.5. Sluggish cognitive tempo growth curve model.

[1] Special thanks to Stephen Becker for granting permission to use a modified version of the power analysis submitted for "Longitudinal Examination of Sluggish Cognitive Tempo and Internalizing Psychopathology in Adolescence," National Institute of Mental Health (NIMH), R01MH122415.

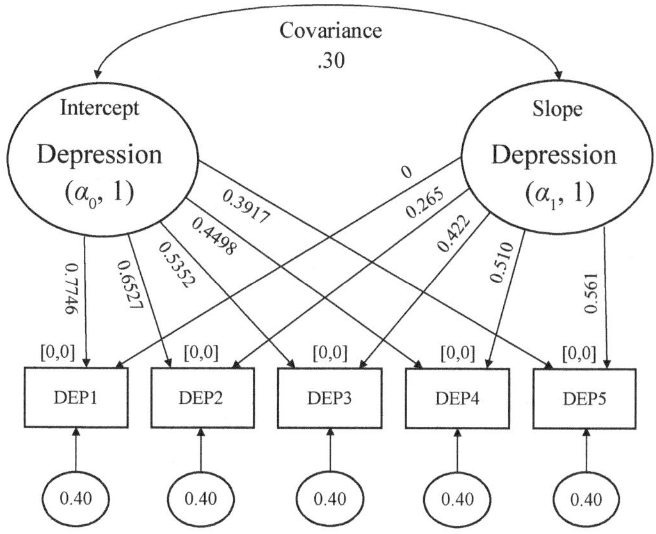

FIGURE 10.6. Depression growth curve model.

recruitment and retention, Becker and colleagues are willing to assume the following estimated values (see Figure 10.8).

Now that estimates have been specified, residual slope variance (shown as '?') for depression can now be calculated using Wright's rules. Assuming standardization, recall that residual variance ($\sigma^2_{\text{RESIDUAL}}$) is equal to one minus variance explained (R^2_{SLOPE}), or ($\sigma^2_{\text{RESIDUAL}} = 1 - R^2_{\text{SLOPE}}$). Furthermore, depression slope variance explained (R^2_{SLOPE}) will be equal to the sum of the depression slope variance explained by each of the three predictors, or ($R^2_{\text{SLOPE}} = R^2_{\text{SLOPE|SCT\_INTERCEPT}} + R^2_{\text{SLOPE|WithDr}} + R^2_{\text{SLOPE|LoneLin}}$).

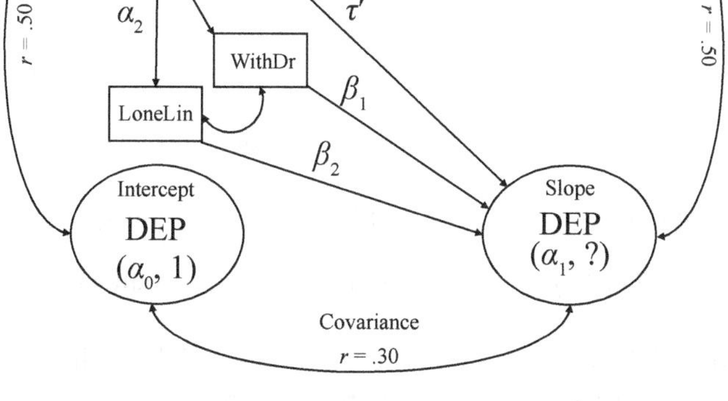

FIGURE 10.7. Mediated parallel-process growth curve model.

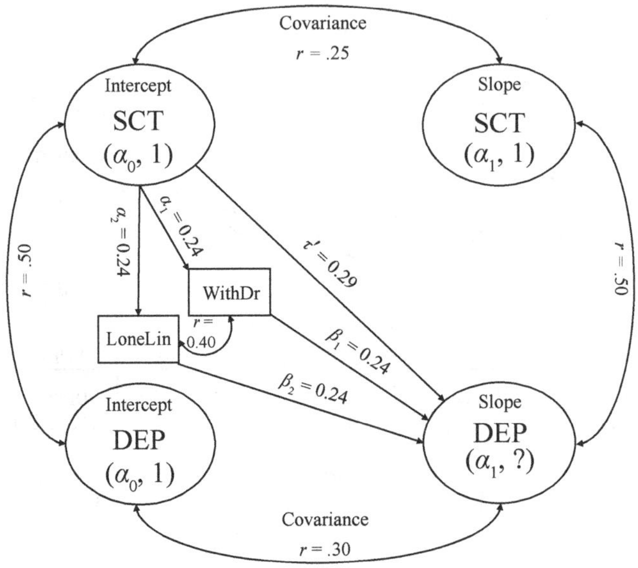

FIGURE 10.8. Specified mediated parallel-process growth curve model.

$$R^2_{\text{SLOPE|SCT\_INTERCEPT}} = (\text{Direct effect} * (\text{Direct effect} + [\text{Sum of indirect effects products}]))$$
$$= (\tau' * (\tau' + [\text{Sum of indirect effects products}]))$$

According to Wright's Rules, there are four admissible indirect pathways between SCT intercept and depression slope (shown in Figure 10.9). The first shows the α_1 and β_1 path. Similarly, the second indirect path (shown in Figure 10.10) involves α_2 and β_2. The third indirect pathway (see Figure 10.11) uses the correlation between social withdrawal and loneliness to connect the α_1 and β_2, paths. Similarly, as shown in Figure 10.12, the last indirect pathway also uses the correlation between social withdrawal and loneliness to connect the α_2 and β_1, paths. So,

$$R^2_{\text{SLOPE|SCT\_INTERCEPT}} = (\tau' * (\tau' + [\text{Sum of indirect effects products}]))$$
$$= (\tau' * (\tau' + [\alpha_1 * \beta_1] + [\alpha_2 * \beta_2] + [\alpha_1 * r * \beta_2] + [\alpha_2 * r * \beta_1]))$$
$$= (0.29 * (0.29 + [0.24 * 0.24] + [0.24 * 0.24] + [0.24 * 0.40 * 0.24] + [0.24 * 0.40 * 0.24]))$$
$$= (0.29 * (0.29 + [0.0576] + [0.0576] + [0.02304] + [0.02304]))$$
$$= (0.29 * 0.45128) = \mathbf{0.1308712}$$

$$R^2_{\text{SLOPE|WithDr}} = (\text{Direct effect} * (\text{Direct effect} + [\text{Sum of indirect effects products}]))$$
$$= (\beta_1 * (\beta_1 + [\text{Sum of indirect effects products}]))$$

According to Wright's Rules, there are three admissible indirect pathways between social withdrawal and depression slope, shown in Figures 10.13 to 10.15. Figure 10.13 uses

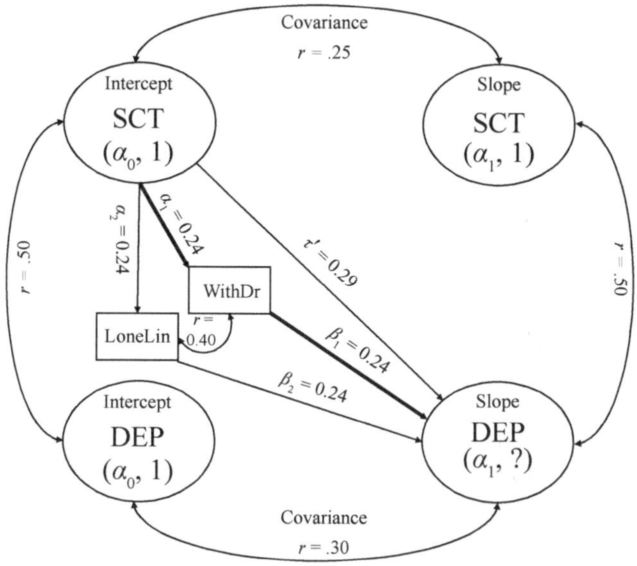

FIGURE 10.9. Mediated parallel-process growth curve model: First depression indirect path.

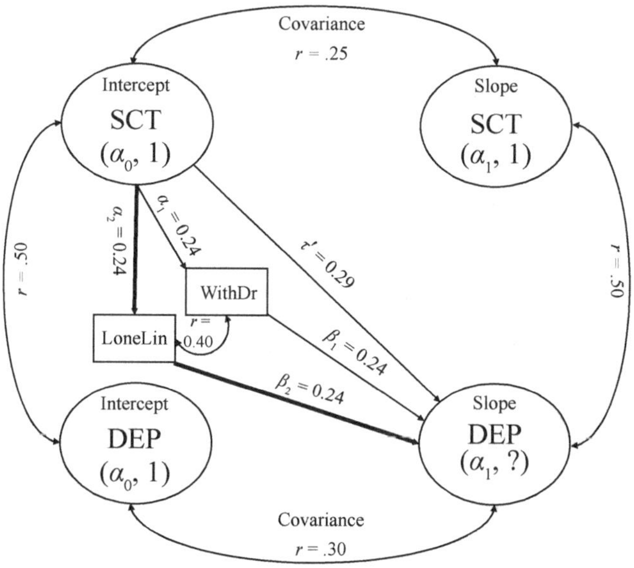

FIGURE 10.10. Mediated parallel-process growth curve model: Second depression indirect path.

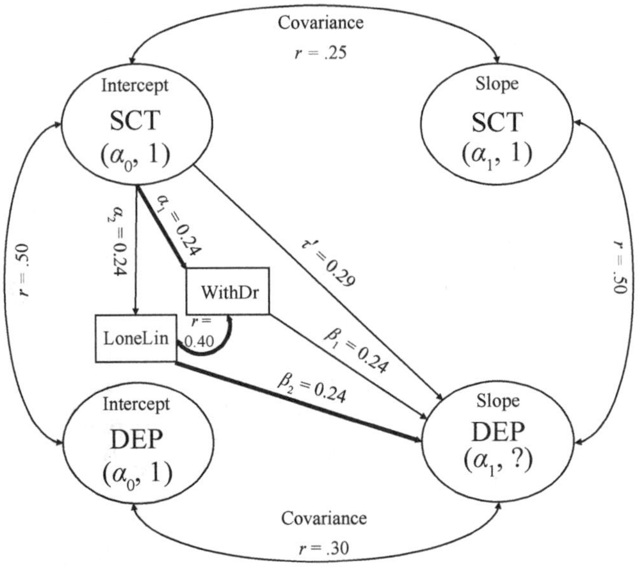

FIGURE 10.11. Mediated parallel-process growth curve model: Third depression indirect path.

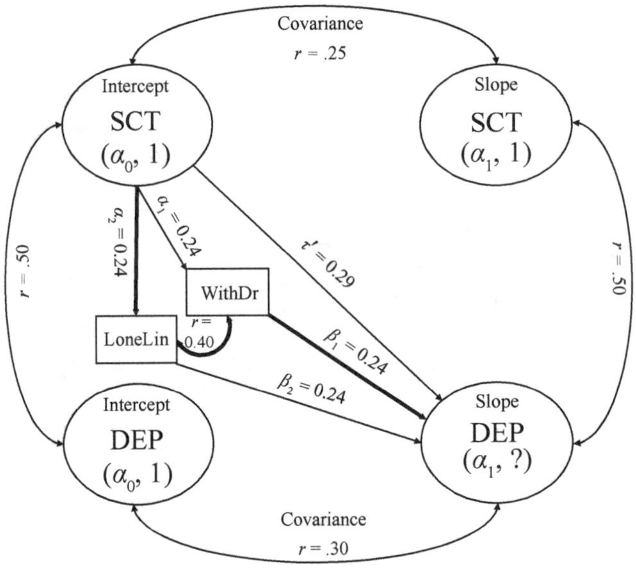

FIGURE 10.12. Mediated parallel-process growth curve model: Final depression indirect path.

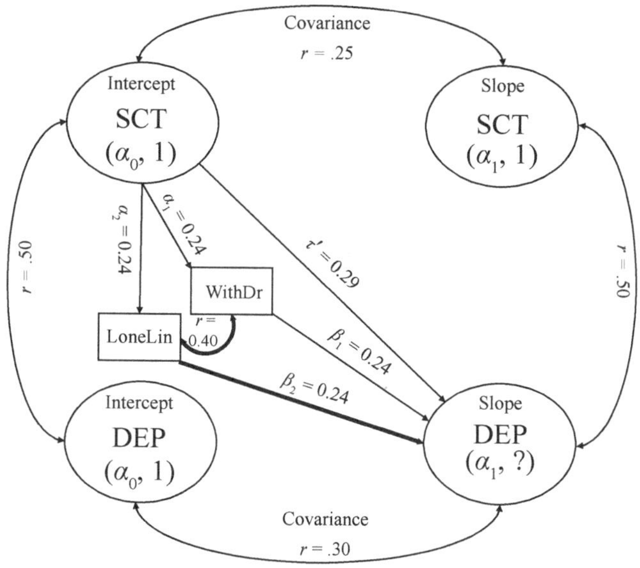

FIGURE 10.13. Mediated parallel-process growth curve model: First withdrawal indirect path.

the correlation between social withdrawal and loneliness and the β_2 path. The second pathway (Figure 10.14) uses α_1 and τ'. The last path (Figure 10.15) uses α_1, α_2 and β_2. So,

$$R^2_{\text{SLOPE|WithDr}} = (\beta_1 * (\beta_1 + [\text{Sum of indirect effects products}]))$$
$$= (0.24 * (0.24 + [0.40 * 0.24] + [0.24 * 0.29] + [0.24 * 0.24 * 0.24]))$$
$$= (0.24 * (0.24 + [0.096] + [0.0696] + [0.013824]))$$
$$= (0.24 * 0.419424) = \mathbf{0.10066176}$$

Again, there are three admissible pathways between loneliness and depression slope (see Figures 10.16 to 10.19). The first (Figure 10.16) involves the correlation between loneliness and social withdrawal and the β_1 path. The second pathway (Figure 10.17) involves α_2 and τ'. The last (Figure 10.18) involves α_2, α_1 and β_1. So,

$$R^2_{\text{SLOPE|LoneLin}} = (\beta_2 * (\beta_2 + [\text{Sum of indirect effects products}]))$$
$$= (0.24 * (0.24 + [0.40 * 0.24] + [0.24 * 0.29] + [0.24 * 0.24 * 0.24]))$$
$$= (0.24 * (0.24 + [0.096] + [0.0696] + [0.013824]))$$
$$= (0.24 * 0.419424) = \mathbf{0.10066176}$$

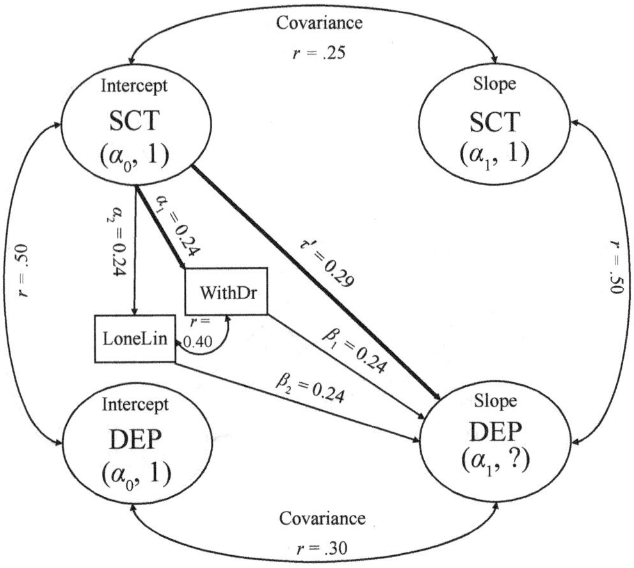

FIGURE 10.14. Mediated parallel-process growth curve model: Second withdrawal indirect path.

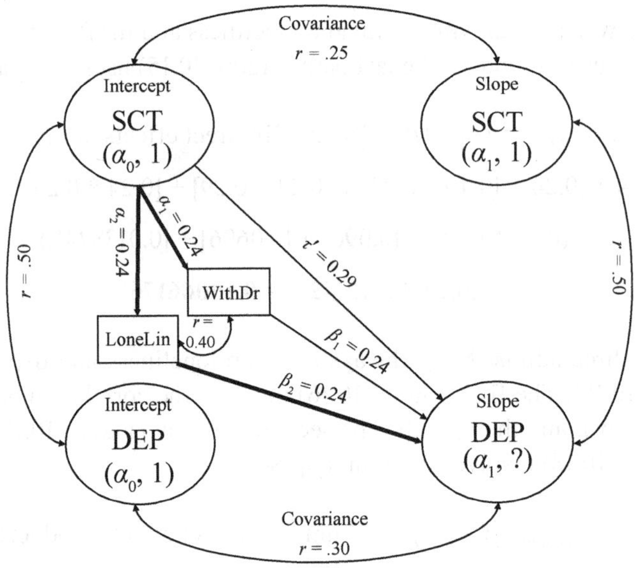

FIGURE 10.15. Mediated parallel-process growth curve model: Last withdrawal indirect path.

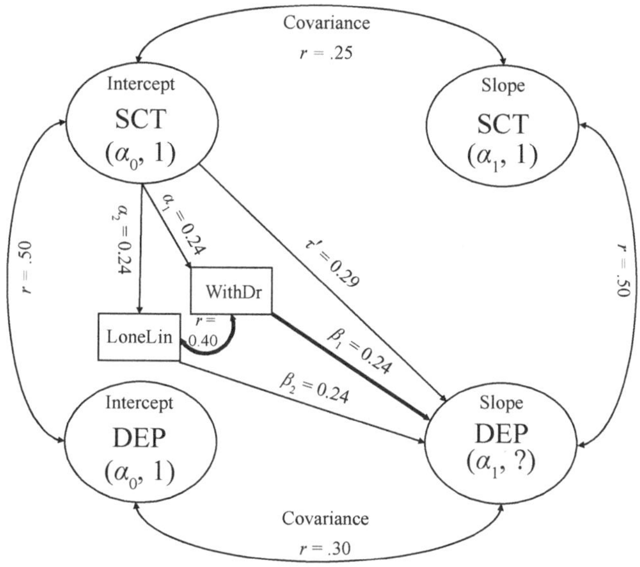

FIGURE 10.16. Mediated parallel-process growth curve model: First loneliness indirect path.

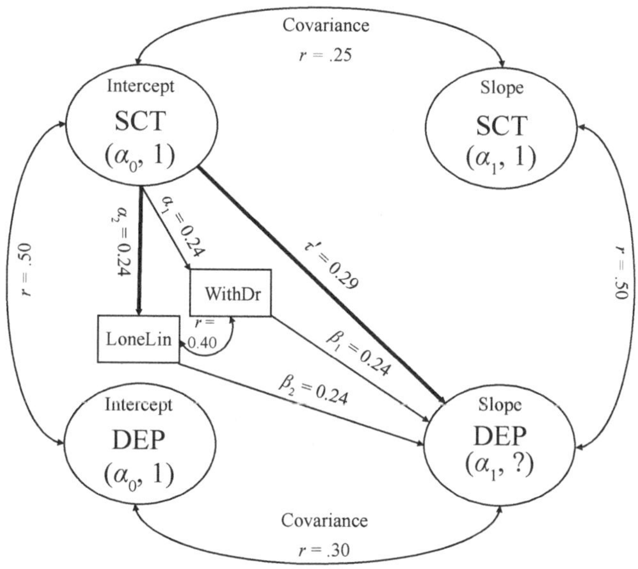

FIGURE 10.17. Mediated parallel-process growth curve model: Second loneliness indirect path.

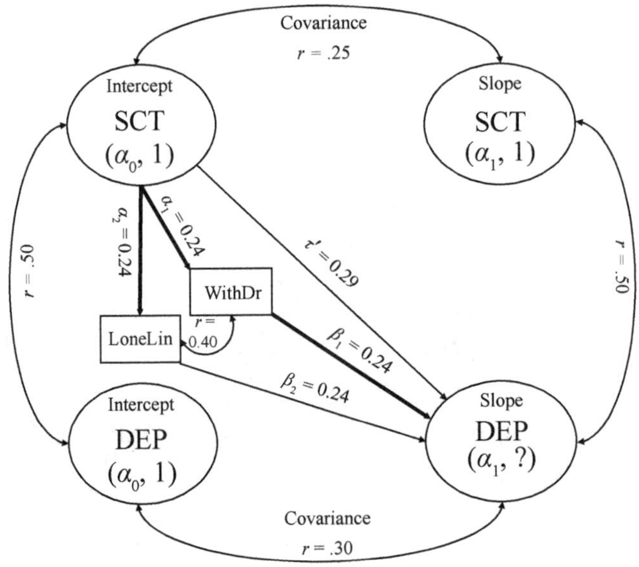

FIGURE 10.18. Mediated parallel-process growth curve model: Final loneliness indirect path.

So,

$$R^2_{\text{SLOPE}} = R^2_{\text{SLOPE|SCT\_INTERCEPT}} + R^2_{\text{SLOPE|WithDr}} + R^2_{\text{SLOPE|LoneLin}}$$

$$R^2_{\text{SLOPE}} = \mathbf{0.1308712 + 0.10066176 + 0.10066176 = 0.33219472}$$

$$\sigma^2_{\text{RESIDUAL}} = 1 - R^2_{\text{SLOPE}} = 1 - \mathbf{0.33219472} = \underline{\mathbf{0.66780528}}$$

So, all that remains is to calculate the residual variances for both social withdrawal and loneliness, which is a straightforward because both are predicted only by the SCT intercept, as shown here:

$$\sigma^2_{\text{RESIDUAL}} = 1 - R^2 = 1 - (0.24)^2 = 0.9424$$

Now that all the needed estimates have been calculated, the model can be checked for admissibility using R syntax by adding the time-invariant covariates social withdrawal and loneliness to the beta (**B**) and psi (**Ψ**) matrices after the observed response variables but before the latent variables as shown in (Equations 10.6–10.11).

B =

	SCT1	SCT2	SCT3	SCT4	SCT5	DEP1	DEP2	DEP3	DEP4	DEP5	WithDr	LoneLin	INT_{SCT}	INT_{DEP}	$SLOPE_{SCT}$	$SLOPE_{DEP}$
SCT1	0	0	0	0	0	0	0	0	0	0	0	0	0.7071	0	0	0
SCT2	0	0	0	0	0	0	0	0	0	0	0	0	0.5927	0	0.265	0
SCT3	0	0	0	0	0	0	0	0	0	0	0	0	0.4716	0	0.422	0
SCT4	0	0	0	0	0	0	0	0	0	0	0	0	0.3786	0	0.510	0
SCT5	0	0	0	0	0	0	0	0	0	0	0	0	0.3125	0	0.561	0
DEP1	0	0	0	0	0	0	0	0	0	0	0	0	0	0.7746	0	0
DEP2	0	0	0	0	0	0	0	0	0	0	0	0	0	0.6527	0	0.265
DEP3	0	0	0	0	0	0	0	0	0	0	0	0	0	0.5352	0	0.422
DEP4	0	0	0	0	0	0	0	0	0	0	0	0	0	0.4498	0	0.510
DEP5	0	0	0	0	0	0	0	0	0	0	0	0	0	0.3917	0	0.561
WithDr	0	0	0	0	0	0	0	0	0	0	0	0	0.24	0	0	0
LoneLin	0	0	0	0	0	0	0	0	0	0	0	0	0.24	0	0	0
INT_{SCT}	0	0	0	0	0	0	0	0	0	0	0	0	0	0	0	0
INT_{DEP}	0	0	0	0	0	0	0	0	0	0	0	0	0	0	0	0
$SLOPE_{SCT}$	0	0	0	0	0	0	0	0	0	0	0	0	0	0	0	0
$SLOPE_{DEP}$	0	0	0	0	0	0	0	0	0	0	0.24	0.24	0.29	0	0	0

(10.6)

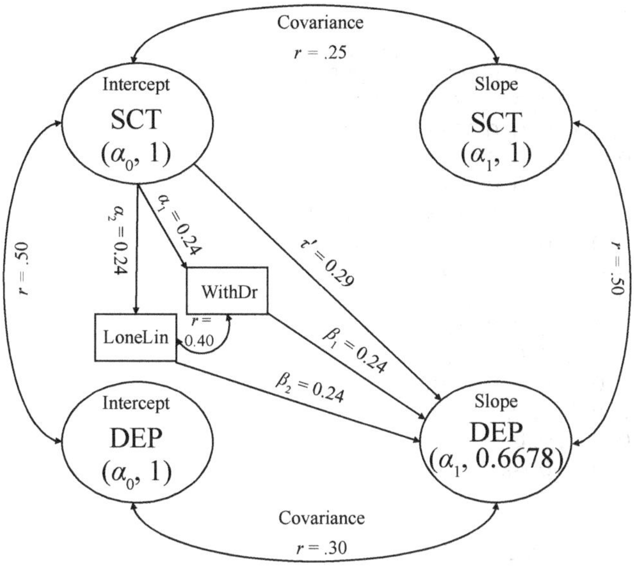

FIGURE 10.19. Fully specified mediated parallel-process growth curve model.

Ψ =

	SCT1	SCT2	SCT3	SCT4	SCT5	DEP1	DEP2	DEP3	DEP4	DEP5	WithDr	LoneLin	INT_{SCT}	INT_{DEP}	$SLOPE_{SCT}$	$SLOPE_{DEP}$
SCT1	0.50	0	0	0	0	0	0	0	0	0	0	0	0	0	0	0
SCT2	0	0.50	0	0	0	0	0	0	0	0	0	0	0	0	0	0
SCT3	0	0	0.50	0	0	0	0	0	0	0	0	0	0	0	0	0
SCT4	0	0	0	0.50	0	0	0	0	0	0	0	0		0	0	0
SCT5	0	0	0	0	0.50	0	0	0	0	0	0	0		0	0	0
DEP1	0	0	0	0	0	0.40	0	0	0	0	0	0	0	0	0	0
DEP2	0	0	0	0	0	0	0.40	0	0	0	0	0	0	0	0	0
DEP3	0	0	0	0	0	0	0	0.40	0	0	0	0	0	0	0	0
DEP4	0	0	0	0	0	0	0	0	0.40	0	0	0		0	0	0
DEP5	0	0	0	0	0	0	0	0	0	0.40	0	0		0	0	0
WithDr	0	0	0	0	0	0	0	0	0	0	0.9424	0.40	0	0	0	0
LoneLin	0	0	0	0	0	0	0	0	0	0	0.40	0.9424	0	0	0	0
INT_{SCT}	0	0	0	0	0	0	0	0	0	0	0	0	1	0.5	0.25	0
INT_{DEP}	0	0	0	0	0	0	0	0	0	0	0	0	0.5	1	0	0.30
$SLOPE_{SCT}$	0	0	0	0	0	0	0	0	0	0	0	0	0.25	0	1	0.50
$SLOPE_{DEP}$	0	0	0	0	0	0	0	0	0	0	0	0	0	0.30	0.50	0.6678

(10.7)

I =

	SCT1	SCT2	SCT3	SCT4	SCT5	DEP1	DEP2	DEP3	DEP4	DEP5	WithDr	LoneLin	INT_{SCT}	INT_{DEP}	$SLOPE_{SCT}$	$SLOPE_{DEP}$
SCT1	1	0	0	0	0	0	0	0	0	0	0	0	0	0	0	0
SCT2	0	1	0	0	0	0	0	0	0	0	0	0	0	0	0	0
SCT3	0	0	1	0	0	0	0	0	0	0	0	0	0	0	0	0
SCT4	0	0	0	1	0	0	0	0	0	0	0	0	0	0	0	0
SCT5	0	0	0	0	1	0	0	0	0	0	0	0	0	0	0	0
DEP1	0	0	0	0	0	1	0	0	0	0	0	0	0	0	0	0
DEP2	0	0	0	0	0	0	1	0	0	0	0	0	0	0	0	0
DEP3	0	0	0	0	0	0	0	1	0	0	0	0	0	0	0	0
DEP4	0	0	0	0	0	0	0	0	1	0	0	0	0	0	0	0
DEP5	0	0	0	0	0	0	0	0	0	1	0	0	0	0	0	0
WithDr	0	0	0	0	0	0	0	0	0	0	1	0	0	0	0	0
LoneLin	0	0	0	0	0	0	0	0	0	0	0	1	0	0	0	0
INT_{SCT}	0	0	0	0	0	0	0	0	0	0	0	0	1	0	0	0
INT_{DEP}	0	0	0	0	0	0	0	0	0	0	0	0	0	1	0	0
$SLOPE_{SCT}$	0	0	0	0	0	0	0	0	0	0	0	0	0	0	1	0
$SLOPE_{DEP}$	0	0	0	0	0	0	0	0	0	0	0	0	0	0	0	1

(10.8)

P =

	SCT1	SCT2	SCT3	SCT4	SCT5	DEP1	DEP2	DEP3	DEP4	DEP5	WithDr	LoneLin	INT_{SCT}	INT_{DEP}	$SLOPE_{SCT}$	$SLOPE_{DEP}$
SCT1	1	0	0	0	0	0	0	0	0	0	0	0	0	0	0	0
SCT2	0	1	0	0	0	0	0	0	0	0	0	0	0	0	0	0
SCT3	0	0	1	0	0	0	0	0	0	0	0	0	0	0	0	0
SCT4	0	0	0	1	0	0	0	0	0	0	0	0	0	0	0	0
SCT5	0	0	0	0	1	0	0	0	0	0	0	0	0	0	0	0
DEP1	0	0	0	0	0	1	0	0	0	0	0	0	0	0	0	0
DEP2	0	0	0	0	0	0	1	0	0	0	0	0	0	0	0	0
DEP3	0	0	0	0	0	0	0	1	0	0	0	0	0	0	0	0
DEP4	0	0	0	0	0	0	0	0	1	0	0	0	0	0	0	0
DEP5	0	0	0	0	0	0	0	0	0	1	0	0	0	0	0	0
WithDr	0	0	0	0	0	0	0	0	0	0	1	0	0	0	0	0
LoneLin	0	0	0	0	0	0	0	0	0	0	0	1	0	0	0	0

(10.9)

$$\Sigma\theta = P(I - B)^{-1}\Psi(I - B)^{-1T}P^{T}$$

```
Beta <- matrix(c(
0, 0, 0, 0, 0, 0, 0, 0, 0, 0, 0, 0, 0.7071, 0, 0, 0,
0, 0, 0, 0, 0, 0, 0, 0, 0, 0, 0, 0, 0.5927, 0, 0.265, 0,
0, 0, 0, 0, 0, 0, 0, 0, 0, 0, 0, 0, 0.4716, 0, 0.422, 0,
0, 0, 0, 0, 0, 0, 0, 0, 0, 0, 0, 0, 0.3786, 0, 0.510, 0,
0, 0, 0, 0, 0, 0, 0, 0, 0, 0, 0, 0, 0.3125, 0, 0.561, 0,
0, 0, 0, 0, 0, 0, 0, 0, 0, 0, 0, 0, 0, 0.7746, 0, 0,
0, 0, 0, 0, 0, 0, 0, 0, 0, 0, 0, 0, 0, 0.6527, 0, 0.265,
0, 0, 0, 0, 0, 0, 0, 0, 0, 0, 0, 0, 0, 0.5352, 0, 0.422,
0, 0, 0, 0, 0, 0, 0, 0, 0, 0, 0, 0, 0, 0.4498, 0, 0.510,
0, 0, 0, 0, 0, 0, 0, 0, 0, 0, 0, 0, 0, 0.3917, 0, 0.561,
0, 0, 0, 0, 0, 0, 0, 0, 0, 0, 0, 0, 0.24, 0, 0, 0,
0, 0, 0, 0, 0, 0, 0, 0, 0, 0, 0, 0, 0.24, 0, 0, 0,
0, 0, 0, 0, 0, 0, 0, 0, 0, 0, 0, 0, 0, 0, 0, 0,
0, 0, 0, 0, 0, 0, 0, 0, 0, 0, 0, 0, 0, 0, 0, 0,
0, 0, 0, 0, 0, 0, 0, 0, 0, 0, 0, 0, 0, 0, 0, 0,
0, 0, 0, 0, 0, 0, 0, 0, 0, 0, 0.24, 0.24, 0.29, 0, 0, 0), ncol = 16, byrow = TRUE)

Psi <- matrix(c(
0.50, 0, 0, 0, 0, 0, 0, 0, 0, 0, 0, 0, 0, 0, 0, 0,
0, 0.50, 0, 0, 0, 0, 0, 0, 0, 0, 0, 0, 0, 0, 0, 0,
0, 0, 0.50, 0, 0, 0, 0, 0, 0, 0, 0, 0, 0, 0, 0, 0,
0, 0, 0, 0.50, 0, 0, 0, 0, 0, 0, 0, 0, 0, 0, 0, 0,
0, 0, 0, 0, 0.50, 0, 0, 0, 0, 0, 0, 0, 0, 0, 0, 0,
0, 0, 0, 0, 0, 0.40, 0, 0, 0, 0, 0, 0, 0, 0, 0, 0,
0, 0, 0, 0, 0, 0, 0.40, 0, 0, 0, 0, 0, 0, 0, 0, 0,
0, 0, 0, 0, 0, 0, 0, 0.40, 0, 0, 0, 0, 0, 0, 0, 0,
0, 0, 0, 0, 0, 0, 0, 0, 0.40, 0, 0, 0, 0, 0, 0, 0,
0, 0, 0, 0, 0, 0, 0, 0, 0, 0.40, 0, 0, 0, 0, 0, 0,
0, 0, 0, 0, 0, 0, 0, 0, 0, 0, 0.9424, 0.40, 0, 0, 0, 0,
0, 0, 0, 0, 0, 0, 0, 0, 0, 0, 0.40, 0.9424, 0, 0, 0, 0,
0, 0, 0, 0, 0, 0, 0, 0, 0, 0, 0, 0, 1, 0.50, 0.25, 0,
0, 0, 0, 0, 0, 0, 0, 0, 0, 0, 0, 0, 0.50, 1, 0, 0.30,
0, 0, 0, 0, 0, 0, 0, 0, 0, 0, 0, 0, 0.25, 0, 1, 0.50,
0, 0, 0, 0, 0, 0, 0, 0, 0, 0, 0, 0, 0, 0.30, 0.50, 0.6678), ncol = 16, byrow = TRUE)

P <- matrix(c(
1, 0, 0, 0, 0, 0, 0, 0, 0, 0, 0, 0, 0, 0, 0, 0,
0, 1, 0, 0, 0, 0, 0, 0, 0, 0, 0, 0, 0, 0, 0, 0,
0, 0, 1, 0, 0, 0, 0, 0, 0, 0, 0, 0, 0, 0, 0, 0,
0, 0, 0, 1, 0, 0, 0, 0, 0, 0, 0, 0, 0, 0, 0, 0,
0, 0, 0, 0, 1, 0, 0, 0, 0, 0, 0, 0, 0, 0, 0, 0,
0, 0, 0, 0, 0, 1, 0, 0, 0, 0, 0, 0, 0, 0, 0, 0,
0, 0, 0, 0, 0, 0, 1, 0, 0, 0, 0, 0, 0, 0, 0, 0,
0, 0, 0, 0, 0, 0, 0, 1, 0, 0, 0, 0, 0, 0, 0, 0,
0, 0, 0, 0, 0, 0, 0, 0, 1, 0, 0, 0, 0, 0, 0, 0,
0, 0, 0, 0, 0, 0, 0, 0, 0, 1, 0, 0, 0, 0, 0, 0,
0, 0, 0, 0, 0, 0, 0, 0, 0, 0, 1, 0, 0, 0, 0, 0,
0, 0, 0, 0, 0, 0, 0, 0, 0, 0, 0, 1, 0, 0, 0, 0), ncol = 16, byrow = TRUE)

I <- matrix(c(
1, 0, 0, 0, 0, 0, 0, 0, 0, 0, 0, 0, 0, 0, 0, 0,
0, 1, 0, 0, 0, 0, 0, 0, 0, 0, 0, 0, 0, 0, 0, 0,
0, 0, 1, 0, 0, 0, 0, 0, 0, 0, 0, 0, 0, 0, 0, 0,
0, 0, 0, 1, 0, 0, 0, 0, 0, 0, 0, 0, 0, 0, 0, 0,
0, 0, 0, 0, 1, 0, 0, 0, 0, 0, 0, 0, 0, 0, 0, 0,
0, 0, 0, 0, 0, 1, 0, 0, 0, 0, 0, 0, 0, 0, 0, 0,
```

```
0, 0, 0, 0, 0, 0, 1, 0, 0, 0, 0, 0, 0, 0, 0, 0,
0, 0, 0, 0, 0, 0, 0, 1, 0, 0, 0, 0, 0, 0, 0, 0,
0, 0, 0, 0, 0, 0, 0, 0, 1, 0, 0, 0, 0, 0, 0, 0,
0, 0, 0, 0, 0, 0, 0, 0, 0, 1, 0, 0, 0, 0, 0, 0,
0, 0, 0, 0, 0, 0, 0, 0, 0, 0, 1, 0, 0, 0, 0, 0,
0, 0, 0, 0, 0, 0, 0, 0, 0, 0, 0, 1, 0, 0, 0, 0,
0, 0, 0, 0, 0, 0, 0, 0, 0, 0, 0, 0, 1, 0, 0, 0,
0, 0, 0, 0, 0, 0, 0, 0, 0, 0, 0, 0, 0, 1, 0, 0,
0, 0, 0, 0, 0, 0, 0, 0, 0, 0, 0, 0, 0, 0, 1, 0,
0, 0, 0, 0, 0, 0, 0, 0, 0, 0, 0, 0, 0, 0, 0, 1), ncol = 16, byrow = TRUE)

corr_matrix <- P %*% (solve(I-Beta)) %*% Psi %*%t(solve(I-Beta)) %*%t(P)

corr_matrix
```

		SCT1	SCT2	SCT3	SCT4	SCT5	DEP1	DEP2	DEP3	DEP4	DEP5	WithDr	LoneLin
	SCT1	1.000	0.466	0.408	0.358	0.320	0.274	0.307	0.310	0.305	0.299	0.170	0.170
	SCT2	0.466	1.000	0.485	0.460	0.438	0.230	0.299	0.327	0.337	0.340	0.158	0.158
	SCT3	0.408	0.485	1.000	0.494	0.483	0.183	0.272	0.314	0.333	0.342	0.139	0.139
	SCT4	0.358	0.460	0.494	1.000	0.497	0.147	0.245	0.295	0.320	0.332	0.121	0.121
	SCT5	0.320	0.438	0.483	0.497	1.000	0.121	0.225	0.279	0.307	0.321	0.109	0.109
$\Sigma\Theta =$	DEP1	0.274	0.230	0.183	0.147	0.121	1.000	0.609	0.579	0.547	0.522	0.093	0.093
	DEP2	0.307	0.299	0.272	0.245	0.225	0.609	1.069	0.669	0.654	0.638	0.188	0.188
	DEP3	0.310	0.327	0.314	0.295	0.279	0.579	0.669	1.089	0.685	0.677	0.239	0.239
	DEP4	0.305	0.337	0.333	0.320	0.307	0.547	0.654	0.685	1.089	0.685	0.265	0.265
	DEP5	0.299	0.340	0.342	0.332	0.321	0.522	0.638	0.677	0.685	1.084	0.279	0.279
	WithDr	0.170	0.158	0.139	0.121	0.109	0.093	0.188	0.239	0.265	0.279	1.000	0.458
	LoneLin	0.170	0.158	0.139	0.121	0.109	0.093	0.188	0.239	0.265	0.279	0.458	1.000

(10.10)

As in the example in Chapter 9, it is again shown that model-reproduced variance values for DEP2–DEP5 exceed a value of one. This is because the residual variance estimates for those variables (all 0.40) were based on an unconditional growth model for depression that does not account for depression slope variance prediction in the current parallel-process growth model example. But as was also shown in Chapter 9, subtracting the amount over a value of one in the model-reproduced matrix above from the residual variance values for DEP2–DEP5 (e.g., DEP2 = 0.40 – 0.06917 = 0.33083; DEP3 = 0.40 – 0.08917 = 0.31083; DEP4 = 0.40 – 0.08953 = 0.31047; & DEP5 = 0.40 – 0.08483 = 0.31517) can be shown to produce a correct correlation matrix and an admissible model.

```
Beta <- matrix(c(
0, 0, 0, 0, 0, 0, 0, 0, 0, 0, 0, 0.7071, 0, 0, 0,
0, 0, 0, 0, 0, 0, 0, 0, 0, 0, 0, 0.5927, 0, 0.265, 0,
0, 0, 0, 0, 0, 0, 0, 0, 0, 0, 0, 0.4716, 0, 0.422, 0,
0, 0, 0, 0, 0, 0, 0, 0, 0, 0, 0, 0.3786, 0, 0.510, 0,
0, 0, 0, 0, 0, 0, 0, 0, 0, 0, 0, 0.3125, 0, 0.561, 0,
0, 0, 0, 0, 0, 0, 0, 0, 0, 0, 0, 0, 0.7746, 0, 0,
0, 0, 0, 0, 0, 0, 0, 0, 0, 0, 0, 0, 0.6527, 0, 0.265,
0, 0, 0, 0, 0, 0, 0, 0, 0, 0, 0, 0, 0.5352, 0, 0.422,
0, 0, 0, 0, 0, 0, 0, 0, 0, 0, 0, 0, 0.4498, 0, 0.510,
0, 0, 0, 0, 0, 0, 0, 0, 0, 0, 0, 0, 0.3917, 0, 0.561,
0, 0, 0, 0, 0, 0, 0, 0, 0, 0, 0, 0.24, 0, 0, 0,
0, 0, 0, 0, 0, 0, 0, 0, 0, 0, 0, 0.24, 0, 0, 0,
0, 0, 0, 0, 0, 0, 0, 0, 0, 0, 0, 0, 0, 0, 0,
0, 0, 0, 0, 0, 0, 0, 0, 0, 0, 0, 0, 0, 0, 0,
```

```
0, 0, 0, 0, 0, 0, 0, 0, 0, 0, 0, 0, 0, 0, 0, 0,
0, 0, 0, 0, 0, 0, 0, 0, 0, 0, 0.24, 0.24, 0.29, 0, 0, 0), ncol = 16, byrow = TRUE)

Psi <- matrix(c(
0.50, 0, 0, 0, 0, 0, 0, 0, 0, 0, 0, 0, 0, 0, 0, 0,
0, 0.50, 0, 0, 0, 0, 0, 0, 0, 0, 0, 0, 0, 0, 0, 0,
0, 0, 0.50, 0, 0, 0, 0, 0, 0, 0, 0, 0, 0, 0, 0, 0,
0, 0, 0, 0.50, 0, 0, 0, 0, 0, 0, 0, 0, 0, 0, 0, 0,
0, 0, 0, 0, 0.50, 0, 0, 0, 0, 0, 0, 0, 0, 0, 0, 0,
0, 0, 0, 0, 0, 0.40, 0, 0, 0, 0, 0, 0, 0, 0, 0, 0,
0, 0, 0, 0, 0, 0, 0.33083, 0, 0, 0, 0, 0, 0, 0, 0, 0,
0, 0, 0, 0, 0, 0, 0, 0.31083, 0, 0, 0, 0, 0, 0, 0, 0,
0, 0, 0, 0, 0, 0, 0, 0, 0.31047, 0, 0, 0, 0, 0, 0, 0,
0, 0, 0, 0, 0, 0, 0, 0, 0, 0.31517, 0, 0, 0, 0, 0, 0,
0, 0, 0, 0, 0, 0, 0, 0, 0, 0, 0.9424, 0.40, 0, 0, 0, 0,
0, 0, 0, 0, 0, 0, 0, 0, 0, 0, 0.40, 0.9424, 0, 0, 0, 0,
0, 0, 0, 0, 0, 0, 0, 0, 0, 0, 0, 0, 1, 0.50, 0.25, 0,
0, 0, 0, 0, 0, 0, 0, 0, 0, 0, 0, 0, 0.50, 1, 0, 0.30,
0, 0, 0, 0, 0, 0, 0, 0, 0, 0, 0, 0, 0.25, 0, 1, 0.50,
0, 0, 0, 0, 0, 0, 0, 0, 0, 0, 0, 0, 0, 0.30, 0.50, 0.6678), ncol = 16, byrow = TRUE)

P <- matrix(c(
1, 0, 0, 0, 0, 0, 0, 0, 0, 0, 0, 0, 0, 0, 0, 0,
0, 1, 0, 0, 0, 0, 0, 0, 0, 0, 0, 0, 0, 0, 0, 0,
0, 0, 1, 0, 0, 0, 0, 0, 0, 0, 0, 0, 0, 0, 0, 0,
0, 0, 0, 1, 0, 0, 0, 0, 0, 0, 0, 0, 0, 0, 0, 0,
0, 0, 0, 0, 1, 0, 0, 0, 0, 0, 0, 0, 0, 0, 0, 0,
0, 0, 0, 0, 0, 1, 0, 0, 0, 0, 0, 0, 0, 0, 0, 0,
0, 0, 0, 0, 0, 0, 1, 0, 0, 0, 0, 0, 0, 0, 0, 0,
0, 0, 0, 0, 0, 0, 0, 1, 0, 0, 0, 0, 0, 0, 0, 0,
0, 0, 0, 0, 0, 0, 0, 0, 1, 0, 0, 0, 0, 0, 0, 0,
0, 0, 0, 0, 0, 0, 0, 0, 0, 1, 0, 0, 0, 0, 0, 0,
0, 0, 0, 0, 0, 0, 0, 0, 0, 0, 1, 0, 0, 0, 0, 0,
0, 0, 0, 0, 0, 0, 0, 0, 0, 0, 0, 1, 0, 0, 0, 0), ncol = 16, byrow = TRUE)

I <- matrix(c(
1, 0, 0, 0, 0, 0, 0, 0, 0, 0, 0, 0, 0, 0, 0, 0,
0, 1, 0, 0, 0, 0, 0, 0, 0, 0, 0, 0, 0, 0, 0, 0,
0, 0, 1, 0, 0, 0, 0, 0, 0, 0, 0, 0, 0, 0, 0, 0,
0, 0, 0, 1, 0, 0, 0, 0, 0, 0, 0, 0, 0, 0, 0, 0,
0, 0, 0, 0, 1, 0, 0, 0, 0, 0, 0, 0, 0, 0, 0, 0,
0, 0, 0, 0, 0, 1, 0, 0, 0, 0, 0, 0, 0, 0, 0, 0,
0, 0, 0, 0, 0, 0, 1, 0, 0, 0, 0, 0, 0, 0, 0, 0,
0, 0, 0, 0, 0, 0, 0, 1, 0, 0, 0, 0, 0, 0, 0, 0,
0, 0, 0, 0, 0, 0, 0, 0, 1, 0, 0, 0, 0, 0, 0, 0,
0, 0, 0, 0, 0, 0, 0, 0, 0, 1, 0, 0, 0, 0, 0, 0,
0, 0, 0, 0, 0, 0, 0, 0, 0, 0, 1, 0, 0, 0, 0, 0,
0, 0, 0, 0, 0, 0, 0, 0, 0, 0, 0, 1, 0, 0, 0, 0,
0, 0, 0, 0, 0, 0, 0, 0, 0, 0, 0, 0, 1, 0, 0, 0,
0, 0, 0, 0, 0, 0, 0, 0, 0, 0, 0, 0, 0, 1, 0, 0,
0, 0, 0, 0, 0, 0, 0, 0, 0, 0, 0, 0, 0, 0, 1, 0,
0, 0, 0, 0, 0, 0, 0, 0, 0, 0, 0, 0, 0, 0, 0, 1), ncol = 16, byrow = TRUE)

corr_matrix <- P %*% (solve(I-Beta)) %*% Psi %*%t(solve(I-Beta)) %*%t(P)

corr_matrix
```

$\Sigma\theta =$

	SCT1	SCT2	SCT3	SCT4	SCT5	DEP1	DEP2	DEP3	DEP4	DEP5	WithDr	LoneLin
SCT1	1	0.4659	0.4081	0.3579	0.3201	0.2739	0.3067	0.3101	0.3052	0.2992	0.1697	0.1697
SCT2	0.4659	1	0.4851	0.4602	0.4377	0.2296	0.2993	0.3272	0.3370	0.3402	0.1581	0.1581
SCT3	0.4081	0.4851	1	0.4938	0.4832	0.1827	0.2718	0.3139	0.3329	0.3419	0.1385	0.1385
SCT4	0.3579	0.4602	0.4938	1	0.4974	0.1466	0.2455	0.2955	0.3198	0.3322	0.1215	0.1215
SCT5	0.3201	0.4377	0.4832	0.4974	1	0.1210	0.2249	0.2794	0.3069	0.3215	0.1087	0.1087
DEP1	0.2739	0.2296	0.1827	0.1466	0.1210	1	0.6087	0.5789	0.5470	0.5218	0.0930	0.0930
DEP2	0.3067	0.2993	0.2718	0.2455	0.2249	0.6087	1	0.6694	0.6541	0.6385	0.1895	0.1895
DEP3	0.3101	0.3272	0.3139	0.2955	0.2794	0.5789	0.6694	1	0.6857	0.6772	0.2412	0.2412
DEP4	0.3052	0.3370	0.3329	0.3198	0.3069	0.5470	0.6541	0.6857	1	0.6857	0.2679	0.2679
DEP5	0.2992	0.3402	0.3419	0.3322	0.3215	0.5218	0.6385	0.6772	0.6857	1	0.2823	0.2823
WithDr	0.1697	0.1581	0.1385	0.1215	0.1087	0.0930	0.1895	0.2412	0.2679	0.2823	1	0.4576
LoneLin	0.1697	0.1581	0.1385	0.1215	0.1087	0.0930	0.1895	0.2412	0.2679	0.2823	0.4576	1

(10.11)

Mplus Monte Carlo Power Analysis for Parallel-Process Mediation

Now that an admissible parallel-process model has been confirmed using model-reproduced matrix calculations, a Monte Carlo simulation power analysis can be performed with the following Mplus syntax.

```
TITLE: MPLUS 10.1 Parallel Process

MONTECARLO:
NAMES ARE
SCT1 SCT2 SCT3 SCT4 SCT5
DEP1 DEP2 DEP3 DEP4 DEP5
WithD LoneL;
OBSERVATIONS = 416;
SEED = 32066;
NREPS = 5000;
MISSING =
SCT2 SCT3 SCT4 SCT5
DEP2 DEP3 DEP4 DEP5
WithD LoneL;
```

All syntax commands are defined as in previous chapters; the only exception is that in addition to the expectation of longitudinal postbaseline response variable missing data, a possibility of missing data on both social withdrawal and loneliness predictor variables is added.

```
MODEL POPULATION:
[SCT1-DEP5@0];

!Lambda Matrix, SCT;
SCT_I BY SCT1@0.7071 SCT2@0.5927 SCT3@0.4716 SCT4@0.3786 SCT5@0.3125;
SCT_S BY SCT1@0 SCT2@0.265 SCT3@0.422 SCT4@0.510 SCT5@0.561;

!Lambda Matrix, Depression;
DEP_I BY DEP1@0.7746 DEP2@0.6527 DEP3@0.5352 DEP4@0.4498 DEP5@0.3917;
DEP_S BY DEP1@0 DEP2@0.265 DEP3@0.422 DEP4@0.510 DEP5@0.561;
```

The first line of syntax following the '`MODEL POPULATION:`' command fixes observed response variable means to zero so that latent intercept and slope variables can be specified, based on values from the lambda ($\mathbf{\Lambda}$) matrices for SCT and depression using '`BY`' statements.

```
!Tau_Prime;
DEP_S ON SCT_I*0.29;

!Beta_One;
DEP_S ON WithD*0.24;
!Beta Two;
DEP_S ON LoneL*0.24;

!Alpha One;
WithD ON SCT_I*0.24;

!Alpha Two;
LoneL ON SCT_I*0.24;
```

The next five lines of Mplus syntax contain prediction information from the beta (**B**) matrix. This information is used to specify the direct (τ') and mediated pathways ($\alpha_1 * \beta_1$ for social withdrawal, $\alpha_2 * \beta_2$ for loneliness) needed to answer the power analysis question.

```
SCT1*0.50;
SCT2*0.50;
SCT3*0.50;
SCT4*0.50;
SCT5*0.50;
DEP1*0.40;
DEP2*0.33083;
DEP3*0.31083;
DEP4*0.31047;
DEP5*0.31517;
```

The next 10 lines of syntax contain residual variances from the respective theta matrices for both SCT and depression.

```
WithD*.9424;
LoneL*.9424;
WithD WITH LoneL*0.40;
```

The following three lines of code specify residual variances and the correlation between the two time-invariant covariates consistent with information from the phi (**Φ**) matrix.

```
[SCT_I*1;
DEP_I*1;
SCT_S*1;
DEP_S*0.6678;

SCT_I WITH DEP_I*0.50;
SCT_I WITH SCT_S*0.25;
DEP_I WITH DEP_S*0.30;
SCT_S WITH DEP_S*0.50;
```

The final eight lines of syntax for the 'MODEL POPULATION:' command specify latent variable variances, correlations, and the residual variance estimate for depression slope, based on information from the psi (Ψ) matrix.

```
MODEL MISSING:
[WithD*-2.945];
[LoneL*-2.945];
```

The first two lines of syntax that follow the 'MODEL MISSING:' command specify a researcher's belief, for example, that missing data will be minimal (i.e., [$\exp^{-2.945}/1 + \exp^{-2.945}$] = 0.05 or 5%) and missing completely at random (MCAR). Reasons for MCAR missing data for social withdrawal and loneliness values could include failure in electronic data collection or a participant exercising their right not to respond for any reason.

```
[SCT2*-2.9444]; !5% MCAR;
[SCT3*-2.1972]; !10% MCAR;
[SCT4*-1.7346]; !15% MCAR;
[SCT5*-1.3862]; !20% MCAR;

[DEP2*-2.9444]; !5% MCAR;
[DEP3*-2.1972]; !10% MCAR;
[DEP4*-1.7346]; !15% MCAR;
[DEP5*-1.3862]; !20% MCAR;
```

The next eight lines of syntax under the 'MODEL MISSING:' command specify MCAR response variable data for postbaseline SCT and depression that increases consistently from 5 to 20% at the final assessment time point.

```
SCT2 ON SCT1*0.0953;
SCT3 ON SCT2*0.0953 SCT1*0.0953;
SCT4 ON SCT3*0.0953 SCT2*0.0953 SCT1*0.0953;
SCT5 ON SCT4*0.0953 SCT3*0.0953 SCT2*0.0953 SCT1*0.0953;

DEP2 ON DEP1*0.1823;
DEP3 ON DEP2*0.1823 DEP1*0.1823;
DEP4 ON DEP3*0.1823 DEP2*0.1823 DEP1*0.1823;
DEP5 ON DEP4*0.1823 DEP3*0.1823 DEP2*0.1823 DEP1*0.1823;
```

The addition of the final eight lines consisting of 'ON' statements now specify MAR; missing data at a given assessment time point now depend on SCT and depression scores at any previous time point. Specifically, the first four 'ON' statements specify a ($\exp^{0.0953}$ = 1.10) 10% increase in the odds of a missing value at a given assessment time point per unit SCT score increase at any previous time point. The final four 'ON' statements specify a ($\exp^{0.1823}$ = 1.20) 20% increase in the odds of a missing value at a given assessment time point per unit depression score increase at any previous time point.

```
MODEL:
[SCT1-DEP5@0];
```

```
SCT_I BY SCT1@0.7071 SCT2@0.5927 SCT3@0.4716 SCT4@0.3786 SCT5@0.3125;
SCT_S BY SCT1@0 SCT2@0.265 SCT3@0.422 SCT4@0.510 SCT5@0.561;

DEP_I BY DEP1@0.7746 DEP2@0.6527 DEP3@0.5352 DEP4@0.4498 DEP5@0.3917;
DEP_S BY DEP1@0 DEP2@0.265 DEP3@0.422 DEP4@0.510 DEP5@0.561;

DEP_S ON SCT_I*0.29;

WithD ON SCT_I*0.24 (a1);
LoneL ON SCT_I*0.24 (a2);

DEP_S ON WithD*0.24 (b1);
DEP_S ON LoneL*0.24 (b2);
```

As stated in previous chapters, only the latent variable loadings (i.e., the 'BY' statements) and time-invariant covariate predictions (i.e., the 'ON' statements) need to be included in the 'MODEL:' statement that specifies how the data generated in the 'MODEL POPULATION:' statement will be analyzed. The only exceptions are the specifications (a1, a2, b1, and b2) listed in parentheses at the end of the final four lines of 'MODEL:' statement syntax. Recall from Chapter 3 that these specifications allow the values of SCT intercept as a predictor of social withdrawal (i.e., the α_1 coefficient) and loneliness (the α_2 coefficient) in each dataset replication to be assigned to variables a1 and a2, respectively; the values for social withdrawal (i.e., the β_1 coefficient) and loneliness (the β_2 coefficient) are similarly assigned to variables b1 and b2, respectively. Mplus allows for the creation of additional variables, based on parameter estimates as follows.

```
MODEL CONSTRAINT:
New (X1*0.0576 X2*0.0576);
X1 = a1*b1;
X2 = a2*b2;
```

Recall from Chapter 3 that the Mplus 'MODEL CONSTRAINT:' command allows 'New' variables to be created from parameters estimates specified in the 'MODEL:' statement. Recall also from Chapter 3 that testing mediation involves testing the joint product coefficient (i.e., the indirect or mediated pathway) for each mediator (i.e., $\alpha_1 * \beta_1$ = a1*b1 for social withdrawal, $\alpha_2 * \beta_2$ = a2*b2 for loneliness) against a null hypothesis that states both indirect pathways are zero. The 'New' specification allows start values (0.0576) to be specified for both indirect pathways based on the effects specified in the 'MODEL POPULATION:' command (i.e., 0.24*0.24 = 0.0576). Listed below is the complete Mplus Monte Carlo simulation power analysis syntax (MPlus 10.1) for a parallel-process mediation model, followed by the results of the syntax and an example power analysis write-up.

```
TITLE: MPLUS 10.1 Parallel Process

MONTECARLO:
NAMES ARE
SCT1 SCT2 SCT3 SCT4 SCT5
DEP1 DEP2 DEP3 DEP4 DEP5
WithD LoneL;
```

```
OBSERVATIONS = 416;
SEED = 32066;
NREPS = 5000;
MISSING =
SCT2 SCT3 SCT4 SCT5
DEP2 DEP3 DEP4 DEP5
WithD LoneL;

MODEL POPULATION:
[SCT1-DEP5@0];

!Lambda Matrix, SCT;
SCT_I BY SCT1@0.7071 SCT2@0.5927 SCT3@0.4716 SCT4@0.3786 SCT5@0.3125;
SCT_S BY SCT1@0 SCT2@0.265 SCT3@0.422 SCT4@0.510 SCT5@0.561;

!Lambda Matrix, Depression;
DEP_I BY DEP1@0.7746 DEP2@0.6527 DEP3@0.5352 DEP4@0.4498 DEP5@0.3917;
DEP_S BY DEP1@0 DEP2@0.265 DEP3@0.422 DEP4@0.510 DEP5@0.561;

!Tau_Prime;
DEP_S ON SCT_I*0.29;

!Beta_One;
DEP_S ON WithD*0.24;
!Beta Two;
DEP_S ON LoneL*0.24;

!Alpha One;
WithD ON SCT_I*0.24;
!Alpha Two;
LoneL ON SCT_I*0.24;

SCT1*0.50;
SCT2*0.50;
SCT3*0.50;
SCT4*0.50;
SCT5*0.50;
DEP1*0.40;
DEP2*0.33083;
DEP3*0.31083;
DEP4*0.31047;
DEP5*0.31517;

WithD*.9424;
LoneL*.9424;
WithD WITH LoneL*0.40;

SCT_I*1;
DEP_I*1;
SCT_S*1;
DEP_S*0.6678;

SCT_I WITH DEP_I*0.50;
SCT_I WITH SCT_S*0.25;
DEP_I WITH DEP_S*0.30;

SCT_S WITH DEP_S*0.50;
```

```
MODEL MISSING:
[WithD*-2.945];
[LoneL*-2.945];

[SCT2*-2.9444]; !5% MCAR;
[SCT3*-2.1972]; !10% MCAR;
[SCT4*-1.7346]; !15% MCAR;
[SCT5*-1.3862]; !20% MCAR;

[DEP2*-2.9444]; !5% MCAR;
[DEP3*-2.1972]; !10% MCAR;
[DEP4*-1.7346]; !15% MCAR;
[DEP5*-1.3862]; !20% MCAR;

SCT2 ON SCT1*0.0953;
SCT3 ON SCT2*0.0953 SCT1*0.0953;
SCT4 ON SCT3*0.0953 SCT2*0.0953 SCT1*0.0953;
SCT5 ON SCT4*0.0953 SCT3*0.0953 SCT2*0.0953 SCT1*0.0953;

DEP2 ON DEP1*0.1823;
DEP3 ON DEP2*0.1823 DEP1*0.1823;
DEP4 ON DEP3*0.1823 DEP2*0.1823 DEP1*0.1823;
DEP5 ON DEP4*0.1823 DEP3*0.1823 DEP2*0.1823 DEP1*0.1823;

MODEL:
[SCT1-DEP5@0];

SCT_I BY SCT1@0.7071 SCT2@0.5927 SCT3@0.4716 SCT4@0.3786 SCT5@0.3125;
SCT_S BY SCT1@0 SCT2@0.265 SCT3@0.422 SCT4@0.510 SCT5@0.561;

DEP_I BY DEP1@0.7746 DEP2@0.6527 DEP3@0.5352 DEP4@0.4498 DEP5@0.3917;
DEP_S BY DEP1@0 DEP2@0.265 DEP3@0.422 DEP4@0.510 DEP5@0.561;

DEP_S ON SCT_I*0.29;

WithD ON SCT_I*0.24 (a1);
LoneL ON SCT_I*0.24 (a2);

DEP_S ON WithD*0.24 (b1);
DEP_S ON LoneL*0.24 (b2);

MODEL CONSTRAINT:
New (X1*0.0576 X2*0.0576);
X1 = a1*b1;
X2 = a2*b2;
```

MODEL RESULTS

	Population	ESTIMATES Average	Std. Dev.	S. E. Average	M. S. E.	95% Cover	% Sig Coeff
New/Additional Parameters							
X1	**0.058**	0.0575	0.0233	0.0229	0.0005	0.929	**0.812**
X2	**0.058**	0.0573	0.0230	0.0229	0.0005	0.934	**0.804**

R Monte Carlo Power Analysis for Parallel-Process Mediation

Unlike in Chapters 8 and 9, the simulation presented here is relatively straightforward because all data are continuous, even though the model is relatively complex. Because of this, we used lavaan to specify the population model and simsem to run the full simulation. The full model is:

```
library(simsem)
library(lavaan)

PopulationModel_Ch10 <- "
 SCT1 ~ 0
 SCT2 ~ 0
 SCT3 ~ 0
 SCT4 ~ 0
 SCT5 ~ 0
 DEP1 ~ 0
 DEP2 ~ 0
 DEP3 ~ 0
 DEP4 ~ 0
 DEP5 ~ 0

 SCT_I =~ 0.7071*SCT1 + 0.5927*SCT2 + 0.4716*SCT3 + 0.3786*SCT4 + 0.3125*SCT5
 SCT_S =~ 0*SCT1 + 0.265*SCT2 + 0.422*SCT3 + 0.510*SCT4 + 0.561*SCT5
 DEP_I =~ 0.7746*DEP1 + 0.6527*DEP2 + 0.5352*DEP3 + 0.4498*DEP4 + 0.3917*DEP5
 DEP_S =~ 0*DEP1 + 0.265*DEP2 + 0.422*DEP3 + 0.510*DEP4 + 0.561*DEP5

 DEP_S ~ .29*SCT_I + .24*WithD + .24*LoneL
 WithD ~ .24*SCT_I
 LoneL ~ .24*SCT_I

 SCT1 ~~ .50*SCT1
 SCT2 ~~ .50*SCT2
 SCT3 ~~ .50*SCT3
 SCT4 ~~ .50*SCT4
 SCT5 ~~ .50*SCT5
 DEP1 ~~ .40*DEP1
 DEP2 ~~ .33083*DEP2
 DEP3 ~~ .31083*DEP3
 DEP4 ~~ .31047*DEP4
 DEP5 ~~ .31517*DEP5

 WithD ~~ .9424*WithD
 LoneL ~~ .9424*LoneL
 WithD ~~ .40*LoneL

 SCT_I ~~ 1*SCT_I + 0.50*DEP_I + 0.25*SCT_S
 DEP_I ~~ 1*DEP_I + 0.30*DEP_S
 SCT_S ~~ 1*SCT_S + 0.50*DEP_S
 DEP_S ~~ .6678*DEP_S
```

```
!New Variables, introduced in the Analysis Model below
X1 := 0.0576
X2 := 0.0576
"
```

The first portion of syntax above, starting with SCT1 ~ 0 to DEP5 ~ 0, reflects the intercepts of SCT and depression. The next portion of syntax,

```
SCT_I =~ 0.7071*SCT1 + 0.5927*SCT2 + 0.4716*SCT3 + 0.3786*SCT4 + 0.3125*SCT5
SCT_S =~ 0*SCT1 + 0.265*SCT2 + 0.422*SCT3 + 0.510*SCT4 + 0.561*SCT5
DEP_I =~ 0.7746*DEP1 + 0.6527*DEP2 + 0.5352*DEP3 + 0.4498*DEP4 + 0.3917*DEP5
DEP_S =~ 0*DEP1 + 0.265*DEP2 + 0.422*DEP3 + 0.510*DEP4 + 0.561*DEP5
```

sets the population parameter factor loadings to the values from the lambda (**Λ**) matrices for SCT and depression.

The third portion of syntax,

```
DEP_S ~ .29*SCT_I + .24*WithD + .24*LoneL
WithD ~ .24*SCT_I
LoneL ~ .24*SCT_I
```

reflects the predictive relationships outlined in the beta (**B**) matrix. Similar to Mplus, this information will be used to specify both the direct and mediated pathways that are necessary to answer the power analysis question relevant for this chapter.

The next portion of syntax, from SCT1 ~~ .50*SCT1 to DEP5 ~~ .31517*DEP5, contain residual variance information, respective to the theta matrices for both SCT and depression, while the following three lines of syntax show the residual variances and correlation from the time-invariant predictors in the phi (**Φ**) matrix.

```
WithD ~~ .9424*WithD
LoneL ~~ .9424*LoneL
WithD ~~ .40*LoneL
```

Two more portions of code are left to describe, and the second to last portion specifies latent variable variances, correlations, and the residual variance estimate for depression slope based on information from the psi (**Ψ**) matrix.

```
SCT_I ~~ 1*SCT_I + 0.50*DEP_I + 0.25*SCT_S
DEP_I ~~ 1*DEP_I + 0.30*DEP_S
SCT_S ~~ 1*SCT_S + 0.50*DEP_S
DEP_S ~~ .6678*DEP_S
```

In the last few lines of syntax, some new variables are introduced that include mediated/indirect effects. Unlike Mplus, which will automatically calculate population values for the mediated/indirect effects of interest, this must be explicitly coded when using lavaan. The calculated indirect effects should equal the product of the $\alpha \times \beta$ effect for each indirect effect of interest. The indirect effects of interest here include the pathway from SCT to WithDr to DEP, and SCT to LoneLin to DEP. The predicted relationship between SCT and WithDr is 0.24, and the predicted relationship between WithDr and DEP is also 0.24. The same is true for LoneLin as mediator. Thus, the expected indirect effects are calculated as $0.24 \times 0.24 = 0.0576$.

```
!New Variable Population Parameters
X1 := 0.0576
X2 := 0.0576
```

After the population model is specified, the missing data model is created to reflect minimal missing data that are missing completely at random (MCAR) at baseline. Missingness over time is expected to be missing at random (MAR), and it is expected to increase to 20% by the final assessment, dependent on SCT and depression scores at any previous time point. Over time, for every one-unit SCT score increase, there is a 10% ($exp^{0.0953} = 1.10$) increase in the odds of a missing value. Similarly, for every one-unit depression score increase, there is a 20% ($exp^{0.1823} = 1.20$) increase in the odds of a missing value at any given assessment point.

```
MissingModel_Ch10 <- "
 #The first value in each equation reflects MCAR intercepts, which is based on known
      probabilities of missingness
 #Following values reflect MAR slopes, which is based on computed logit values from
      missingness at prior time points
 WithD ~ -2.945
 LoneL ~ -2.945

 SCT2 ~ -2.9444 + .0953*SCT1
 SCT3 ~ -2.1972 + .0953*SCT2 + .0953*SCT1
 SCT4 ~ -1.7346 + .0953*SCT3 + .0953*SCT2 + .0953*SCT1
 SCT5 ~ -1.3862 + .0953*SCT4 + .0953*SCT3 + .0953*SCT2 + .0953*SCT1

 DEP2 ~ -2.9444 + .1823*DEP1
 DEP3 ~ -2.1972 + .1823*DEP2 + .1823*DEP1
 DEP4 ~ -1.7346 + .1823*DEP3 + .1823*DEP2 + .1823*DEP1
 DEP5 ~ -1.3862 + .1823*DEP4 + .1823*DEP3 + .1823*DEP2 + .1823*DEP1 "
```

Using lavaan specification, the sample analysis model shown in this chapter was specified.

```
AnalysisModel_Ch10 <- "
 SCT_I =~ 0.7071*SCT1 + 0.5927*SCT2 + 0.4716*SCT3 + 0.3786*SCT4 + 0.3125*SCT5
 SCT_S =~ 0*SCT1 + 0.265*SCT2 + 0.422*SCT3 + 0.510*SCT4 + 0.561*SCT5
 DEP_I =~ 0.7746*DEP1 + 0.6527*DEP2 + 0.5352*DEP3 + 0.4498*DEP4 + 0.3917*DEP5
 DEP_S =~ 0*DEP1 + 0.265*DEP2 + 0.422*DEP3 + 0.510*DEP4 + 0.561*DEP5

 DEP_S ~ SCT_I
 DEP_S ~ b1*WithD
 DEP_S ~ b2*LoneL
 WithD ~ a1*SCT_I
 LoneL ~ a2*SCT_I

 SCT1 ~~ SCT1
 SCT2 ~~ SCT2
 SCT3 ~~ SCT3
```

```
SCT4 ~~ SCT4
SCT5 ~~ SCT5
DEP1 ~~ DEP1
DEP2 ~~ DEP2
DEP3 ~~ DEP3
DEP4 ~~ DEP4
DEP5 ~~ DEP5

WithD ~~ WithD
LoneL ~~ LoneL
WithD ~~ LoneL

SCT_I ~~ 1*SCT_I + DEP_I + SCT_S
DEP_I ~~ 1*DEP_I + DEP_S
SCT_S ~~ 1*SCT_S + DEP_S
DEP_S ~~ .6678*DEP_S

!New Variables, introduced in the Analysis Model below
X1 := a1*b1
X2 := a2*b2
"
```

The first four lines of code constrains, or fixes, the factor loadings to identify the intercept and slope latent variables. The next five lines of code:

```
DEP_S ~ SCT_I
DEP_S ~ b1*WithD
DEP_S ~ b2*LoneL
WithD ~ a1*SCT_I
LoneL ~ a2*SCT_I
```

identify the regressions among variables of interest and assign a name to each parameter. Recall from Chapter 3 that assigning a name to a parameter allows the values of the parameters to be used in additional model constraints.

The next three chunks of code, from SCT1 ~~ SCT1 to DEP_S ~~ .6678*DEP_S, reflect the estimated residual variances, variances, and covariances. The last section of code is used to create the estimate of the indirect effect.

```
X1 := a1*b1
X2 := a2*b2
```

Recall from the population model that the calculated indirect effects should equal the product of $\alpha \times \beta$. Rather than directly calculating these values from the known population parameters, we assigned names to the relevant simulation parameters (e.g., DEP_S ~ b1*WithD), creating four new variables that represent the a_1, a_2, b_1, and b_2 pathways. These variables can be used to construct an estimate of each relevant indirect effect, which we named X1 and X2. X1 and X2 are each compared against the population variable with the same name to examine statistical power for the indirect effect.

After specifying the population and sample models, we evaluated the Monte Carlo simulation using the 'sim()' command.

```
output_Ch10 <- sim(nRep = 5000,                        #number of replications
               n = 416,                                 #target sample size
               model = AnalysisModel_Ch10,              #Analysis Model
               generate = PopulationModel_Ch10,         #Population Model
               miss = MissingModel_Ch10,                #Missing data model
               std.lv = FALSE,
               seed = 32066,
               silent = TRUE)
```

and examined an overall summary of the simulation results.

```
summary(output_Ch10)
```

This overall summary contains two elements: A summary of the model fit and convergence, and a dataframe that contains the Monte Carlo simulation model estimate(s). There is a column called Power, which reflects the power estimates for all parameters in the model. Only the two rows that reflect the indirect effects are shown in Table 10.1.

Like the Mplus output, these results show that a sample size of 416, with the anticipated level of missingness, and moderate effects among variables, has power ≥ .80 for the joint product coefficient where either social withdrawal or loneliness is a mediator of the relationship between SCT and depression.

Parallel-Process Simulation Power Analysis Write-Up

"The power analysis question involves the sample size needed to achieve power ≥ .80 to reject the null hypothesis for either social withdrawal or loneliness as potential mediators of sluggish cognitive tempo (SCT) intercept as a predictor of depression score change over time (slope) in a parallel-process growth model with $T = 5$ assessment time points. A Monte Carlo simulation power analysis involving 5,000 dataset replications was conducted using Mplus (version 8.5) assuming: (1) standardization of all observed SCT and depression observed response variables included in the parallel-process model, (2) linear trend that explains ($R^2 = 0.50$) 50% of SCT and ($R^2 = 0.60$) 60% of depression observed response variable variance, respectively, (3) SCT intercept as a predictor that explain ($R^2 = 0.0576$) 5.76% of both social withdrawal and loneliness variance, (4) social withdrawal and loneliness, together with the direct effect of SCT intercept, that explains ($R^2 = 0.3322$) 33.22% of depression slope variance, (5) missing

TABLE 10.1. Indirect Effect Power Results for Parallel-Process Mediation

	Estimate average	Estimate SD	Average SE	Power (not equal to 0)
X1: a1*b1	0.058	0.023	0.023	0.818
X2: a2*b2	0.057	0.022	0.023	0.817

data for social withdrawal and loneliness data that is minimal (i.e., 5%) and missing completely at random (MCAR), (6) missing data for both SCT and depression observed response variable scores expected to increase between 5 and 20% from postbaseline to the study conclusion, and is assumed to be MAR as SCT and depression score increases at any assessment time point are expected to increase the odds of missing data 10 and 20%, respectively, at a subsequent assessment time point. Results from 5,000 dataset replications showed power ≥ .80 for any joint product coefficient ($\alpha * \beta \geq 0.0576$; 95% CI = 0.013, 0.103) for either social withdrawal or loneliness as a mediator if SCT intercept as a predictor of depression slope if proper missing data handling makes $N = 416$ available for analysis."

SUGGESTED READINGS

- Grubbs, J. B., Kraus, S. W., Perry, S. L., Lewczuk, K., & Gola, M. (2020). Moral incongruence and compulsive sexual behavior: Results from cross-sectional interactions and parallel growth curve analyses. *Journal of Abnormal Psychology, 129,* 266–278.
- Koo, N., Leite, W. L., & Algina, J. (2016). Mediated effects with the parallel process latent growth model: An evaluation of methods for testing mediation in the presence of non-normal data. *Structural Equation Modeling: A Multidisciplinary Journal, 23*(1), 32–44.
- Lee, Y. K., & Ju, U. (2021). Joint trajectories of extrinsic motivation and competence beliefs: A parallel-process growth mixture modeling approach. *Contemporary Educational Psychology, 65,* 101944.
- Liu, J., & Perera, R. A. (2021). Estimating knots and their association in parallel bilinear spline growth curve models in the framework of individual measurement occasions. *Psychological Methods, 27*(5), 703–729.
- Liu, X., Zhang, Z., Valentino, K., & Wang, L. (2024). The impact of omitting confounders in parallel process latent growth curve mediation models: Three sensitivity analysis approaches. *Structural Equation Modeling: A Multidisciplinary Journal, 31*(1), 132–150.
- Nazari, S., Leite, W. L., & Huggins-Manley, A. C. (2023). A comparison between the piecewise and parallel-process piecewise latent growth models. *The Journal of Experimental Education, 91*(1), 62–81.
- Zhu, J., & Chen, Y. (2021). Developmental Pathways from Parental Rejection to Adolescent Internet Gaming Disorder: A Parallel Process Latent Growth Model. *Children and Youth Services Review, 128*(3), 106128.

11

Power Analysis for Complex Longitudinal Designs

Randomized control trials, even those with numerous covariates, typically involve relatively straightforward power analysis models because the research question often proposes one or more specific hypotheses about the effect of treatment on one or more outcomes of interest. Observational studies are also a popular research design for many reasons, not the least of which is that many research questions are not practically or morally amenable to random assignment. Unlike randomized control trials that tend to pose specific research questions that test specific effects, observational studies often seek to understand the nature and direction of how multiple constructs may be related. The power analysis model from Chapter 10 illustrates this idea well: Becker and colleagues (2016) sought to understand both how depression and sluggish cognitive tempo (SCT) changed over time, and if social withdrawal and loneliness mediated the relationship between SCT initial status and depression changes over time, in a sample of adolescent research participants. The point to be made is that, in seeking to understand possible relationships among numerous variables, observational research questions can get somewhat elaborate, and the subsequent power analyses needed to answer them can become very complex. Not only do complex longitudinal power analysis models that are based on elaborate research questions pose a stern test of many of the guiding themes presented here (such as standardization simplifies and admissibility verification through model-reproduced correlation matrix calculations), but they also offer an opportunity to illustrate an additional power analysis technique: If power estimates for a complex longitudinal model are needed, a helpful simplifying strategy involves working with manageable sections of the analysis model, and moving systematically from the *endogenous* to the *exogenous*, or from the inside out.

A Complex Longitudinal Power Analysis Model Based on Beal et al. (2020)

Research by Beal and colleagues (2020) examined the relationships between retrospective childhood maltreatment (defined as abuse or neglect), psychological distress, and self-reported adult pain. Specifically, the authors hypothesized that maltreatment would produce increased psychological distress, which would, in turn, result in increased self-reported pain. Results showed that various indices of psychological distress were significant mediators of the relationship between maltreatment and binary ("Have you experienced more than 'every day' pain in the last week? [1 = Yes, 0 = No]"), count (number of specific pain locations), and continuous (average pain intensity) indices of self-reported pain. Beal and colleagues (2020) subsequently proposed a larger research study that investigated: (1) changes in adolescent (ages 13–17) psychological functioning over time (measured by the Child Depression Inventory; CDI), (2) effect of childhood maltreatment (MalTx) on adolescent psychological functioning over time, (3) adolescent psychological functioning as a predictor of adult quality of life (QOL), and (4) childhood maltreatment as a predictor of later (a) self-reported pain (measured by qualitative sensory testing and self-report; Pain), (b) stress reactions (measured by cortisol levels; Stress), and (c) acute inflammation (measured by C-reactive protein; Inflam), and (d) QOL, pain, stress, and inflammation as predictors of whether (= 1) or not (= 0) participants meet subsequent diagnostic criteria for opioid abuse disorder. A complex longitudinal analysis model consistent with these proposed relationships is shown in Figure 11.1.

Two observations are immediately apparent from the longitudinal analysis model in Figure 11.1. First, Beal and colleagues are willing to assume that linear trend best describes CDI scores over time and will explain (R^2 = 0.70) 70% of CDI variance. Second, a complex set of predictions involving linear CDI trend, maltreatment, QOL, biological markers (inflame, stress, and pain), and the probability of an opioid misuse diagnosis (opioid) are being tested. At this point, though, what is missing from the model in Figure 11.1 are both

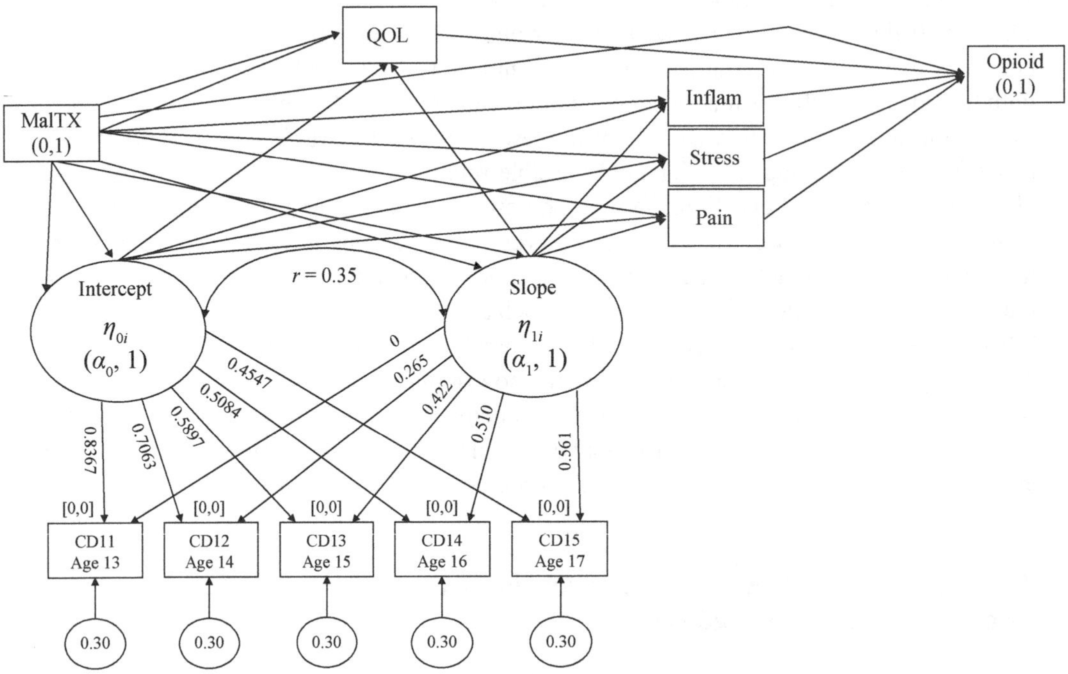

FIGURE 11.1. A complex longitudinal model. Data from Beal et al. (2020).

parameter estimates for this complex set of relationships and a systematic way of computing residual variances for CDI trajectory, QOL, and the biological markers that would allow a model admissibility check and a subsequent Monte Carlo power analysis. However, first, after consulting a number of relevant meta-analytic (Bernard, Frost, Bennett, & Lindhiem, 2017; Davis, Luecken, & Zautra, 2005; Fischer, Macare, & Cleare, 2017; Horn et al., 2018; Kennis et al., 2020; Kuhlman, Horn, Chiang, & Bower, 2020; Pitharouli et al., 2022; Stubbs et al., 2017) and empirical publications (Beal et al., 2019, 2020; Kugler et al., 2019; Kuhlman, Geiss, Vargas, & Lopez-Duran, 2015; Kuhlman, Chiang, Horn, & Bower, 2017; Olson, Shenk, Noll, & Allen, 2022; Palmos et al., 2019; Peckins, Susman, Negriff, Noll, & Trickett, 2015; Rivera, Bray, Guastaferro, Kugler, & Noll, 2018; Shenk, Noll, Peugh, Griffin, & Bensman, 2016), a reasonable set of parameter estimates can be specified for all the complex relationships tested in the model in Figure 11.1. Second, and more importantly, distinct response variables (CDI trajectory, QOL, the biological markers, and opioid misuse diagnosis) are being predicted at different points in the longitudinal model. This allows for a partitioning of the analysis model to calculate residual variances by moving systematically from the *endogenous* predicted variables to the *exogenous* predicted variables, or from the inside to the outside.

Maltreatment Predicting CDI Trajectory Variance

The process of computing residual variances using a systematic methodology between sections of the analytic model from the inside to the outside means starting with any predictors of trajectory component variation in CDI score changes over time (the endogenous response variables). The only predictor of CDI change over time is the binary maltreatment indicator variable. Based on previous research, the authors theorize that maltreatment will explain ($R^2 = 0.10$) 10% of CDI intercept variance, and ($R^2 = 0.1,5$) 15% of CDI linear slope variance. As the only predictor of CDI trajectory variance, the authors, by definition, are specifying a standardized coefficient of ($\beta_1 = \sqrt{0.10} = 0.31623$) $\beta = 0.31623$ for maltreatment as a predictor of intercept variance, and a standardized coefficient of ($\beta_2 = \sqrt{0.15} = 0.3873$) $\beta = 0.3873$ for maltreatment as a predictor of linear slope variance, as shown in Figure 11.2.

CDI Trajectories and Maltreatment Predict Quality of Life (QOL)

Based on prior research, Beal and colleagues (2019, 2020) hypothesize the following standardized coefficients quantifying the effects of CDI trajectory component variances and maltreatment as a predictor of later adult quality of life, as shown in Figure 11.3.

As shown in previous chapters and assuming standardization, residual QOL variance ($\sigma^2_{\text{RESIDUAL}}$) will equal one minus variance explained by predictors (R^2), or $\sigma^2_{\text{RESIDUAL}} = 1{-}R^2$. Furthermore, QOL variance explained (R^2) can be calculated as the sum of the variance explained by CDI intercept, CDI linear slope, and maltreatment as predictors, or ($R^2 = R^2_{\text{CDI\_Intercept}} + R^2_{\text{CDI\_Slope}} + R^2_{\text{Maltreatment}}$). As also shown previously, each of the three variance explained components ($R^2_{\text{CDI\_Intercept}}$, $R^2_{\text{CDI\_Slope}}$, and $R^2_{\text{Maltreatment}}$) can be computed using Wright's path tracing rules.

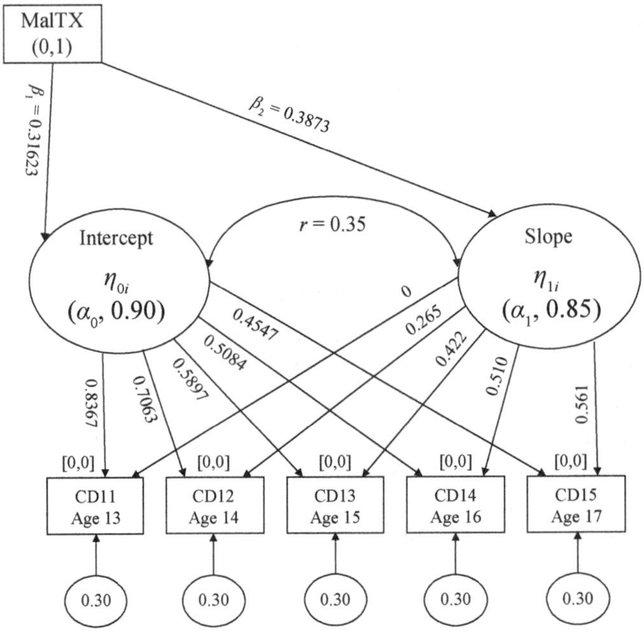

FIGURE 11.2. Maltreatment predicting CDI trajectory variance.

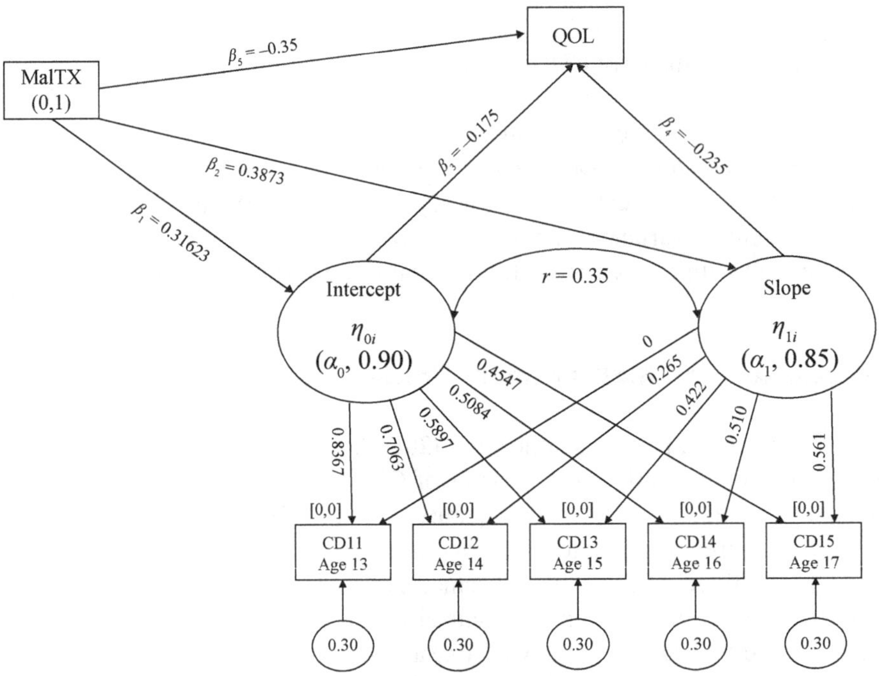

FIGURE 11.3. QOL predicted by CDI trajectory and maltreatment.

$$R^2_{\text{Stress|CDI\_Slope}} = (\text{Direct effect} * (\text{Direct effect} + [\text{Sum of indirect effects products}]))$$
$$= (\beta_3 * (\beta_3 + [\text{Sum of indirect effects products}]))$$

According to Wright's rules, there are four admissible indirect effects from the CDI intercept to QOL. The first is from the CDI intercept to the CDI slope, and from the CDI slope to QOL, as shown in Figure 11.4. The second admissible indirect path is from the CDI intercept to maltreatment, and from maltreatment to QOL, as shown in Figure 11.5. The third admissible indirect path is from the CDI intercept to the CDI slope, from the CDI slope to maltreatment, and from maltreatment to QOL, as shown in Figure 11.6. The final admissible indirect path is from the CDI intercept to maltreatment, from maltreatment to the CDI slope, and from the CDI slope to QOL, as shown in Figure 11.7. So,

$$R^2_{\text{Stress|CDI\_Slope}} = (\beta_3 * (\beta_3 + [\text{Sum of indirect effects products}]))$$
$$= (\beta_3 * (\beta_3 + [r * \beta_4] + [\beta_1 * \beta_5] + [r * \beta_2 * \beta_5] + [\beta_1 * \beta_2 * \beta_4]))$$
$$= (-0.175 * (-0.175 + [0.35 * -0.235] + [0.31623 * -0.35]$$
$$+ [0.35 * 0.3873 * -0.35] [+ 0.31623 * 0.3873 * -0.235]))$$
$$= (-0.175 * (-0.175 + [-0.08225] + [-0.11068] + [-0.04744425] + [-0.0287818]))$$
$$= (-0.175 * (-0.444156581565)) = \mathbf{0.077727401773875}$$

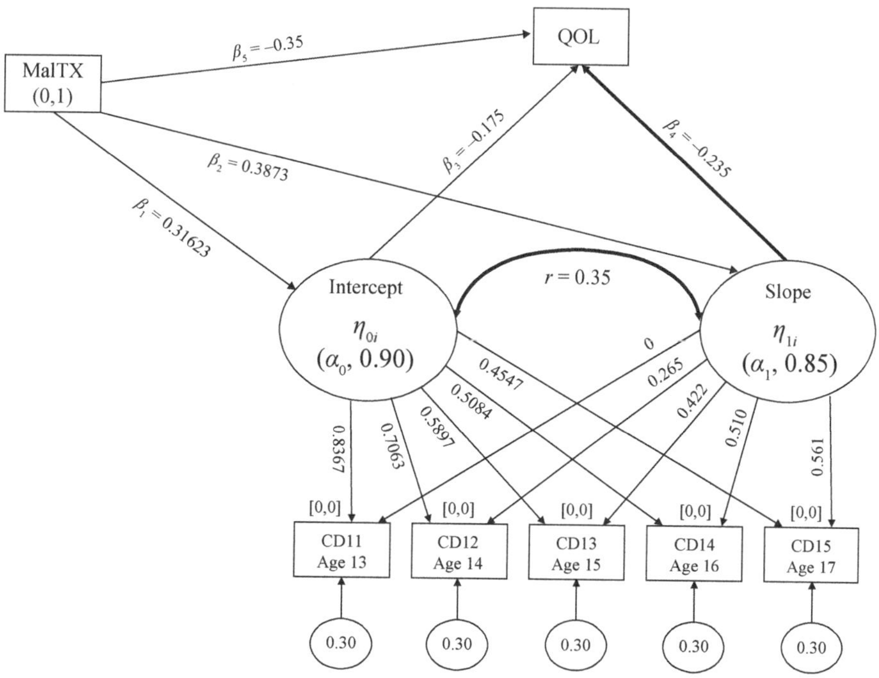

FIGURE 11.4. QOL predicted by CDI intercept: First indirect path.

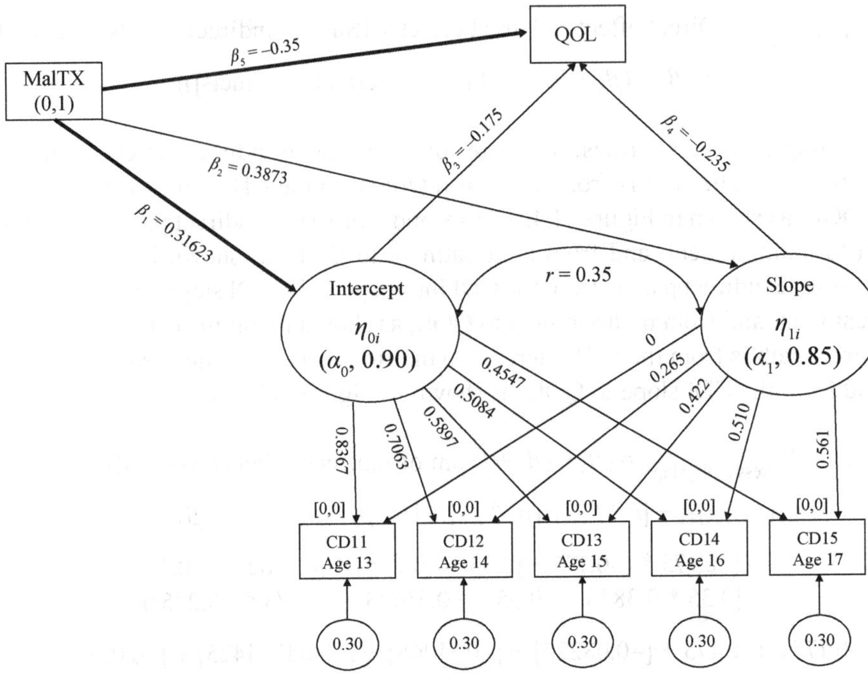

FIGURE 11.5. QOL predicted by CDI intercept: Second indirect path.

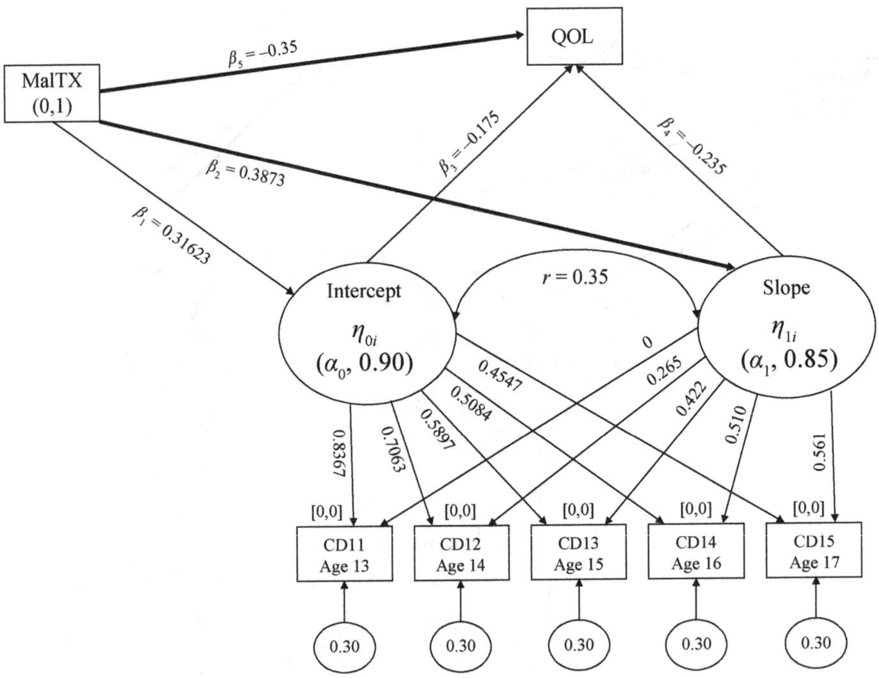

FIGURE 11.6. QOL predicted by CDI intercept:: Third indirect path.

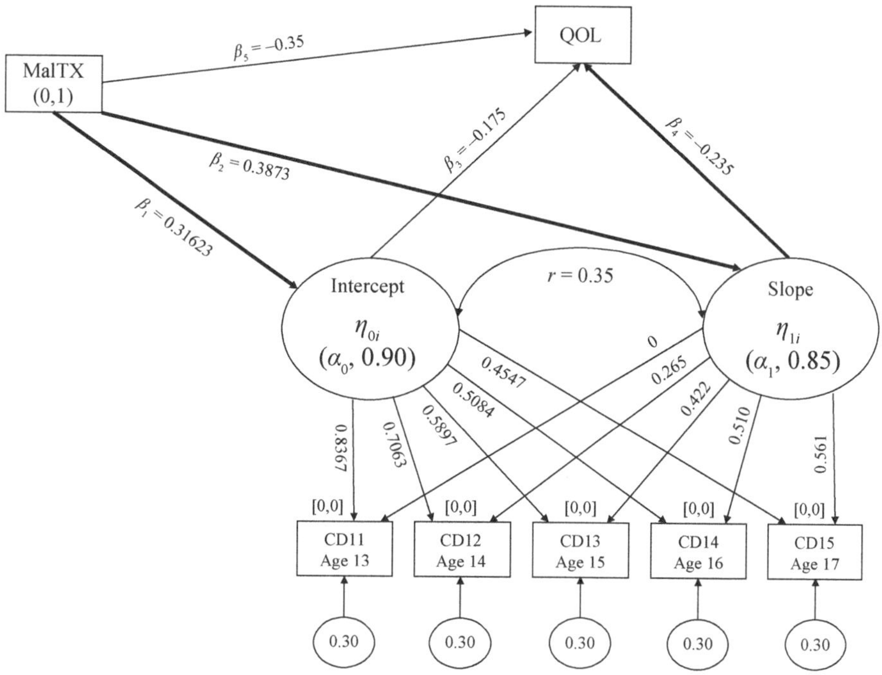

FIGURE 11.7. QOL predicted by CDI intercept: Final indirect path.

$$R^2_{\text{CDI\_Slope}} = (\text{Direct effect} * (\text{Direct effect} + [\text{Sum of indirect effects products}]))$$
$$= (\beta_4 * (\beta_4 + [\text{Sum of indirect effects products}]))$$

There are three admissible indirect pathways from the CDI linear slope to QOL. The first is from the CDI slope to the CDI intercept, and then from the CDI intercept to QOL, as shown in Figure 11.8. The second admissible indirect pathway is from the CDI slope to the CDI intercept, from the CDI intercept to maltreatment, and from maltreatment to QOL, as shown in Figure 11.9. The final admissible pathway is from the CDI slope to maltreatment, and then from maltreatment to QOL, as shown in Figure 11.10. So,

$$R^2_{\text{CDI\_Slope}} = (\beta_4 * (\beta_4 + [\text{Sum of indirect effects products}]))$$
$$= (\beta_4 * (\beta_4 + [r * \beta_3] + [r * \beta_1 * \beta_5] + [\beta_2 * \beta_5]))$$
$$= (-0.235 * (-0.235 + [0.35 * -0.175] + [0.35 * 0.31625 * -0.35] + [0.3875 * -0.35]))$$
$$= (-0.235 * (-0.470615625)) = \mathbf{0.110594671875}$$

$$R^2_{\text{Maltreatment}} = (\text{Direct effect} * (\text{Direct effect} + [\text{Sum of indirect effects products}]))$$
$$= (\beta_5 * (\beta_5 + [\text{Sum of indirect effects products}]))$$

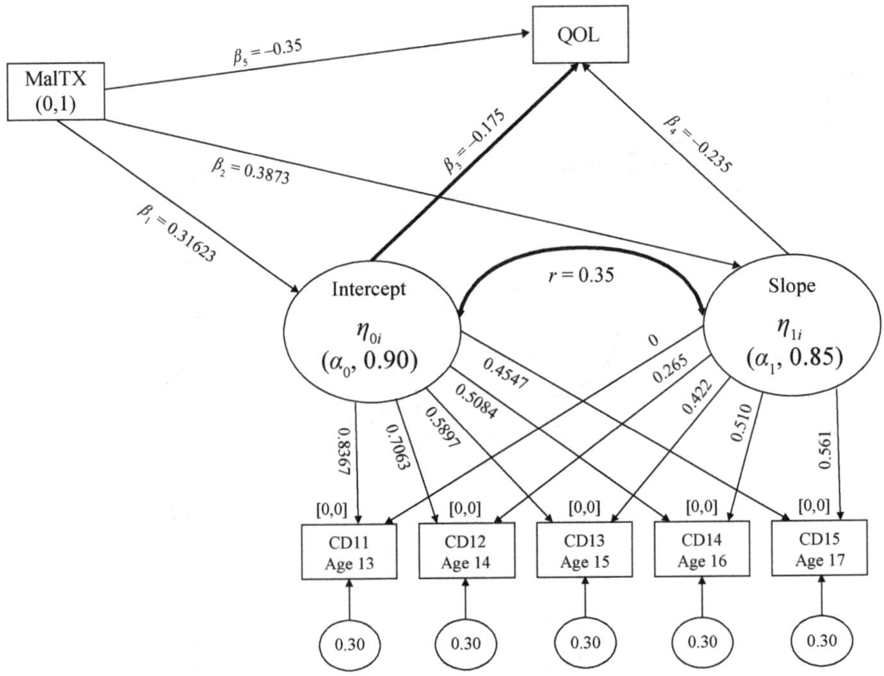

FIGURE 11.8. QOL predicted by CDI slope: First indirect path.

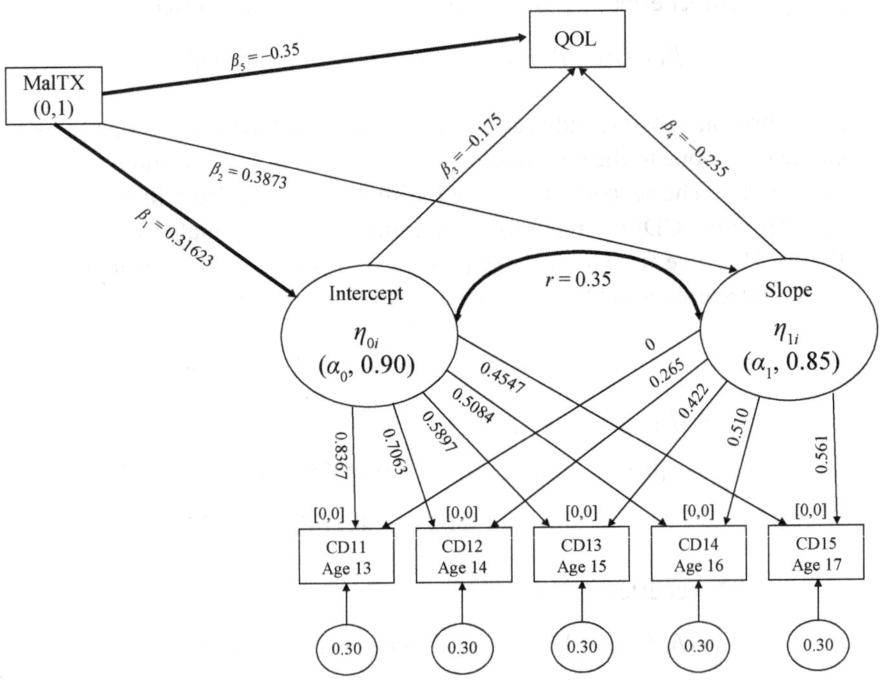

FIGURE 11.9. QOL predicted by CDI slope: Second indirect path.

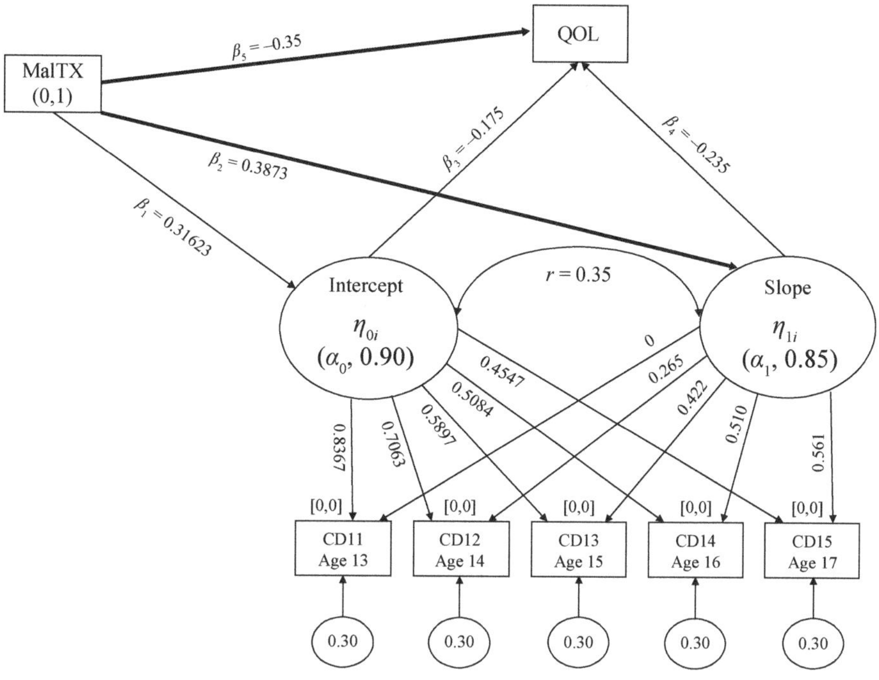

FIGURE 11.10. QOL predicted by CDI slope: Final indirect path.

There are three admissible indirect pathways from maltreatment to QOL. The first is from maltreatment to the CDI intercept and from the CDI intercept to QOL, as shown in Figure 11.11. The second admissible indirect path is from maltreatment to the CDI intercept, from the CDI intercept to the CDI slope, and then from the CDI slope to QOL, as shown in Figure 11.12. The final admissible indirect path is from maltreatment to the CDI slope and then from the CDI slope to QOL, as shown in Figure 11.13. So,

$$R^2_{\text{Maltreatment}} = (\beta_5 * (\beta_5 + [\text{Sum of indirect effects products}]))$$
$$= (\beta_5 * (\beta_5 + [\beta_1 * \beta_3] + [\beta_1 * r * \beta_4] + [\beta_2 * \beta_4]))$$
$$= (-0.35 * (-0.35 + [0.31623 * -0.175] + [0.31623 * 0.35 * -0.235] + [0.3873 * -0.235]))$$
$$= (-0.35 * (-0.5223656675)) = \mathbf{0.182827983625}$$

And,

$$(R^2 = R^2_{\text{CDI\_Intercept}} + R^2_{\text{CDI\_Slope}} + R^2_{\text{Maltreatment}})$$
$$= (R^2 = \mathbf{0.077727401773875} + \mathbf{0.110594671875} + \mathbf{0.182827983625})$$
$$= R^2 = \mathbf{0.37115}$$

So,

$$(\sigma^2_{\text{RESIDUAL}} = 1 - R^2) = 1 - 0.37115 = \underline{\mathbf{0.62885}}$$

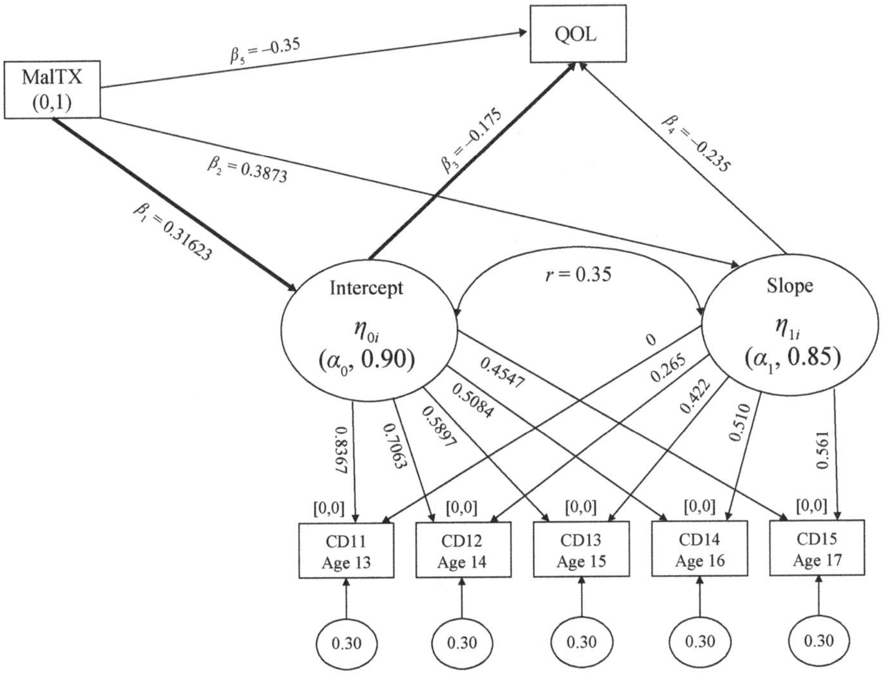

FIGURE 11.11. QOL predicted by maltreatment: First indirect path.

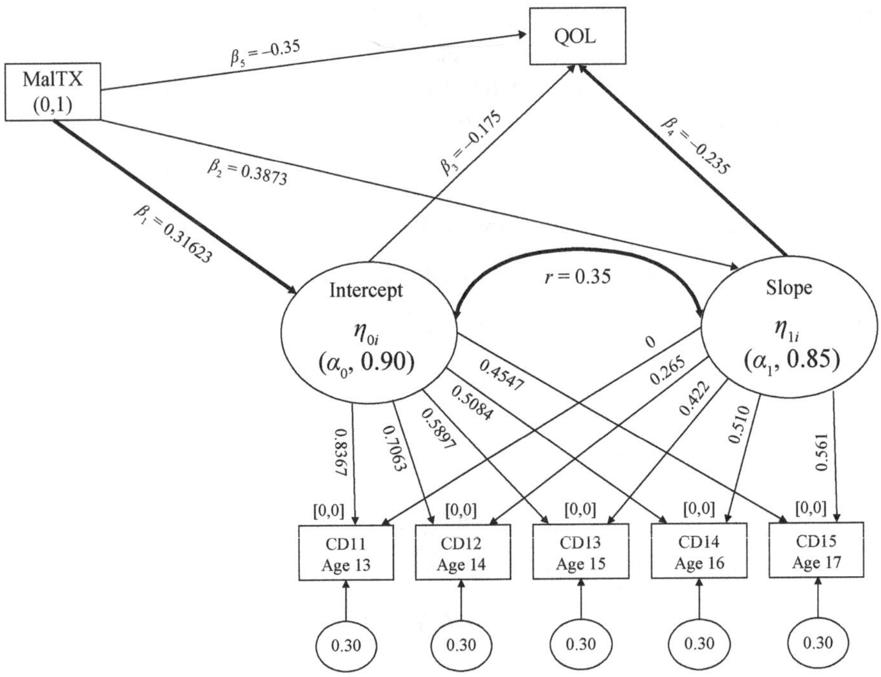

FIGURE 11.12. QOL predicted by maltreatment: Second indirect path.

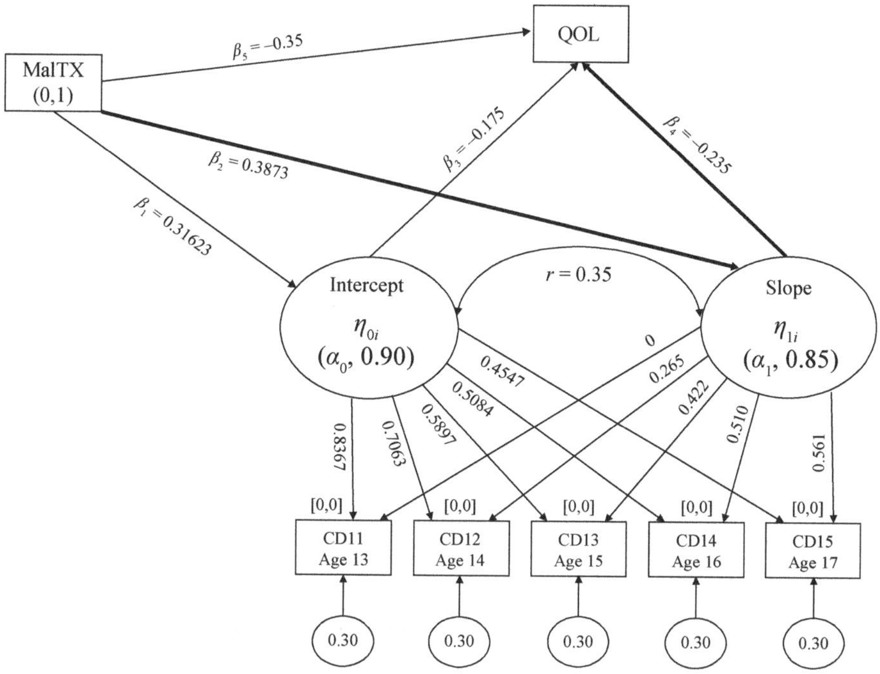

FIGURE 11.13. QOL predicted by maltreatment: Final indirect path.

CDI Trajectory and Maltreatment Predict Biomarkers

Furthermore, also based on previous research, are the following standardized effects for the CDI trajectory and maltreatment that predicts the three biomarkers, as shown in Figure 11.14. Prior to undertaking the task of computing residual variances in the three biomarkers using Wright's rules, it is important to point out that an additional, and not readily apparent, assumption is being made in the analysis model shown here. Notice that there are no curved, double-headed arrows connecting any of the three biomarkers. This means that, conditional on the CDI intercept, the CDI slope, and maltreatment as predictors, the residual variances among the three biomarkers are assumed to be uncorrelated. Just as in the previous section, Wright's rules will be used to compute residual variances assuming, under standardization:

$$(\sigma^2_{\text{RESIDUAL}} = 1 - R^2),$$

and

$$(R^2 = R^2_{\text{CDI}_{\text{Intercept}}} + R^2_{\text{CDI}_{\text{Slope}}} + R^2_{\text{Maltreatment}})$$

for all three biomarkers, beginning with inflammation (inflam), followed by stress, and then by pain.

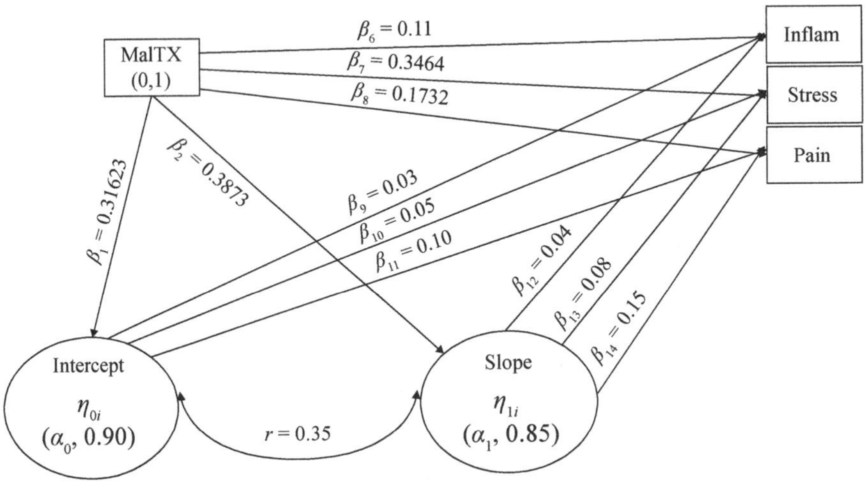

FIGURE 11.14. Biomarkers predicted by CDI trajectory and maltreatment.

$$R^2_{\text{Inflam|CDI\_Intercept}} = (\text{Direct effect} * (\text{Direct effect} + [\text{Sum of indirect effects products}]))$$
$$= (\beta_9 * (\beta_9 + [\text{Sum of indirect effects products}]))$$

There are four admissible indirect effects from the CDI intercept to inflammation. The first is from the CDI intercept to the CDI slope and from the CDI slope to inflammation, as shown in Figure 11.15. The second admissible indirect pathway is from the CDI intercept to maltreatment and from maltreatment to inflammation, as shown in Figure 11.16. The third admissible indirect pathway is from the CDI intercept to the CDI slope, from the CDI slope to maltreatment, and from maltreatment to inflammation, as shown in Figure 11.17. The final admissible indirect pathway is from the CDI intercept to maltreatment, from maltreatment to the CDI slope, and from the CDI slope to inflammation, as shown in Figure 11.18.

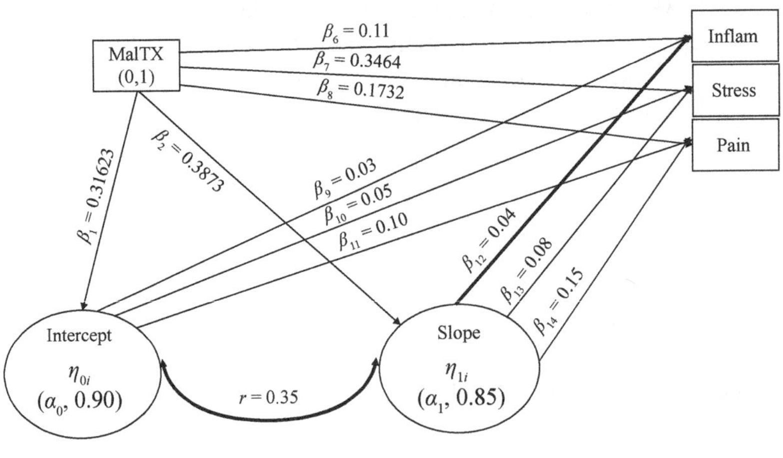

FIGURE 11.15. Inflammation predicted by CDI intercept: First indirect path.

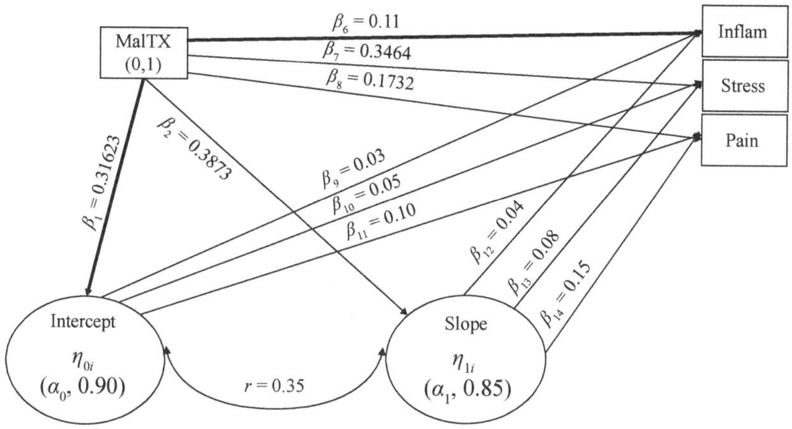

FIGURE 11.16. Inflammation predicted by CDI intercept: Second indirect path.

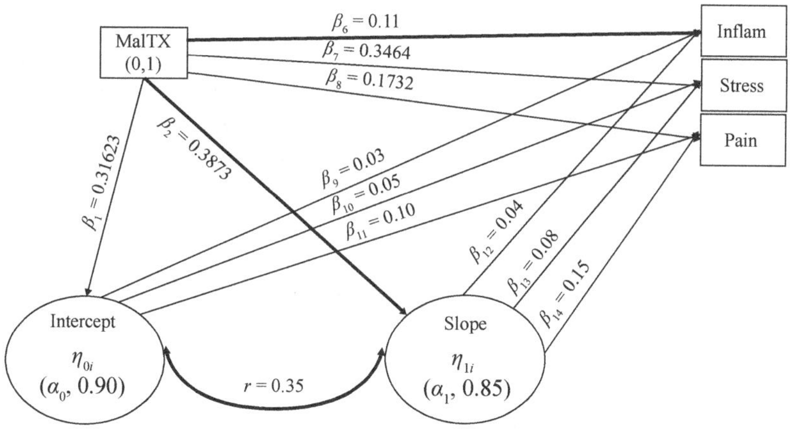

FIGURE 11.17. Inflammation predicted by CDI intercept: Third indirect path.

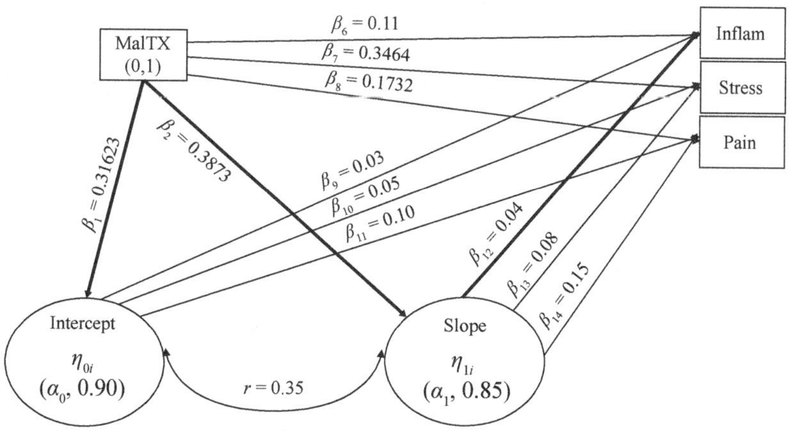

FIGURE 11.18. Inflammation predicted by CDI intercept: Final indirect path.

So,

$$R^2_{\text{Inflam|CDI\_Intercept}} = (\beta_9 * (\beta_9 + [\text{Sum of indirect effects products}]))$$
$$= (\beta_9 * (\beta_9 + [r * \beta_{12}] + [\beta_1 * \beta_6] + [r * \beta_2 * \beta_6] + [\beta_1 * \beta_2 * \beta_{12}]))$$
$$= (0.03 * (0.03 + [0.35 * 0.04] + [0.31623 * 0.11]$$
$$+ [0.35 * 0.3873 * 0.11][+ 0.31623 * 0.3873 * 0.04]))$$
$$= (0.03 * (0.09859538516)) = \mathbf{0.0029578615548}$$

$$R^2_{\text{Inflam|CDI\_Slope}} = (\text{Direct effect} * (\text{Direct effect} + [\text{Sum of indirect effects products}]))$$
$$= (\beta_{12} * (\beta_{12} + [\text{Sum of indirect effects products}]))$$

There are also four admissible indirect paths from CDI slope to inflammation. The first admissible indirect path is from the CDI slope to the CDI intercept and then from the CDI intercept to inflammation, as shown in Figure 11.19. The second admissible indirect path is from the CDI slope to maltreatment and from maltreatment to inflammation, as shown in Figure 11.20. The third admissible indirect path is from the CDI slope to the CDI intercept, from the CDI intercept to maltreatment, and from maltreatment to inflammation, as shown in Figure 11.21. The final admissible indirect path is from the CDI slope to maltreatment, from maltreatment to the CDI intercept, and from the CDI intercept to inflammation, as shown in Figure 11.22. So,

$$R^2_{\text{Inflam|CDI\_Slope}} = (\beta_{12} * (\beta_{12} + [\text{Sum of indirect effects products}]))$$
$$= (\beta_{12} * (\beta_{12} + [r * \beta_9] + [\beta_2 * \beta_6] + [r * \beta_1 * \beta_6] + [\beta_2 * \beta_1 * \beta_9]))$$
$$= (0.04 * (0.04 + [0.35 * 0.03] + [0.3873 * 0.11]$$
$$+ [0.35 * 0.31623 * 0.11][+ 0.3873 * 0.31623 * 0.03]))$$
$$= (0.04 * (0.10895213137)) = \mathbf{0.0043580852548}$$

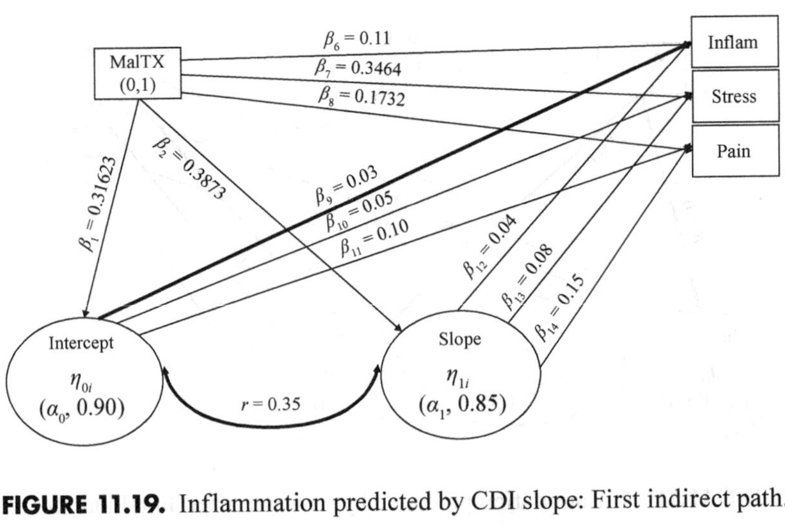

FIGURE 11.19. Inflammation predicted by CDI slope: First indirect path.

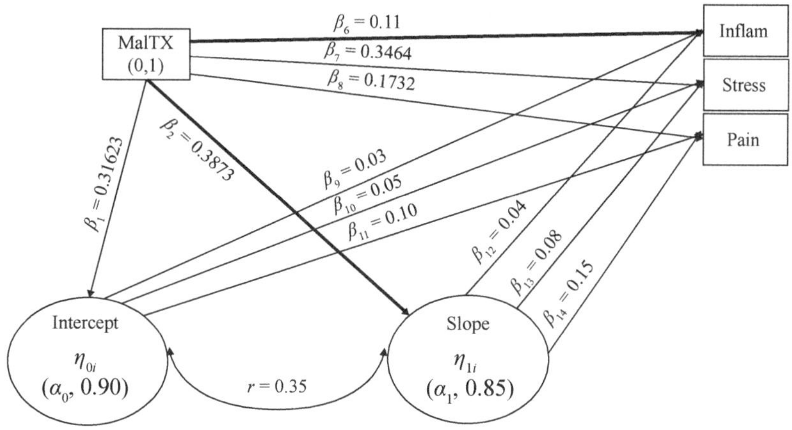

FIGURE 11.20. Inflammation predicted by CDI slope: Second indirect path.

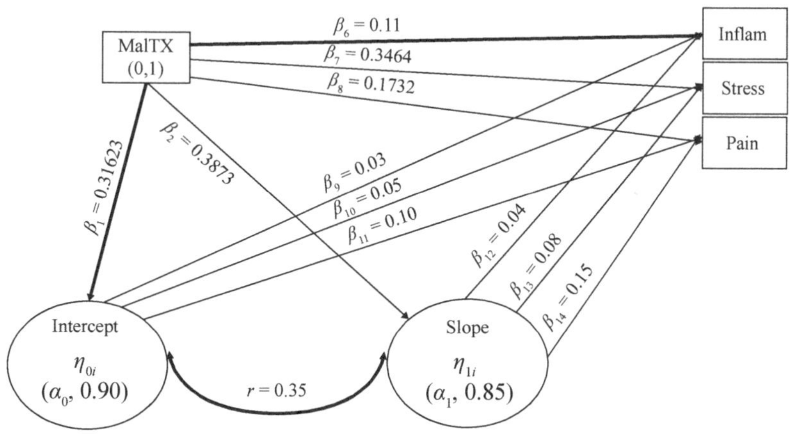

FIGURE 11.21. Inflammation predicted by CDI slope: Third indirect path.

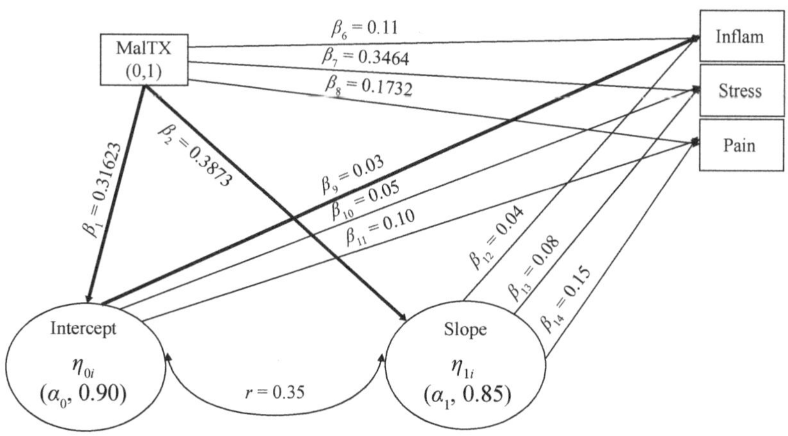

FIGURE 11.22. Inflammation predicted by CDI slope: Final indirect path.

$$R^2_{\text{Inflam|Maltreatment}} = (\text{Direct effect} * (\text{Direct effect} + [\text{Sum of indirect effects products}]))$$
$$= (\beta_6 * (\beta_6 + [\text{Sum of indirect effects products}]))$$

There are also four indirect pathways from maltreatment to inflammation. The first admissible indirect pathway is from maltreatment to the CDI slope and from the CDI slope to inflammation, as shown in Figure 11.23. The second admissible indirect pathway is from maltreatment to the CDI intercept and then from the CDI intercept to inflammation, as shown in Figure 11.24. The third admissible indirect pathway is from maltreatment to the CDI slope, then from the CDI slope to the CDI intercept, and then from the CDI intercept to inflammation, as shown in Figure 11.25. The final admissible indirect pathway is from maltreatment to the CDI intercept, then from the CDI intercept to the CDI slope, and then from the CDI slope to inflammation, as shown in Figure 11.26. So,

$$R^2_{\text{Inflam|Maltreatment}} = (\beta_6 * (\beta_6 + [\text{Sum of indirect effects products}]))$$
$$= (\beta_6 * (\beta_6 + [\beta_2 * \beta_{12}] + [\beta_1 * \beta_9] + [\beta_2 * r * \beta_9] + [\beta_1 * r * \beta_{12}]))$$
$$= (0.11 * (0.11 + [0.3873 * 0.04] + [0.31623 * 0.03]$$
$$+ [0.3873 * 0.35 * 0.03][0.31623 * 0.35 * 0.04]))$$
$$= (0.11 * (0.14347277)) = \mathbf{0.0157820047}$$

And,

$$R^2_{\text{Inflam}} = R^2_{\text{CDI\_Intercept}} + R^2_{\text{CDI\_Slope}} + R^2_{\text{Maltreatment}}$$
$$R^2_{\text{Inflam}} = \mathbf{0.0029578615548} + \mathbf{0.0043580852548} + \mathbf{0.0157820047} = \mathbf{0.023098}$$

So,

$$\sigma^2_{\text{RESIDUAL}} = 1 - R^2 = 1 - \mathbf{0.023098} = \underline{\mathbf{0.9769}}$$

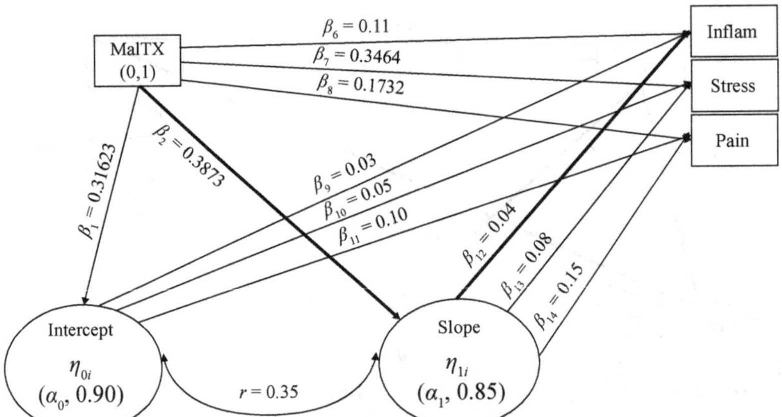

FIGURE 11.23. Inflammation predicted by maltreatment: First indirect path.

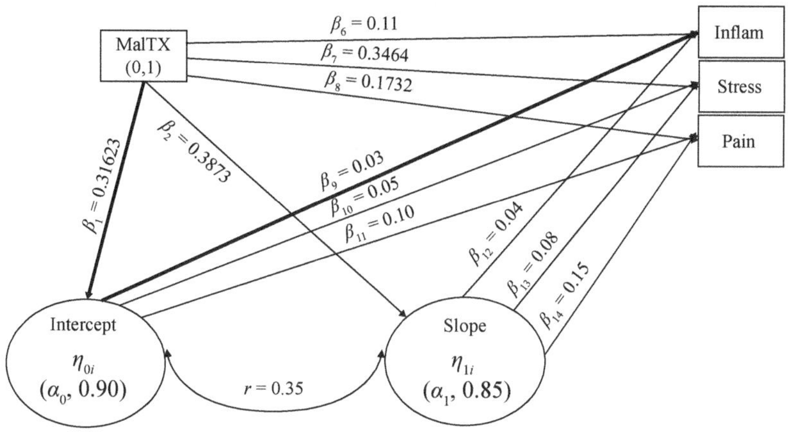

FIGURE 11.24. Inflammation predicted by maltreatment: Second indirect path.

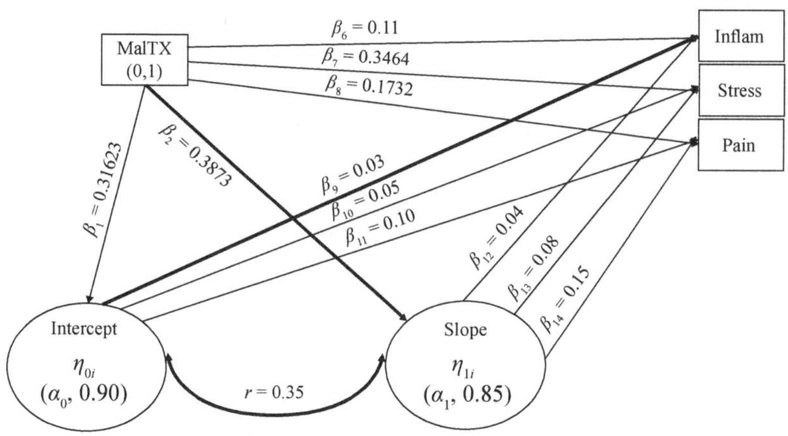

FIGURE 11.25. Inflammation predicted by maltreatment: Third indirect path.

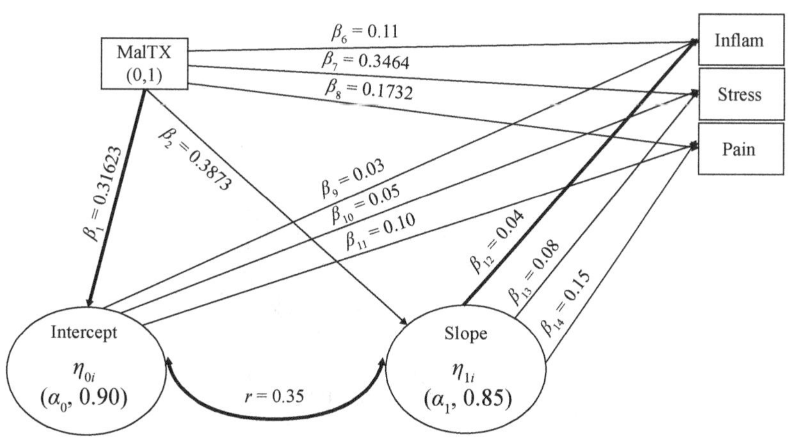

FIGURE 11.26. Inflammation predicted by maltreatment: Final indirect path.

Computing stress residual variance follows the same pattern assuming

$$\sigma^2_{\text{RESIDUAL}} = 1 - R^2$$

and

$$R^2_{\text{Stress}} = R^2_{\text{CDI}_{\text{Intercept}}} + R^2_{\text{CDI}_{\text{Slope}}} + R^2_{\text{Maltreatment}}$$

and will start with CDI intercept.

$$\begin{aligned} R^2_{\text{Stress|CDI\_Intercept}} &= (\text{Direct effect} * (\text{Direct effect} + [\text{Sum of indirect effects products}])) \\ &= (\beta_{10} * (\beta_{10} + [\text{Sum of indirect effects products}])) \end{aligned}$$

Again, there are four admissible indirect pathways from the CDI intercept to the stress biomarker. The first is from the CDI intercept to the CDI slope and then from the CDI slope to stress, as shown in Figure 11.27. The second admissible indirect pathway is from the CDI intercept to maltreatment and then from maltreatment to the stress biomarker, as shown in Figure 11.28. The third admissible indirect pathway is from the CDI intercept to the CDI slope, from the CDI slope to maltreatment, and then from maltreatment to the stress biomarker, as shown in Figure 11.29. The final admissible indirect pathway is from the CDI intercept to maltreatment, from maltreatment to the CDI slope, and then from the CDI slope to the stress biomarker, as shown in Figure 11.30. So,

$$\begin{aligned} R^2_{\text{Stress|CDI\_Intercept}} &= (\beta_{10} * (\beta_{10} + [\text{Sum of indirect effects products}])) \\ &= (\beta_{10} * (\beta_{10} + [r * \beta_{13}] + [\beta_1 * \beta_7] + [r * \beta_2 * \beta_7] + [\beta_1 * \beta_2 * \beta_{13}])) \\ &= (0.05 * (0.05 + [0.35 * 0.08] + [0.31623 * 0.3464] \\ &\quad + [0.35 * 0.3873 * 0.3464][0.31623 * 0.3873 * 0.08])) \\ &= (0.05 * (0.24429639432)) = \mathbf{0.012214819716} \end{aligned}$$

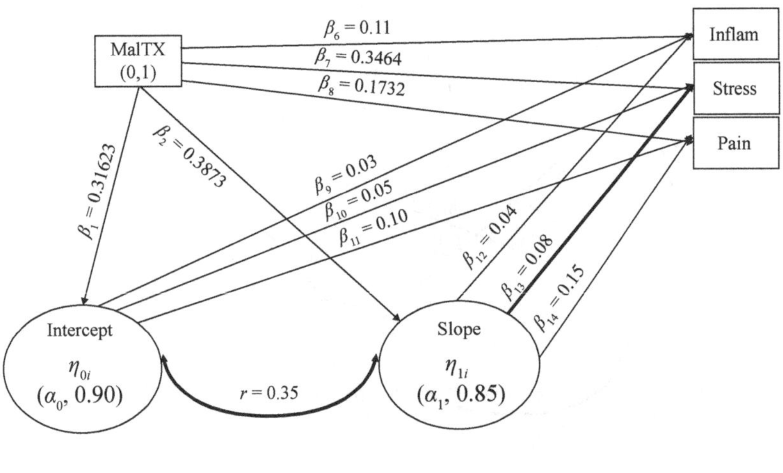

FIGURE 11.27. Stress predicted by CDI intercept: First indirect path.

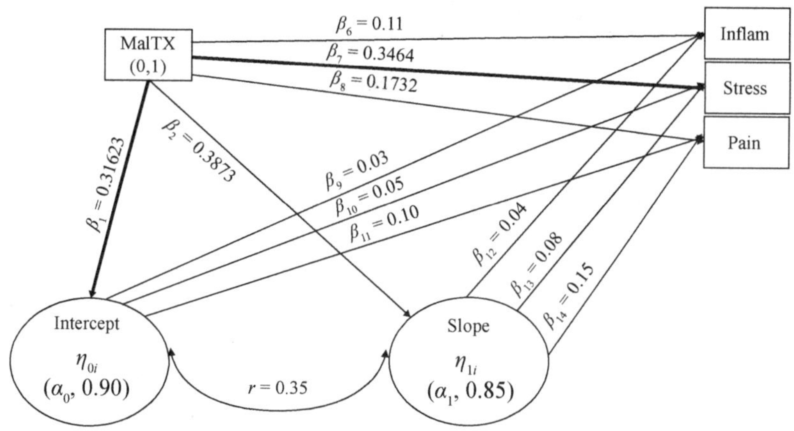

FIGURE 11.28. Stress predicted by CDI intercept: Second indirect path.

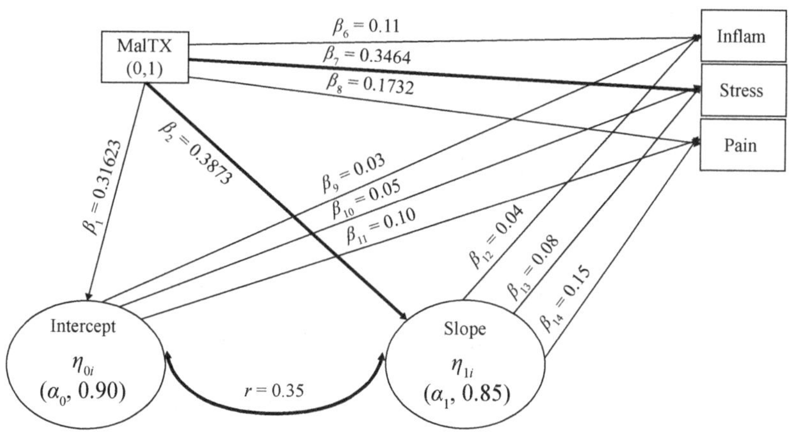

FIGURE 11.29. Stress predicted by CDI intercept: Third indirect path.

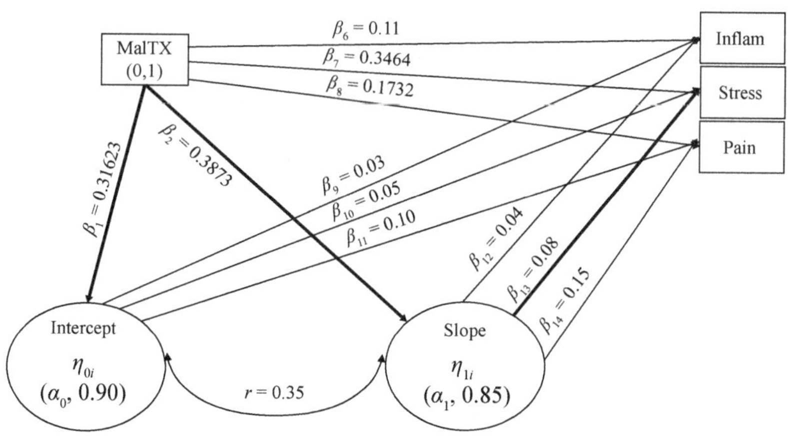

FIGURE 11.30. Stress predicted by CDI intercept: Final indirect path.

$$R^2_{Stress|CDI\_Slope} = (\text{Direct effect} * (\text{Direct effect} + [\text{Sum of indirect effects products}]))$$
$$= (\beta_{13} * (\beta_{13} + [\text{Sum of indirect effects products}]))$$

The four admissible indirect pathways between the CDI slope and the stress biomarker mirror closely the four admissible pathways between the CDI intercept and stress. The first admissible indirect pathway is from the CDI slope to the CDI intercept and then from the CDI intercept to stress, as shown in Figure 11.31. The second admissible indirect pathway is from the CDI slope to maltreatment and then from maltreatment to stress, as shown in Figure 11.32. The third admissible indirect pathway is from the CDI slope to the CDI intercept, from the CDI intercept to maltreatment, and then from maltreatment to stress, as shown in Figure 11.33. The final admissible indirect pathway is from the CDI slope to maltreatment, from maltreatment to the CDI intercept, and then from the CDI intercept to stress, as shown in Figure 11.34. So,

$$R^2_{Stress|CDI\_Slope} = (\beta_{13} * (\beta_{13} + [\text{Sum of indirect effects products}]))$$
$$= (\beta_{13} * (\beta_{13} + [r * \beta_{10}] + [\beta_2 * \beta_7] + [r * \beta_1 * \beta_7] + [\beta_2 * \beta_1 * \beta_{10}]))$$
$$= (0.08 * (0.08 + [0.35 * 0.05] + [0.3873 * 0.3464]$$
$$+ [0.35 * 0.31623 * 0.3464][+ 0.3873 * 0.31623 * 0.05]))$$
$$= (0.08 * (0.27612423915)) = \mathbf{0.022089939132}$$

$$R^2_{Stress|Maltreatment} = (\text{Direct effect} * (\text{Direct effect} + [\text{Sum of indirect effects products}]))$$
$$= (\beta_7 * (\beta_7 + [\text{Sum of indirect effects products}]))$$

Finally, there are also four admissible indirect pathways between maltreatment and stress. The first admissible indirect pathway is from maltreatment to the CDI intercept and then from the CDI intercept to stress, as shown in Figure 11.35. The second admissible indi-

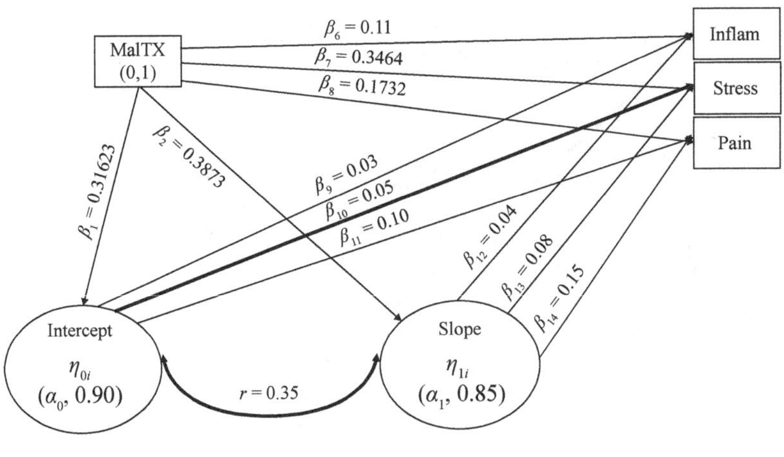

FIGURE 11.31. Stress predicted by CDI slope: First indirect path.

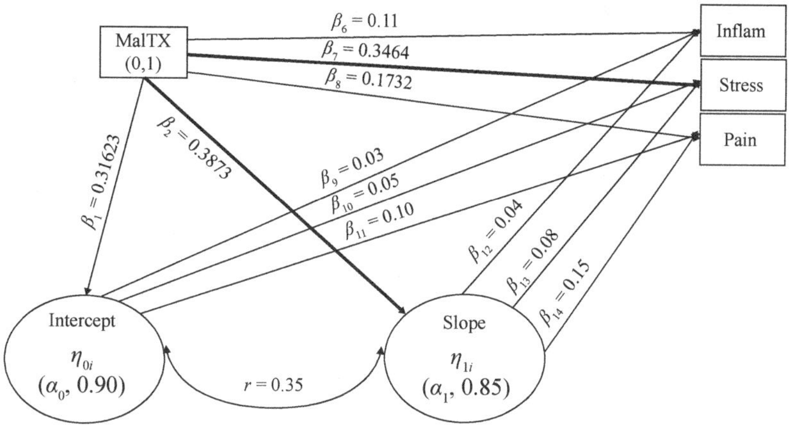

FIGURE 11.32. Stress predicted by CDI slope: Second indirect path.

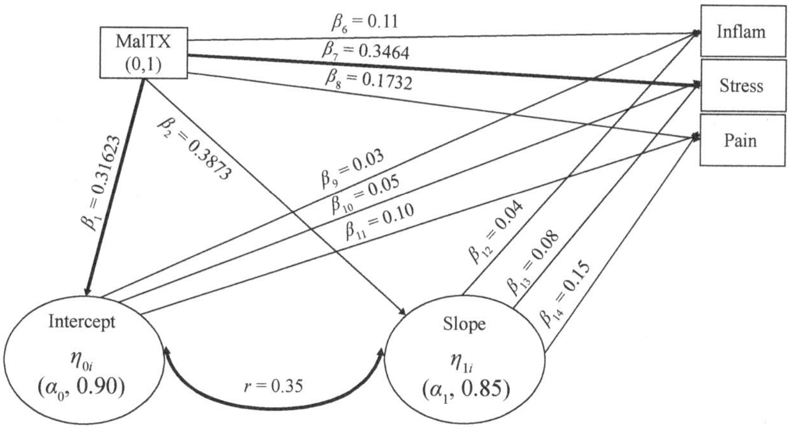

FIGURE 11.33. Stress predicted by CDI slope: Third indirect path.

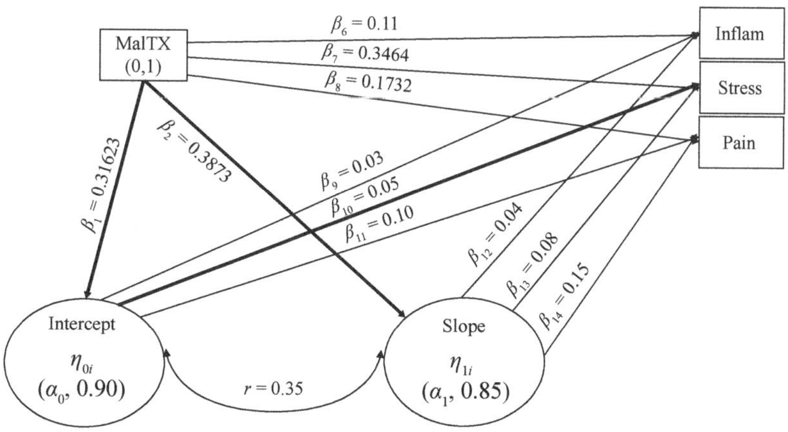

FIGURE 11.34. Stress predicted by CDI slope: Final indirect path.

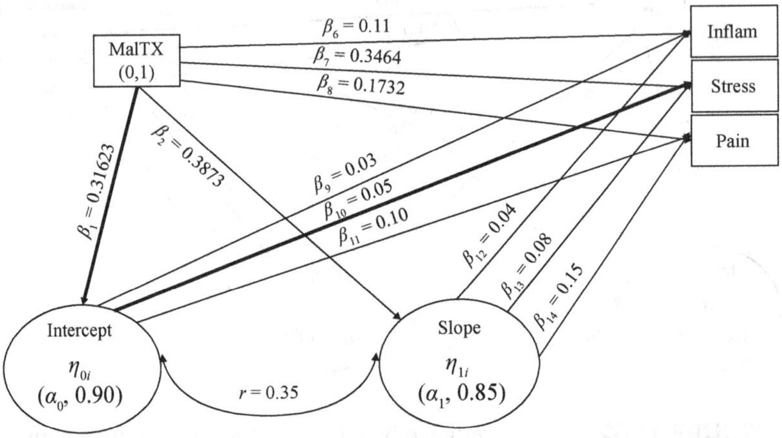

FIGURE 11.35. Stress predicted by maltreatment: First indirect path.

rect pathway is from maltreatment to the CDI slope and then from the CDI slope to stress, as shown in Figure 11.36. The third admissible indirect pathway is from maltreatment to the CDI intercept, from the CDI intercept to the CDI slope, and then from the CDI slope to stress, as shown in Figure 11.37. The final admissible indirect pathway is from maltreatment to the CDI slope, from the CDI slope to the CDI intercept, and then from the CDI intercept to stress, as shown in Figure 11.38. So,

$$R^2_{\text{Stress|Maltreatment}} = (\beta_7 * (\beta_7 + [\text{Sum of indirect effects products}]))$$

$$= (\beta_7 * (\beta_7 + [\beta_1 * \beta_{10}] + [\beta_2 * \beta_{13}] + [\beta_1 * r * \beta_{13}] + [\beta_2 * r * \beta_{10}]))$$

$$= (0.3464 * (0.3464 + [0.31623 * 0.05] + [0.3873 * 0.08] + [0.31623 * 0.35 * 0.08][+ 0.3873 * 0.35 * 0.05]))$$

$$= (0.3464 * (0.40882769)) = \mathbf{0.141617911816}$$

And,

$$R^2_{\text{Stress}} = R^2_{\text{CDI\_Intercept}} + R^2_{\text{CDI\_Slope}} + R^2_{\text{Maltreatment}}$$

$$= \mathbf{0.012214819716} + \mathbf{0.022089939132} + \mathbf{0.141617911816} = \mathbf{0.175922670664}$$

$$\sigma^2_{\text{RESIDUAL}} = 1 - R^2 = 1 - \mathbf{0.175922670664} = \underline{\mathbf{0.8241}}$$

Finally, computing pain residual variance will also follow the same pattern by assuming $\sigma^2_{\text{RESIDUAL}} = 1 - R^2$ and

$$R^2_{\text{Pain}} = R^2_{\text{CDI\_Intercept}} + R^2_{\text{CDI\_Slope}} + R^2_{\text{Maltreatment}}$$

and will start with the CDI intercept.

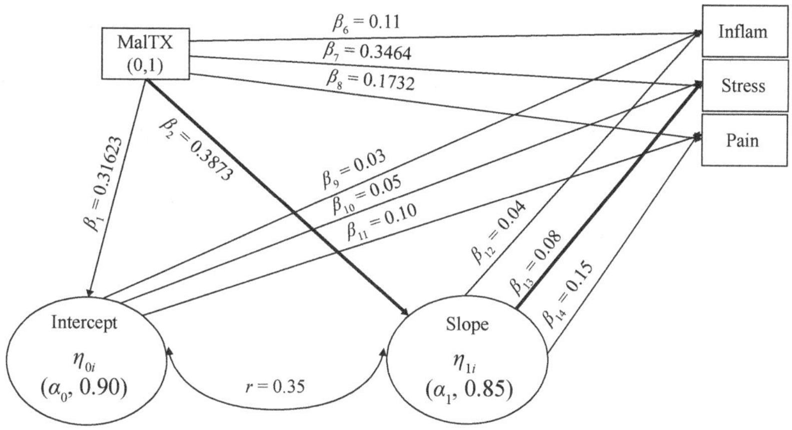

FIGURE 11.36. Stress predicted by maltreatment: Second indirect path.

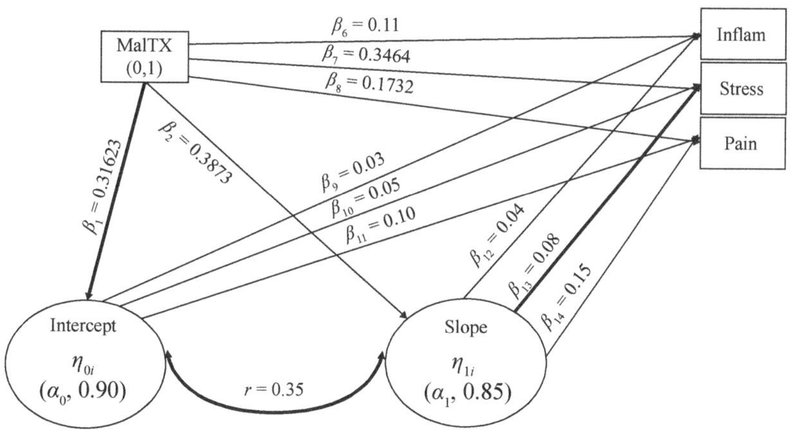

FIGURE 11.37. Stress predicted by maltreatment: Third indirect path.

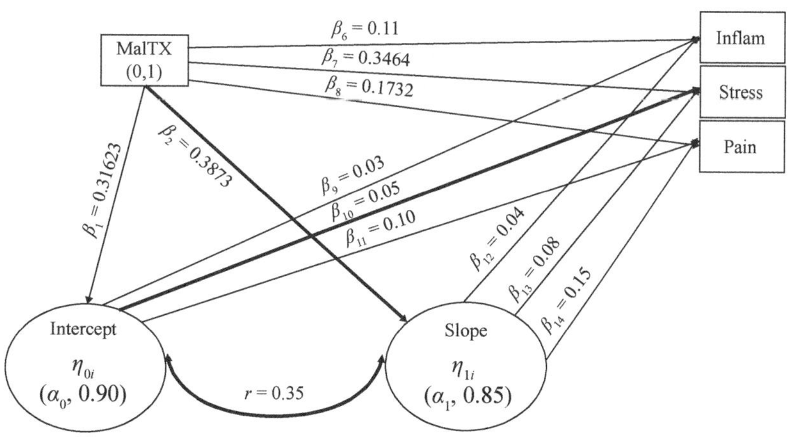

FIGURE 11.38. Stress predicted by maltreatment: Final indirect path.

$$R^2_{\text{Pain|CDI\_Intercept}} = (\text{Direct effect} * (\text{Direct effect} + [\text{Sum of indirect effects products}]))$$
$$= (\beta_{11} * (\beta_{11} + [\text{Sum of indirect effects products}]))$$

Again, there are four admissible indirect pathways between the CDI intercept and the pain biomarker. The first is from the CDI intercept to the CDI slope and then from the CDI slope to the pain biomarker, as shown in Figure 11.39. The second admissible indirect pathway is from the CDI intercept to maltreatment and then from maltreatment to the pain biomarker, as shown in Figure 11.40. The third admissible indirect pathway is from the CDI intercept to the CDI slope, from the CDI slope to maltreatment, and then from maltreatment to the pain biomarker, as shown in Figure 11.41. The final admissible indirect pathway is from the CDI intercept maltreatment, then from maltreatment to the CDI slope, and then from the CDI slope to the pain biomarker, as shown in Figure 11.42. So,

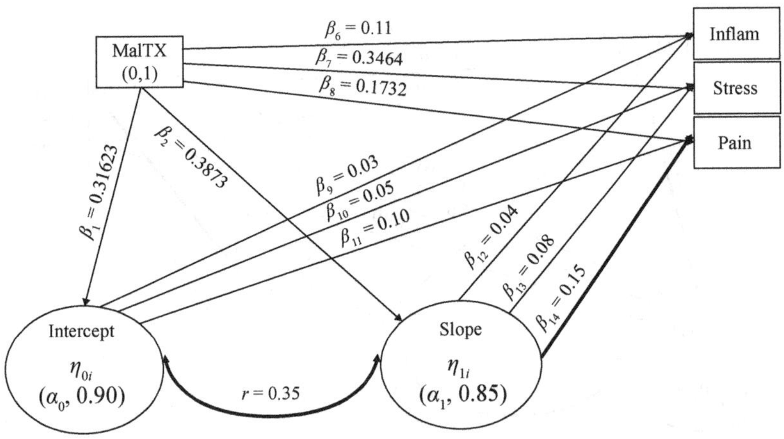

FIGURE 11.39. Pain predicted by CDI intercept: First indirect path.

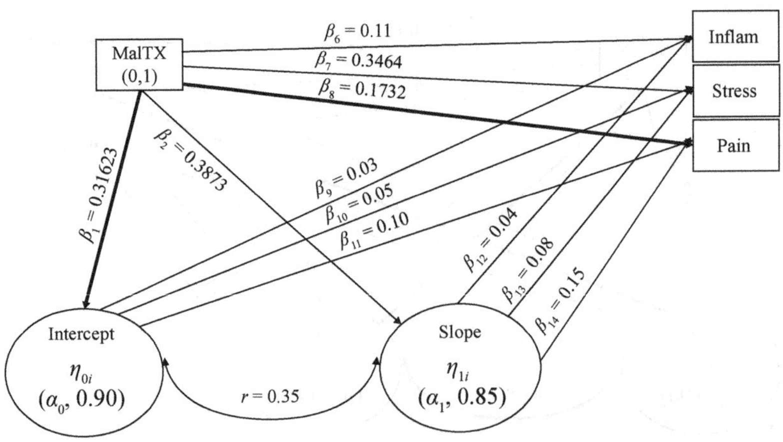

FIGURE 11.40. Pain predicted by CDI intercept: Second indirect path.

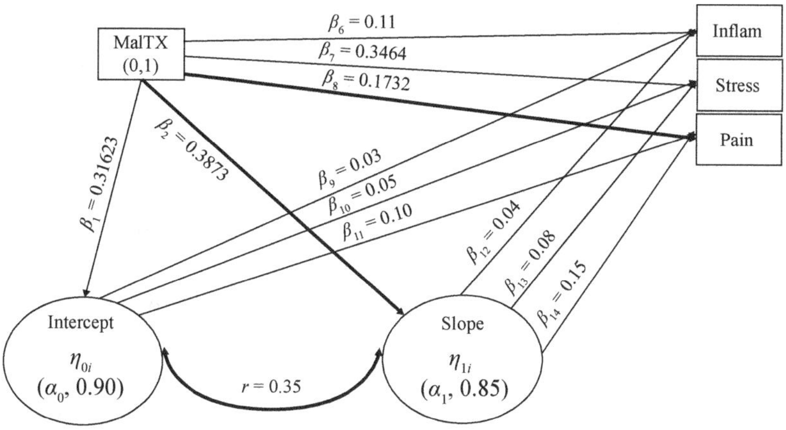

FIGURE 11.41. Pain predicted by CDI intercept: Third indirect path.

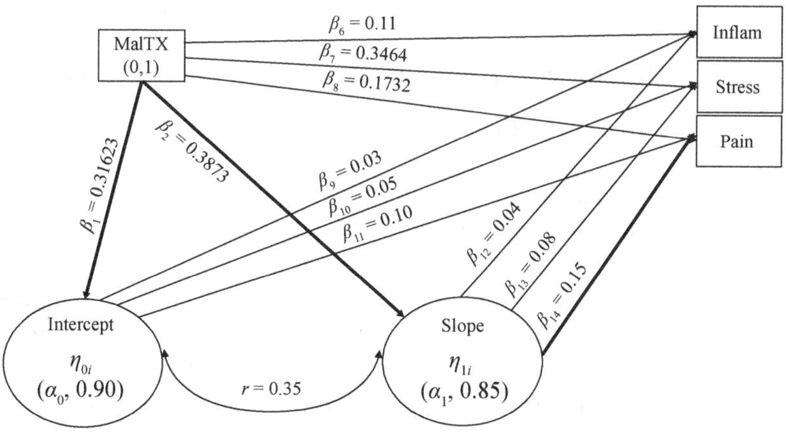

FIGURE 11.42. Pain predicted by CDI intercept: Final indirect path.

$$R^2_{\text{Pain|CDI\_Intercept}} = (\beta_{11} * (\beta_{11} + [\text{Sum of indirect effects products}]))$$

$$= (\beta_{11} * (\beta_{11} + [r * \beta_{14}] + [\beta_1 * \beta_8] + [r * \beta_2 * \beta_8] + [\beta_1 * \beta_2 * \beta_{14}]))$$

$$= (0.11 * (0.11 + [0.35 * 0.15] + [0.31623 * 0.1732] + [0.35 * 0.3873 * 0.1732] + [0.31623 * 0.3873 * 0.15]))$$

$$= (0.11 * (0912054385)) = \mathbf{0.0285032598235}$$

$$R^2_{\text{Pain|CDI\_Slope}} = (\text{Direct effect} * (\text{Direct effect} + [\text{Sum of indirect effects products}]))$$

$$= (\beta_{14} * (\beta_{14} + [\text{Sum of indirect effects products}]))$$

There are, once again, four admissible indirect effect pathways from the CDI slope to the pain biomarker. The first is from the CDI slope to the CDI intercept and then from the CDI intercept to the pain biomarker, as shown in Figure 11.43. The second admissible indirect pathway is from the CDI slope to maltreatment and then then from maltreatment to the pain biomarker, as shown in Figure 11.44. The third admissible indirect pathway is from the CDI slope to the CDI intercept, then from the CDI intercept to maltreatment, and then from maltreatment to the pain biomarker, as shown in Figure 11.45. The final admissible indirect pathway is from the CDI slope to maltreatment, then from maltreatment to the CDI intercept, and then from the CDI intercept to the pain biomarker, as shown in Figure 11.46. So,

$$R^2_{\text{Pain|CDI\_Slope}} = (\beta_{14} * (\beta_{14} + [\text{Sum of indirect effects products}]))$$

$$= (\beta_{14} * (\beta_{14} + [r * \beta_{11}] + [\beta_2 * \beta_8][r * \beta_1 * \beta_8] + [\beta_2 * \beta_1 * \beta_{11}]))$$

$$= (0.15 * (0.15 + [0.35 * 0.10] + [0.3873 * 0.1732]$$
$$+ [0.35 * 0.31623 * 0.1732][+ 0.3873 * 0.31623 * 0.10]))$$

$$= (0.15 * (0.2834978105)) = \mathbf{0.042524671575}$$

$$R^2_{\text{Pain|Maltreatment}} = (\text{Direct effect} * (\text{Direct effect} + [\text{Sum of indirect effects products}]))$$

$$= (\beta_8 * (\beta_8 + [\text{Sum of indirect effects products}]))$$

Again, there are four admissible indirect pathways from maltreatment to the pain biomarker. The first admissible indirect pathway is from maltreatment to the CDI intercept and then from the CDI intercept to the pain biomarker, as shown in Figure 11.47. The second admissible indirect pathway is from maltreatment to the CDI slope and then from the CDI slope to the pain biomarker, as shown in Figure 11.48. The third admissible indirect pathway is from maltreatment to the CDI intercept, from the CDI intercept to the CDI slope, and then from the CDI slope to the pain biomarker, as shown in Figure 11.49). The final admissible indirect pathway is from maltreatment to the CDI slope, from the CDI slope to the CDI

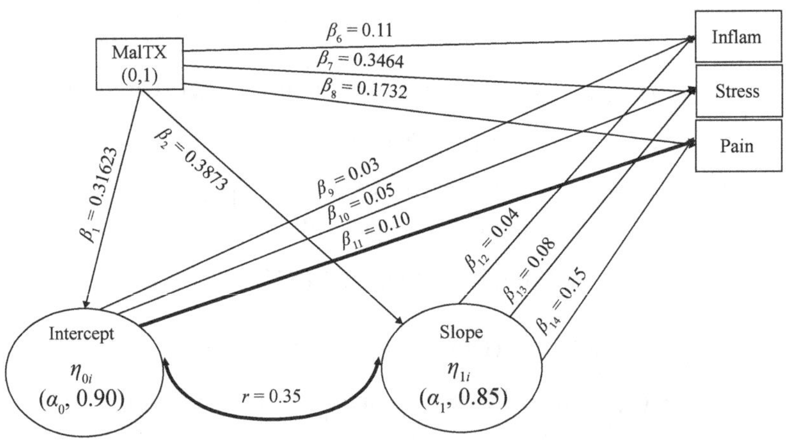

FIGURE 11.43. Pain predicted by CDI slope: First indirect path.

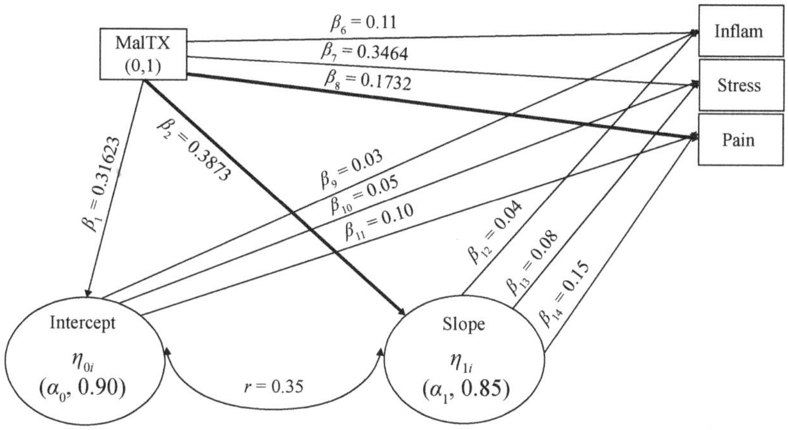

FIGURE 11.44. Pain predicted by CDI slope: Second indirect path.

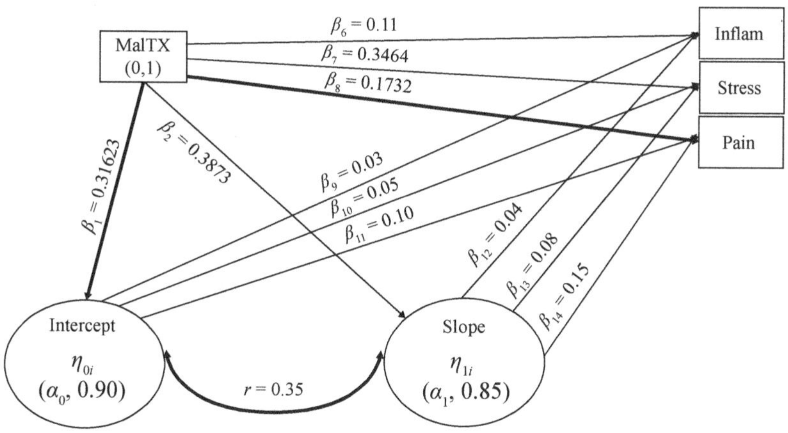

FIGURE 11.45. Pain predicted by CDI slope: Third indirect path.

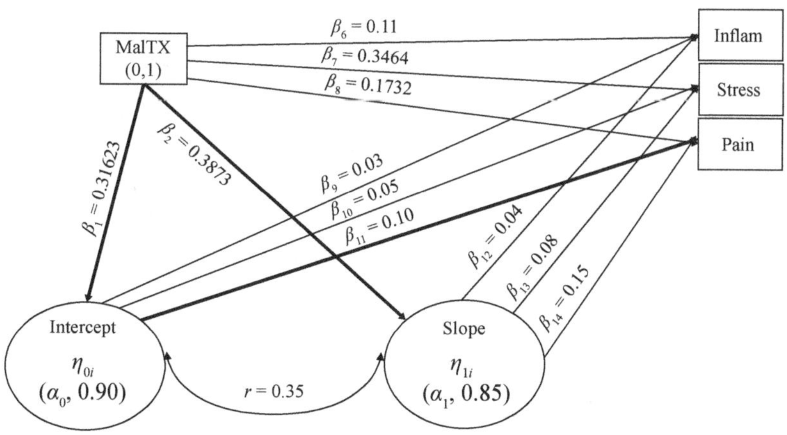

FIGURE 11.46. Pain predicted by CDI slope: Final indirect path.

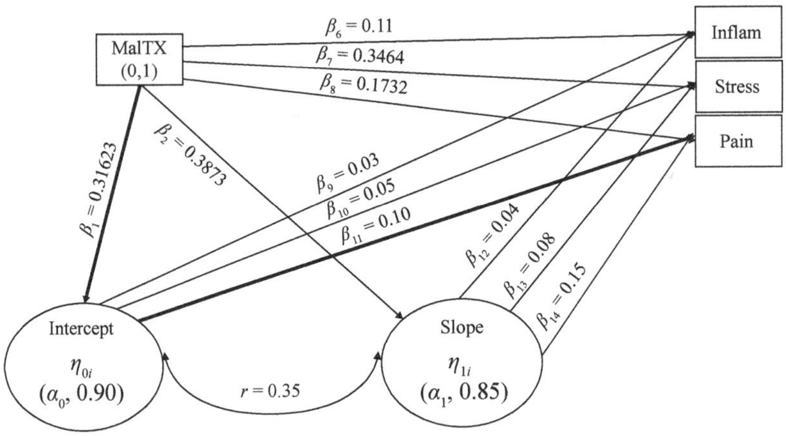

FIGURE 11.47. Pain predicted by maltreatment. First indirect path.

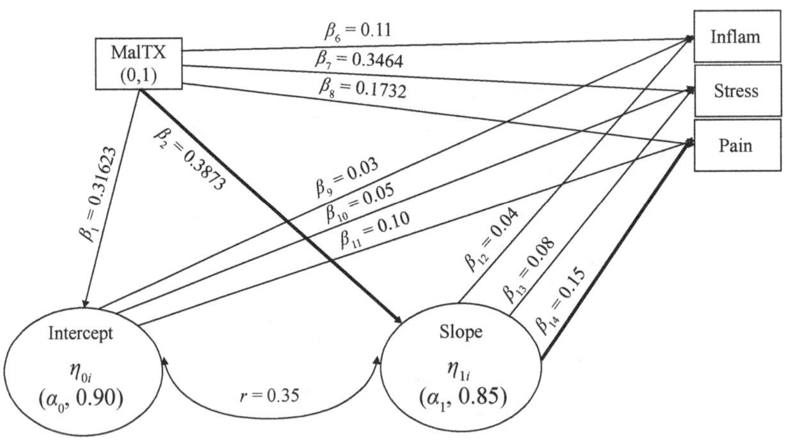

FIGURE 11.48. Pain predicted by maltreatment: Second indirect path.

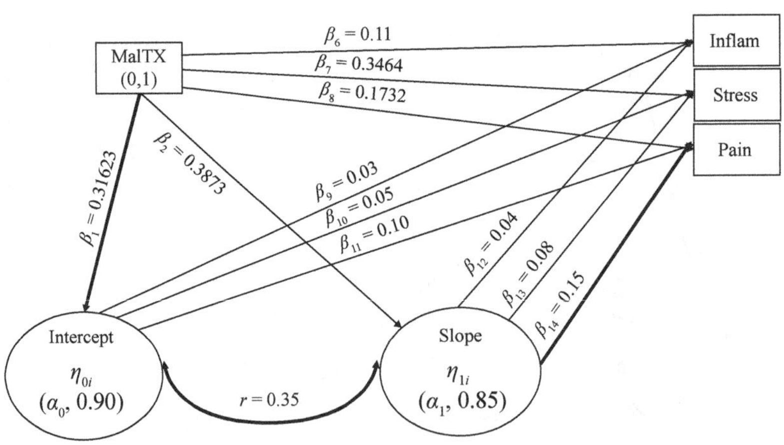

FIGURE 11.49. Pain predicted by maltreatment: Third indirect path.

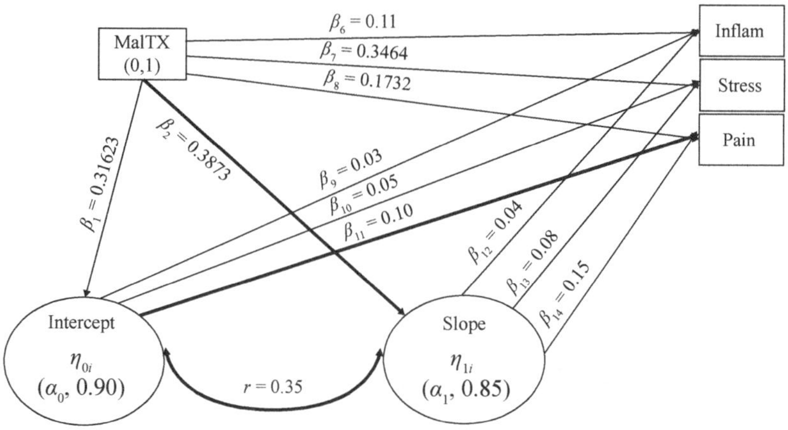

FIGURE 11.50. Pain predicted by maltreatment: Final indirect path.

intercept, and then from the CDI intercept to the pain biomarker, as shown in Figure 11.50. So,

$$R^2_{\text{Pain|Maltreatment}} = (\beta_8 * (\beta_8 + [\text{Sum of indirect effects products}]))$$
$$= (\beta_8 * (\beta_8 + [\beta_1 * \beta_{11}] + [\beta_2 * \beta_{14}] + [\beta_1 * r * \beta_{14}] + [\beta_2 * r * \beta_{11}]))$$
$$= (0.1732 * (0.1732 + [0.31623 * 0.10] + [0.3873 * 0.15] + [0.31623 * 0.35 * 0.15][+ 0.3873 * 0.35 * 0.10]))$$
$$= (0.1732 * (0.293075575)) = \mathbf{0.05076068959}$$

And,

$$R^2_{\text{Pain}} = R^2_{\text{CDI\_Intercept}} + R^2_{\text{CDI\_Slope}} + R^2_{\text{Maltreatment}}$$
$$R^2_{\text{Pain}} = 0.0285032598235 + 0.042524671575 + 0.05076068959$$
$$= \mathbf{0.1217886209885}$$

and

$$\sigma^2_{\text{RESIDUAL}} = 1 - R^2 = 1 - \mathbf{0.1217886209885} = \underline{\mathbf{0.8782}}$$

Prediction of Opioid Misuse Disorder

The last distinct prediction section of the analysis model involves the logistic prediction of opioid misuse disorder. Based on previous research, the authors specify the logistic hypotheses shown in Figure 11.51. Specifically, the authors hypothesize that (exp[–2.19722] / 1 + exp[–2.19722] = 0.10) 10% of nonmaltreated (MalTX = 0) participants will meet diagnostic

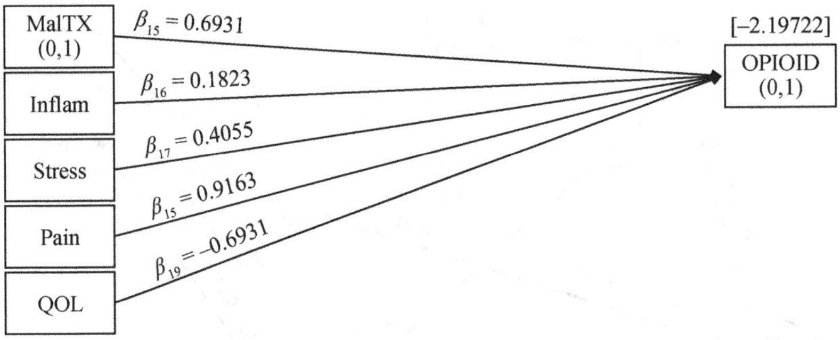

FIGURE 11.51. Binary opioid use prediction.

criteria for opioid misuse disorder. More specifically, the authors suspect that 20% of maltreated participants and 10% of matched control participants will meet diagnostic criteria for opioid misuse disorder, and this is reflected as a logit slope of (0.6931), which specifies a ($\exp^{0.6931} = 2.0$) doubling of the odds of a misuse disorder diagnosis for maltreated participants compared to matched control condition participants. The remaining logistic slopes specify the odds for opioid misuse disorder: (1) increase ($\exp^{0.1823} = 1.20$) 20% per unit increase in inflammation, (2) increase ($\exp^{0.4055} = 1.50$) 50% per unit increase in stress, (3) double ($\exp^{-0.6931} = 0.50$; $1/0.50 = 2.0$) per unit *decrease* in QOL, and (4) experience ($\exp^{0.9163} = 2.5$) 2.5 times greater per unit increase in pain intensity.

For demonstration purposes, it is assumed that the research question of interest involves a complex indirect pathway: the effect of maltreatment on changes in depression over time, depression changes over time as a predictor of pain, and pain as a predictor of subsequent opioid misuse, as shown in Figure 11.52. The power analysis question under consideration involves the sample size needed for power ≥ .80 to detect the complex indirect effect.

However, before building the needed Mplus syntax, readers may have already spotted a problem with how this analysis model, in general, and the complex indirect effect, in particular, have been specified. Maltreatment as a predictor of linear changes in depression over time (MalTx → CDI_{SLOPE}), and linear changes in depression over time as a predictor of pain (CDI_{SLOPE} → Pain) are both linear regression slopes because both endogenous variables are continuous. However, pain as a predictor of a binary indicator of opioid misuse (Pain → Opioid) is a logistic slope coefficient. The product of the three prediction coefficients defines the complex indirect effect, but linear regression slopes and logistic slopes are not measured on the same scale. The question now becomes: Can logistic coefficients be converted to a scale that is equivalent to linear regression coefficients? The answer is yes, if a *probit* rather than a *logistic* model parameterization specification is used. The answer to the question of *how* logistic coefficients can be converted to a scale equivalent to linear regression coefficients is shown quickly below. The answer to the question of *why* they are considered equivalent for complex indirect effect power estimation purposes is explained in the Mplus syntax assembly section that immediately follows.

Among other similarities, linear regression coefficients and logistic regression coefficients can both be interpreted in terms of proportions or probabilities. Based on properties of the logistic distribution, and as was shown in Chapter 5, logistic threshold/intercept

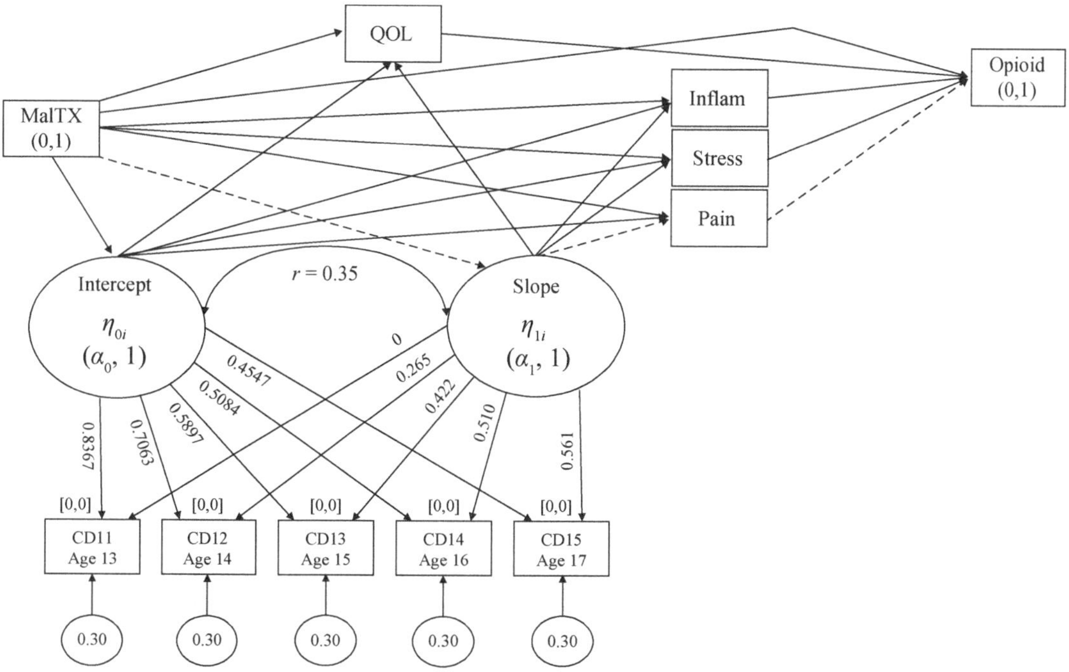

FIGURE 11.52. Complex indirect path of theoretical interest.

estimates and slope estimates could both be converted to proportions or probabilities. Probit threshold/intercept estimates and slope estimates can also be converted to proportions or probabilities based on properties of the unit normal (standardized score or *z*-score) distribution. Specifically, the unit normal distribution has a standard deviation of one, the logistic distribution has a standard deviation of $\sqrt{\pi^2/3}$; this means that the needed conversion is: $\beta_{\text{PROBIT}} = \beta_{\text{LOGISTIC}}/\sqrt{\pi^2/3}$ (Muthén et al., 2017, pp. 211–240 and Equation 5.59). Converting the logistic coefficient values shown in Figure 11.51 to probit coefficient values, based on the above conversion, results in a new probit parameterization specification as shown in Figure 11.53.

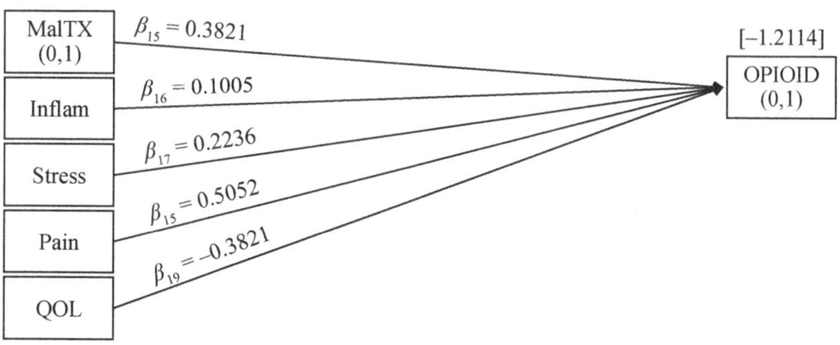

FIGURE 11.53. New probit specification for opioid misuse prediction.

Assembling the Mplus Syntax

```
TITLE: MPLUS 11.1 Complex Designs

MONTECARLO:
NAMES =
MalTX QOL Opioid
Inflam Stress Pain
CDI1 CDI2 CDI3 CDI4 CDI5;

CUTPOINTS = MalTX (0);

CATEGORICAL = Opioid;
GENERATE = Opioid(1);

MISSING = CDI2 CDI3 CDI4 CDI5
Inflam Stress Pain;
```

The 'NAMES' statement contains the names of the longitudinal response variables (CDI1 – CDI5), the biomarker variables (Inflam, Stress, Pain), quality of life (QOL), the binary predictor variable indicating maltreatment (MalTX), and the binary response variable indicating opioid misuse (Opioid). The 'CUTPOINTS' keyword is used to specify binary predictor variables, and the value of zero (0) specifies the intent of the researcher to sample an equal proportion of nonmaltreated (MalTX = 0) and maltreated (MalTX = 1) participants. Zero is the mean of a unit normal distribution; 50% of binary generated values will occur below the mean (MalTX = 0) and 50% will occur above the mean (MalTX = 1). The 'CATEGORICAL' keyword specifies 'Opioid' to be a categorical response variable; the 'GENERATE' keyword with a (1) after 'Opioid' indicates the response variable is binary with a single threshold. The 'MISSING' command declares the intent of the researcher to generate missing data for the response variables (CDI1 – CDI5) and the biomarker variables (Inflam, Stress, Pain).

```
NREPS = 5000;
SEED = 8675309;
NOBS = 1604;
```

The 'NREPS' keyword requests 5,000 datasets be generated and analyzed, the 'SEED' keyword provides a starting point for the random number generator that begins the data generation process. The 'NOBS' statement tests $N = 1{,}604$ for acceptable statistical power.

```
MODEL POPULATION:
[CDI1 – CDI5@0];
I_CDI BY CDI1@0.8367 CDI2@0.7063 CDI3@0.5897 CDI4@0.5084
    CDI5@0.4547;
S_CDI BY CDI1@0 CDI2@0.265 CDI3@0.422 CDI4@0.510 CDI5@0.561;
I_CDI WITH S_CDI*0.35;
CDI1 – CDI5*0.30;
```

The five lines of Mplus syntax above specify a linear growth curve analysis model that explains 70% of longitudinal CDI variance, as shown previously in Chapter 7.

```
I_CDI*0.90;
S_CDI*0.85;

I_CDI ON MalTX*0.31623;
S_CDI ON MalTX*0.3873;
```

The first two lines of Mplus syntax specify residual variances for latent CDI intercept and CDI slope at 0.90 and 0.85, respectively. The reason for this is shown in the next two lines of syntax: assuming CDI standardization, and because maltreatment (`MalTX`) is the only trajectory predictor, intercept and slope residual variances ($\sigma^2_{\text{Residual}}$) can be computed as ($\sigma^2_{\text{CDI\_I}} = 1 - [0.31623]^2$; $\sigma^2_{\text{CDI\_S}} = 1 - [0.3873]^2$), respectively.

```
QOL ON MalTX*-0.35;
QOL ON I_CDI*-0.175;
QOL ON S_CDI*-0.235;

Inflam ON MalTX*0.11;
Inflam ON I_CDI*0.3464;
Inflam ON S_CDI*0.1732;

Stress ON MalTX*0.03;
Stress ON I_CDI*0.05;
Stress ON S_CDI*0.10;

Pain ON MalTX*0.04;
Pain ON I_CDI*0.08;
Pain ON S_CDI*0.15;
```

All of the prediction values shown in the syntax above are based on a cursory search of the applicable literature and transformations of the published effects.

```
[QOL*0 Inflam*0 Stress*0 Pain*0];
QOL*0.62885;
Inflam*0.9769;
Stress*0.8241;
Pain*0.8782;
MalTX*1;
```

Consistent with the standardization assumption, the means for quality of life (`QOL`) and the three biomarker variables (`Inflam, Stress, Pain`) are given starting values of zero. The next four lines of Mplus syntax specify residual variance values for the four variables as determined by path tracing. The variance for the binary maltreatment (`MalTX`) variable was set to one (Mplus creates categorical variables from threshold cutpoints based on the unit normal distribution).

```
[Opioid$1*-1.2114];
Opioid ON MalTX*0.3821;
Opioid ON Inflam*0.1005;
Opioid ON Stress*0.0.2236;
Opioid ON Pain*0.5052;
Opioid ON QOL*-0.3821;
```

The previous `'CUTPOINTS'` and `'GENERATE'` keywords under the `'MONTECARLO:'` declared `Opioid` misuse to be a binary response variable. All values are probit coefficients (converted from the logistic coefficients obtained from the literature), as shown in Figure 11.53.

```
MODEL MISSING:
[CDI2*-2.9444]; !5% MCAR;
[CDI3*-2.1972]; !10% MCAR;
[CDI4*-1.7346]; !15% MCAR;
[CDI5*-1.3862]; !20% MCAR;

CDI2 ON CDI1*0.0953;
CDI3 ON CDI2*0.0953 CDI1*0.0953;
CDI4 ON CDI3*0.0953 CDI2*0.0953 CDI1*0.0953;
CDI5 ON CDI4*0.0953 CDI3*0.0953 CDI2*0.0953 CDI1*0.0953;

CDI2-CDI5 ON MalTx*0.0488;

[Inflam*-2.19715];
[Stress*-2.19715];
[Pain*-2.19715];
```

The first four lines of Mplus syntax beneath the `'MODEL MISSING;'` command specify missing completely at random (MCAR) missing data at all four postbaseline assessments that increases from $\exp^{-2.944}/(1 + \exp^{-2.944}) = 0.05$, or 5% MCAR at the first postbaseline assessment to $\exp^{-1.3862}/(1 + \exp^{-1.3862}) = 0.20$, or 20% MCAR at the final assessment. The next five lines of Mplus syntax specify MAR missing data; the probability of a missing data point will increase ($\exp^{0.0953} = 1.10$) 10% at any assessment time point per unit CDI increase at any previous time point, and will increase ($\exp^{0.0488} = 1.05$) 5% at any postbaseline assessment time point for maltreated (`MalTX = 1`) participants. The final three lines of syntax specify $\exp^{-2.19115}/(1 + \exp^{-2.19115}) = 0.10$, 10% MCAR missing data for the three biomarker variables due to completely random phenomena (equipment failure, laboratory processing errors, reluctance to respond, etc.).

```
ANALYSIS:
ESTIMATOR = ML;
LINK = PROBIT;
PROCESSORS = 24;
ALGORITHM = INTEGRATION EM;
INTEGRATION = MONTECARLO;
```

Both the estimation (`ESTIMATOR = ML;`) and link function (`LINK = PROBIT;`) are both critically important for accurately testing the complex indirect path proposed above for reasons that will be described below. Monte Carlo integration (`INTEGRATION = MONTECARLO;`) is needed because the ultimate endogenous observed response variable (`OPIOID`) is binary. The '`PROCESSORS = 24;`' and '`ALGORITHM = INTEGRATION EM;`' statements are included because they can decrease the Monte Carlo simulation runtime.

```
MODEL:
[CDI1 – CDI5@0];
I_CDI BY CDI1@0.8367 CDI2@0.7063 CDI3@0.5897 CDI4@0.5084 CDI5@0.4547;
S_CDI BY CDI1@0 CDI2@0.265 CDI3@0.422 CDI4@0.510 CDI5@0.561;
I_CDI WITH S_CDI*0.35;
CDI1 – CDI5*0.30;

I_CDI*0.90;
S_CDI*0.85;

I_CDI ON MalTX*0.31623;
S_CDI ON MalTX*0.3873;

QOL ON MalTX*-0.35;
QOL ON I_CDI*-0.175;
QOL ON S_CDI*-0.235;

Inflam ON MalTX*0.11;
Inflam ON I_CDI*0.3464;
Inflam ON S_CDI*0.1732;

Stress ON MalTX*0.03;
Stress ON I_CDI*0.05;
Stress ON S_CDI*0.10;

Pain ON MalTX*0.04;
Pain ON I_CDI*0.08;
Pain ON S_CDI*0.15;

[QOL*0 Inflam*0 Stress*0 Pain*0];
QOL*0.62885;
Inflam*0.9769;
Stress*0.8241;
Pain*0.8782;

[Opioid$1*-1.2114];
Opioid ON MalTX*0.3821;
Opioid ON Inflam*0.1005;
Opioid ON Stress*0.2236;
Opioid ON Pain*0.5052;
Opioid ON QOL*-0.3821;
```

The data-generation model specified under the '`MODEL POPULATION:`' command can be copied and pasted into the '`MODEL:`' command in its entirety with one exception: the syntax line specifying maltreatment variance ('`MalTX*1;`') needed for data generation in the '`MODEL POPULATION:`' command is not needed in the data analysis '`MODEL:`' command and will generate an error message if included.

```
MODEL INDIRECT:
Opioid IND Pain S_CDI MalTx;
```

At this point, an answer to the question of *why* probit and linear coefficients can be combined into a mediated effect can be offered: Mplus is able to estimate a latent continuous variable (call it `Opioid*`) underlying the observed binary Opioid variable, but only if two specific syntax specifications are included: (1) add '`LINK = PROBIT`' to the `ANALYSIS:` command and (2) use '`MODEL INDIRECT:`' to test the complect mediated path under consideration. Specifically, these two model specifications allow the complex indirect effect to be estimated and tested as a product of linear coefficient estimates on similar scales. The combined Mplus syntax is given below, followed by the Monte Carlo simulation results and an example write-up.[1]

```
TITLE: MPLUS 11.1 Complex Designs

MONTECARLO:
NAMES =
MalTX QOL Opioid
Inflam Stress Pain
CDI1 CDI2 CDI3 CDI4 CDI5;

CUTPOINTS = MalTX (0);

CATEGORICAL = Opioid;
GENERATE = Opioid(1);

MISSING = CDI2 CDI3 CDI4 CDI5
Inflam Stress Pain;

NREPS = 5000;
SEED = 1234;
NOBS = 1604;

MODEL POPULATION:
[CDI1 – CDI5@0];
I_CDI BY CDI1@0.8367 CDI2@0.7063 CDI3@0.5897 CDI4@0.5084 CDI5@0.4547;
S_CDI BY CDI1@0 CDI2@0.265 CDI3@0.422 CDI4@0.510 CDI5@0.561;
I_CDI WITH S_CDI*0.35;
CDI1 – CDI5*0.30;

I_CDI*0.90;
S_CDI*0.85;

I_CDI ON MalTX*0.31623;
S_CDI ON MalTX*0.3873;

QOL ON MalTX*-0.35;
QOL ON I_CDI*-0.175;
QOL ON S_CDI*-0.235;
```

---

[1]The authors wish to extend their appreciation and gratitude to Linda Muthén of Mplus statmodel support for her help in clarifying how this feature is specified. Many thanks.

```
Inflam ON MalTX*0.11;
Inflam ON I_CDI*0.3464;
Inflam ON S_CDI*0.1732;

Stress ON MalTX*0.03;
Stress ON I_CDI*0.05;
Stress ON S_CDI*0.10;

Pain ON MalTX*0.04;
Pain ON I_CDI*0.08;
Pain ON S_CDI*0.15;

[QOL*0 Inflam*0 Stress*0 Pain*0];
QOL*0.62885;
Inflam*0.9769;
Stress*0.8241;
Pain*0.8782;
MalTX*1;

[Opioid$1*-1.2114];
Opioid ON MalTX*0.3821;
Opioid ON Inflam*0.1005;
Opioid ON Stress*0.2236;
Opioid ON Pain*0.5052;
Opioid ON QOL*-0.3821;

MODEL MISSING:
[CDI2*-2.9444]; !5% MCAR;
[CDI3*-2.1972]; !10% MCAR;
[CDI4*-1.7346]; !15% MCAR;
[CDI5*-1.3862]; !20% MCAR;

CDI2 ON CDI1*0.0953;
CDI3 ON CDI2*0.0953 CDI1*0.0953;
CDI4 ON CDI3*0.0953 CDI2*0.0953 CDI1*0.0953;
CDI5 ON CDI4*0.0953 CDI3*0.0953 CDI2*0.0953 CDI1*0.0953;

CDI2-CDI5 ON MalTx*0.0488;

[Inflam*-2.19715];
[Stress*-2.19715];
[Pain*-2.19715];

ANALYSIS:
ESTIMATOR = ML;
LINK = PROBIT;
PROCESSORS = 24;
ALGORITHM = INTEGRATION EM;
INTEGRATION = MONTECARLO;

MODEL:
[CDI1 – CDI5@0];
I_CDI BY CDI1@0.8367 CDI2@0.7063 CDI3@0.5897 CDI4@0.5084 CDI5@0.4547;
S_CDI BY CDI1@0 CDI2@0.265 CDI3@0.422 CDI4@0.510 CDI5@0.561;
I_CDI WITH S_CDI*0.35;
CDI1 – CDI5*0.30;
```

```
I_CDI*0.90;
S_CDI*0.85;

I_CDI ON MalTX*0.31623;
S_CDI ON MalTX*0.3873;

QOL ON MalTX*-0.35;
QOL ON I_CDI*-0.175;
QOL ON S_CDI*-0.235;

Inflam ON MalTX*0.11;
Inflam ON I_CDI*0.3464;
Inflam ON S_CDI*0.1732;

Stress ON MalTX*0.03;
Stress ON I_CDI*0.05;
Stress ON S_CDI*0.10;

Pain ON MalTX*0.04;
Pain ON I_CDI*0.08;
Pain ON S_CDI*0.15;

[QOL*0 Inflam*0 Stress*0 Pain*0];
QOL*0.62885;
Inflam*0.9769;
Stress*0.8241;
Pain*0.8782;

[Opioid$1*-1.2114];
Opioid ON MalTX*0.3821;
Opioid ON Inflam*0.1005;
Opioid ON Stress*0.2236;
Opioid ON Pain*0.5052;
Opioid ON QOL*-0.3821;

MODEL INDIRECT:
Opioid IND Pain S_CDI MalTx;
```

```
                                ESTIMATES              S. E.     M. S. E.  95%   % Sig
                   Population   Average    Std. Dev.   Average             Cover Coeff

Effects from MALTX to OPIOID

  Sum indirect        0.053      0.0289     0.0116      0.0115     0.0007  0.412 0.816

 Specific indirect 1
  OPIOID
  PAIN
  S_CDI
  MALTX               0.053      0.0289     0.0116      0.0115     0.0007  0.412 0.816
```

A Note on R Syntax for This Design

The same issue arose here as in Chapter 5: It was not possible to simulate both a binary predictor (i.e., treatment) variable and a binary outcome (i.e., opioid use) in the same SEM model in R. This highlights a major limitation of current R packages at the time of writing this book; standard R SEM packages were unable to handle seemingly common research designs that incorporated combinations of binary and continuous variables. Although the example in this chapter is relatively complex, it was the combination of binary predictors and binary outcome variables that impeded our ability to fully evaluate a power analysis in either lavaan or simsem. More details about what could be accomplished can be found in the online supplemental materials at *www.guilford.com/peugh-materials*.

Complex Longitudinal Simulation Power Analysis Write-Up

> "The power analysis question involved the smallest sample size needed to achieve power ≥ .80 to detect the complex sequential mediator (maltreatment → depression change over time → pain → opioid misuse) indirect pathway. A Monte Carlo simulation power analysis was conducted using Mplus (version 8.11) assuming: (1) recruitment of equal sample sizes for maltreated and nonmaltreated participants, (2) maltreatment will explain ($R^2 = 0.10$) 10% of depression variance at initial status and ($R^2 = 0.15$) 15% of variance in depression score linear changes over time, (3) maltreatment and depression trajectory together will explain ($R^2 = 0.37$) 37% of variance in quality of life, (4) maltreatment and depression trajectory together will also explain ($R^2 = 0.03 - 0.18$) between 3 and 18% of the variance in the three biomarker variables (inflammation, stress, and pain), (5) maltreatment status is expected to double the odds of opioid misuse disorder diagnosis, (6) unit increases in pain are expected to increase the odds of an opioid misuse disorder diagnosis by 250% (assumptions 5 and 6 parameterized as probit coefficients), (7) missing data on longitudinal depression assessments are expected to be MAR, increase from 5 to 20% over the course of the study, increase 10% at a given assessment time point per unit increase in depression scores at any previous time point, and will be 5% higher for maltreated participants at any post-baseline assessment, and (8) 10% MCAR missing data for the three biomarker variables are expected owing to random equipment malfunction or laboratory processing error. Monte Carlo simulation power analysis results aggregated over 5,000 replications showed power ≥ .80 for the complex sequential mediation pathway if a probit link function is used with '`MODEL INDIRECT:`' in Mplus to test mediation and $N = 1{,}604$ is available for analysis following acceptable missing data handling."

SUGGESTED READINGS

- Ma, Z. W., & Zeng, W. N. (2014). A multiple mediator model: Power analysis based on Monte Carlo simulation. *American Journal of Applied Psychology, 3,* 72–79.
- McCormick, E. M., Curran, P. J., & Hancock, G. R. (2024). Latent growth factors as predictors of distal outcomes. *Psychological Methods.* Advance online publication. *https://dx.doi.org/10.1037/met0000642*
- Nguyen, T. Q., Webb-Vargas, Y., Koning, I. M., & Stuart, E. A. (2016). Causal mediation analysis with a binary outcome and multiple continuous or ordinal mediators: Simulations and application to an alcohol intervention. *Structural Equation Modeling, 23,* 368–383.

- Schoemann, A. M., Boulton, A. J., & Short, S. D. (2017). Determining power and sample size for simple and complex mediation models. *Social Psychological and Personality Science, 8*, 379–386.
- Sim, M., Kim, S. Y., & Suh, Y. (2021). Sample size requirements for simple and complex mediation models. *Educational and Psychological Measurement, 82*(1), 76–106.
- Thoemmes, F., MacKinnon, D. P., & Reiser, M. R. (2010). Power analysis for complex mediational designs using Monte Carlo methods. *Structural Equation Modeling, 17*, 510–534.

Part III
Conclusion

12

Statistical Power in a "Post-$p < .05$" World

Ringing the Alarm Bell

All of the power analyses in the previous 11 chapters (as well as the additional power analyses in Appendices A–D in the supplemental online materials at *www.guilford.com/peugh-materials*) have followed the same four-step formula for computing statistical power: (1) specify theoretically defensible parameters for the analysis model of interest, (2) generate a sufficiently high number of replication datasets (such as 5,000) at a given sample size that mimics random samples from a population consistent with the central limit theorem, (3) analyze all generated datasets taking note of the number of times across all replications the effect of interest was statistically significant, and (4) divide the observed frequency of statistical significance by 5,000 replications to obtain a statistical power estimate. This four-step computational procedure makes two notable assumptions. First, the null hypothesis value against which all effects of interest are tested is zero. Second, *statistical significance* is defined as a probability of occurrence for the effect of interest at the prespecified magnitude of less than 5% if the null hypothesis in the population is assumed to be true, or $p < .05$. However, fairly recently, both assumptions have been called into question, and many believe both may ultimately be headed the way of the dinosaur:

> The process of turning data into insight is central to the scientific enterprise. It is therefore remarkable that the most widely used approach—null hypothesis significance testing (NHST)—has been subjected to devastating criticism for so long to so little effect. The emergence of the so-called replication crisis has catalyzed widespread debate about NHST in general and the use of *p*-values in particular (e.g., Nuzzo 2014; Baker 2016). This debate reached a turning-point in March 2016 with the publication of an unprecedented statement by the American Statistical Association (ASA) stating that *p*-values are "commonly misused and misinterpreted" (Wasserstein & Lazar 2016) and calling for researchers to move toward a "post-$p < .05$ era." (Matthews, 2019, p. 202)

It is important to note that despite documenting the fact that decades old warnings about the misuse of *p*-values have not been heeded and *p*-value misinterpretations have been ignored, "The ASA Statement of *p*-values and Statistical Significance" (Wasserstein & Lazar, 2016) stopped just short of calling for the elimination of *p*-values in general and "statistical significance" declarations in particular. In response to the ASA Statement, the journal *The American Statistician* published a special issue in 2019, asking contributing researchers not only to ponder a "World Beyond $p < .05$", but to also speculate as to what procedures would then be involved in research science and what standard for declaring a novel scientific finding might be. But the premises behind both the ASA statement and the special issue of *The American Statistician* beg several questions. For example, if it is true of the *p*-value that, ". . . tool has become the tyrant" (Wasserstein, Schirm, & Lazar, 2019, p. 2; see also Halsey, 2019), then: Why are *p*-values so deeply entrenched in scientific research, and why have reform efforts essentially been reduced to exercises in abject futility? According to Calin-Jageman & Cumming, 2019):

> The inertia behind *p*-values is considerable, and 60+ years of incisive criticism has not yet dethroned NHST (*null hypothesis significance testing*) as the dominant approach to inference in many fields of science. (p. 277)

Recall from Chapter 1 of this book that not only have 60+ years of criticism not done away with NHST as noted by Calin-Jageman and Cumming (2019) above, but 60+ years have also failed to produce an appreciable increase in sample sizes (Holmes, 1979, 1983; Marszalek et al., 2011) or statistical power levels (Schimmack, 2012; Smaldino & McElreath, 2016). Chapter 1 also outlined three possible causes for these phenomena: (1) a publication bias, (2) Campbell's Law, and (3) questionable research practices, but perhaps a more succinct explanation has been offered by Goodman (2019, p. 20):

> The basic explanation is neither philosophical nor scientific, but sociologic; everyone uses them, . . . It's the same reason we can use money. When everyone believes in something's value, we can use it for real things; money for food, and *p*-values for knowledge claims, publication, funding, and promotion. It doesn't matter if the *p*-value doesn't mean what people think it means; it becomes valuable because of what it buys.

Within this context, the critical question facing all of research science becomes: Should *p*-values (and statistical significance claims by extension) go the way of the dinosaur, or should *p*-value critical regions be reconsidered, and *p*-values be accompanied by additional statistical indices that meaningfully inform the probability of an inferential error? To be sure, not all in the scientific research community agree with the premise, let alone what any possible remedy might be. Even the authors of the 43 papers included in the special issue of *The American Statistician* disagreed on both the premise and possible solutions. Several special issue authors did call for the outright elimination of both NHST and *p*-values (Calin-Jageman & Cumming, 2019; Goodman, 2019; Hubbard, 2019; McShane, Gall, Gelman, Robert, & Tackett, 2019; Pogrow, 2019; Trafimow, 2019). Many other contributing authors advocated for keeping *p*-values, but minimizing their importance, changing the criteria that defines a critical region under the null hypothesis distribution, and adding additional information that speaks to either evidence against the null hypothesis, or evidence of the likelihood that the alternative hypothesis is true (Amrhein, Trafimow, & Greenland, 2019; Anderson, 2019; Benjamin & Berger, 2019; Betensky, 2019; Blume et al., 2019; Colquhoun, 2019; Gannon et al., 2019; Goodman et al., 2019; Greenland, 2019; Johnson, 2019; Krueger & Heck, 2019; Lazzeroni, Lu, & Belitskaya-Lévy, 2016; Matthews, 2019). However, in addition to the need to eliminate the ubiquitous, "statistical significance does not equal scientific relevance" problem, even the special issue contributors who favor retaining *p*-values in an altered and supplemented form agree that change proposals should address two additional questions: (1) chance capitalization and (2) strength of evidence.

Possible Paths toward a "Post-*p* < .05" World

Lazzeroni et al. (2016; *Side Note: Lazzeroni, et al. [2016] was not included in the special issue of The American Statistician*), in addressing both questions, state that *p*-values themselves are variables that vary widely, even among replication studies conducted with a sample of the same size drawn randomly from the same population, so researchers should not be surprised when results are not replicated. To expand upon and supplement their argument, the authors offer an Excel spreadsheet (available at: *https://doi.org/10.1038/nmeth.3741*) that computes a 95% CI around the *p*-value from a specific study to estimate π, or the hypothetical population *p*-value that would be observed if the sample data were perfectly generated by the population reality. Furthermore, while not calling for the elimination of the $p < .05$ standard for statistical significance, the authors use their π calculating Excel spreadsheet to call it into question. Specifically, the authors show how, for example, if a researcher alleges "statistical significance" based on a two-tailed $p = .049$ *regardless of the sample size on which it is based*, the 95% CI upper bound value for π is 0.99; assuming a two-tailed significance test, a value of 1 is the assumed null hypothesis value. The authors also show using the Excel calculation spreadsheet that an observed *p*-value of $p = .00001$ would be required before a researcher could be 95% certain that a replication study at the same sample size would have a priori power $\geq .80$. In a response, Halsey, Curran-Everett, Vowler, and Drummond (2016) further asserted that that *p*-values from a single study should be viewed as unreliable unless the researcher can document a priori statistical power $\geq$ *.90*.

In keeping with questioning a $p < .05$ standard for statistical significance declarations (Ioannidis, 2018), Amrhein et al. (2019) advocate for converting *p*-values to "Shannon information transforms," or s, defined as $s = -\log_2(p)$, which would provide binary information units against the null hypothesis. For example, keeping with Lazzeroni et al.'s (2016) example of a researcher declaring statistical significance based on $p = .049$, it can be shown that $s = -\log_2(0.049) = 4.35$, or that there are roughly four binary units of information *against the null hypothesis*, which can be further explained by a simple hypothetical experiment. Suppose a researcher wanted to test whether a coin was a "fair" coin (i.e., the null hypothesis, or H_0:) or a coin improperly weighted or balanced in order to influence the result of a flip (i.e., the alternative hypothesis, or H_A:). A Shannon information transform value of $s = 4.35$ is roughly equivalent to flipping the hypothetical test coin four times and observing four consecutive tails, which the authors characterize as less than convincing evidence in favor of rejecting the null hypothesis. Taking the example a step further, and using Lazzeroni et al.'s, study replication standard of $p = .00001$, such a *p*-value would result in $s = -\log_2(0.00001)$

= 16.61, or roughly the equivalent of observing *17 consecutive* tails—far more convincing evidence against the null hypothesis.

Blume, Greevy, Welty, Smith, and Dupont (2019) recommend replacing $p < .05$ with a second-generation *p*-value (SGPV), which under the null hypothesis, represents a range of effects that that are clinically, scientifically, or practically meaningless. SGPV is further defined by the authors as a proportion that summarizes all zero and nonzero meaningless effects. SGPVs differ from a traditional $p < .05$ null hypothesis assumption in that $p < .05$ refers to an area in the tail of the null hypothesis distribution whose mean is zero. SGPVs can be conceptualized as a confidence interval null hypothesis that covers zero but also includes all irrelevant effects that surround zero. If the confidence interval for the effect of interest in a given study does not include the SGPV interval, the authors suggest that a researcher is far less likely at risk of a false discovery. Blume et al. (2019) offer online SGPV computational resources available at: *www.statisticalevidence.com* or *https://github.com/weltybiostat/sgpv*. In a similar vein, Colquhoun (2019) recommends supplementing an observed *p*-value with a false-positive risk (FPR) statistic. Continuing further with an example assuming statistical significance at $p = .049$, Colquhoun showed that such a declaration carries a 20–30% false positive risk and also offers an online FPR calculator at *http://fpr-calc.ucl.ac.uk/*.

Finally, Benjamin and Berger (2019; see also Halsey, 2019) address both the chance capitalization and strength of evidence question by recommending a twofold remedy: (1) changing the critical alpha level for declaring statistical significance from $p < .05$ to .005, and classifying results of $.05 > p > .005$ as questionable and (2) supplement all observed *p*-values with a Bayes factor bound (BFB) estimate, computed as $\text{BFB} = 1 / (-ep*\ln[p])$, where p is the observed *p*-value, ln is the natural logarithm, and e is a mathematical constant ($e = 2.71828$). BFB is defined as the maximum odds in favor of the alternative hypothesis versus the null hypothesis. To further illustrate the need for both a more stringent *p*-value for statistical significance declarations along with the addition of BFB estimates, the authors show: (1) $p < .05$ has BFB = 2.44, or 2.44 to 1 odds favoring the alternative hypothesis and a 29% chance that the null hypothesis is true; (2) $p < .005$ has a BFB = 13.9, or 13.9 to 1 odds favoring the alternative hypothesis, but more importantly, only a 6.7% chance that the null hypothesis is true, which is much closer to the nominal Type 1 error rate of a 5% chance that the null hypothesis is true; and (3) $p < .001$ has a BFB = 52.9, or 52.9 to 1 odds favoring the alternative hypothesis and a only a 1.9% chance that the null hypothesis is true. This twofold change, according to Benjamin and Berger, is needed to address both the scientific meaningfulness versus statistical significance question and the need to minimize false discoveries by providing the maximum odds favoring the alternative hypothesis.

What Does *All of This* Mean?

As detailed in Chapter 1, neither sample sizes nor statistical power estimates in empirical research have changed much in 60 years due to the convergence of a publication bias with Campbell's Law to produce "questionable research practices." As noted by Calin-Jageman and Cumming (2019), the same 60-year span has also failed to topple NHST or $p < .05$ from their positions of primacy in empirical inference. Questionable research practices, NHST, and $p < .05$ continue to persist because they are collectively systemic and self-sustaining. Furthermore, $p < .05$ as a standard for declaring novel discovery in empirical research has been shown to be mathematically questionable, and this comes after decades of publications strongly suggesting it to be empirically and theoretically cancerous. What is the point to be made? *Change is coming.* "Momentum, though, seems to be finally on the side of reform." (Calin-Jageman & Cumming, 2019, p. 277).

Throughout the book, we have used the standards of power ≥ .80 based on $p < .05$. We could rightly be accused of perpetuating the very problems we have outlined both in this chapter and in Chapter 1. However, a straightforward interim remedy can be gleaned from Halsey et al. (2016): If it is true that *p*-values from studies that have a priori statistical power less than .90 are unreliable, then the statistical power standard could be (should be?) raised to power > .90. If Halsey et al. (2016) are correct, and *p*-values from studies with a priori power > .90 are more reliable, especially if the evidence standard of $p < .05$ for claiming statistical significance is lowered (i.e., $p < .005$), then supplementing *p*-values with any of the above suggestions (a 95% CI estimate for π, Shannon information transforms [*s*], SGPV, FPR, or BFB) would provide greater transparency and allow the research consumer to judge the accuracy, strength, and reliability of the research "discovery" being proposed by using a declaration of statistical significance. Such changes in standards, increasing power to .90, and dropping *p* significance criterion to .005, would also bring about a welcome side effect: An increase in research study sample sizes by up to 70% or more (Benjamin, et al., 2018).

It bears repeating that not all in the scientific research community agree with either "The ASA Statement of *p*-values and Statistical Significance" (Wasserstein & Lazar, 2016) or the premise behind the special issue of *The American Statistician.* Many of the criticisms are documented by Benjamin et al. (2018) and include: (1) a lack of acknowledgment of potentially more serious scientific issues such as the "curse of multiplicity" for significance testing, HARK-ing, *p*-hacking, institutional perpetuation of questionable research practices, and publication biases; (2) the argument that a different *p*-value standard is needed for different fields of scientific inquiry, and (3) the argument that lowering *p*-values is a drop in the proverbial bucket relative to the need to do away with NHST altogether. Possibly the biggest criticism of the movement toward a "Post-$p < .05$ World," in general, and suggestions that $p < .05$ as a statistical significance standard is too low, is lacking in the requisite scientific rigor, and must be lowered specifically, is the criticism that is most statistically and mathematically readily apparent: Lowering the $p < .05$ standard will inevitably produce an increase in Type II inferential errors, and could well be the death knell for so-called "discovery science." The response to this criticism given by Benjamin and Berger (2019, p. 10, *italics added*) can be both simple and straightforward: "Moreover, the false negative rate will not increase *if sample sizes are increased so that statistical power is held constant.*" Which is exactly why this book was written.

SUGGESTED READINGS

- Artman, W. J., Nahum-Shani, I., Wu, T., McKay, J. R., & Ertefaie, A. (2020). Power analysis in a SMART design: Sample size estimation for determining the best embedded dynamic treatment regime. *Biostatistics, 21*(3), 432–448.

- Dziak, J. J., Dierker, L. C., & Abar, B. (2020). The interpretation of statistical power after the data have been gathered. *Current Psychology, 39,* 870–877.
- Smaldino, P. E., & McElreath, R. (2016). The natural selection of bad science. *Royal Society Open Science, 3*(9), 1–17.
- Stewart, A. J., & Plotkin, J. B. (2021). The natural selection of good science. *Nature Human Behaviour, 5*(11), 1510–1518.

References

Abraham, W. T., & Russell, D. W. (2008). Statistical power analysis in psychological research. *Social and Personality Psychology Compass, 2*, 283–301.

Agresti, A. (2013). *Categorical data analysis* (3rd ed.). Wiley.

Amrhein, V., Trafimow, D., & Greenland, S. (2019). Inferential statistics as descriptive statistics: There is no replication crisis if we don't expect replication. *The American Statistician, 73*(Supp. 1), 262–270.

Anderson, A. A. (2019). Assessing statistical results: Magnitude, precision, and model uncertainty. *The American Statistician, 73*(Supp. 1), 118–121.

Anderson, S. F., Kelley, K., & Maxwell, S. E. (2017). Sample-size planning for more accurate statistical power: A method adjusting sample effect sizes for publication bias and uncertainty. *Psychological Science, 28*, 1547–1562.

Arend, M. G., & Schäfer, T. (2019). Statistical power in two-level models: A tutorial based on Monte Carlo simulation. *Psychological Methods, 24*, 1–19.

Asparouhov, T., & Muthén, B. O. (2014). Continuous-time survival analysis in Mplus. *Technical appendix*. Muthén & Muthén.

Baker, D. H., Vilidaite, G., Lygo, F. A., Smith, A. K., Flack, T. R., Gouws, A. D., et al. (2020). Power contours: Optimising sample size and precision in experimental psychology and human neuroscience. *Psychological Methods, 26*, 295–314.

Baker, M. (2016). 1,500 Scientists lift the lid on reproducibility. *Nature, 533*, 452–454.

Bakker, M., van Dijk, A., & Wicherts, J. M. (2012). The rules of the game called psychological science. *Perspectives on Psychological Science, 7*, 543–554.

Baron, R. M., & Kenny, D. A. (1986). The moderator–mediator variable distinction in social psychological research: Conceptual, strategic, and statistical considerations. *Journal of Personality and Social Psychology, 51*(6), 1173–1182.

Basu, A. P., & Ebrahimi, N. (1996). Basic distributional results and properties. In N. Balakrishnan & A. P. Basu (Eds.), *The exponential distribution: Theory, methods, and applications* (pp. 7–16). CRC Press.

Bauer, D. J., & Curran, P. J. (2004). The integration of continuous and discrete latent variable models: Potential problems and promising opportunities. *Psychological Methods, 9*, 3–29.

Beal, S. J., Kashikar-Zuck, S., King, C., Black, W., Barnes, J., & Noll, J. G. (2020). Heightened risk for pain in young adult women with a history of childhood maltreatment: A prospective longitudinal study. *Pain, 161*, 156–165.

Beal, S. J., Wingrove, T., Mara, C. A., Lutz, N., Noll, J. G., & Greiner, M. V. (2019, June). Childhood adversity and associated psychosocial function in adolescents with complex trauma. In *Child & youth care forum* (Vol. 48, No. 3, pp. 305–322). Springer US.

Becker, S. P., Leopold, D. R., Burns, G. L., Jarrett, M. A., Langberg, J. M., Marshall, S. A., et al. (2016). The internal, external, and diagnostic validity of sluggish cognitive tempo: A meta-analysis and critical review. *Journal of the American Academy of Child and Adolescent Psychiatry, 55*, 163–178.

Benjamin, D., Berger, J., Johannesson, M., Nosek, B. A., Wagenmakers, E.-J., Berk, R., et al. (2018). Redefine statistical significance. *Nature Human Behaviour, 2*, 6–10.

Benjamin, D. J., & Berger, J. O. (2019). Three recommendations for improving the use of *p*-values. *The American Statistician, 73*(Supp. 1), 186–191.

Bernard, K., Frost, A., Bennett, C. B., & Lindhiem, O. (2017). Maltreatment and diurnal cortisol regulation: A meta-analysis. *Psychoneuroendocrinology, 78*, 57–67.

Betensky, R. A. (2019). The p-value requires context, not a threshold. *The American Statistician, 73*(1), 115–117.

Bezeau, S., & Graves, R. (2001). Statistical power and effect sizes of clinical neuropsychology research. *Journal of Clinical and Experimental Neuropsychology, 23*, 399–406.

Bhattacharyya, G. K. (1996). Inferences under two-sample and multi-sample situations. In N. Balakrishnan & A. P. Basu (Eds.), *The exponential distribution: Theory, methods, and applications* (pp. 93–118). CRC Press.

Biesanz, J. C., Deeb-Sossa, N., Papadakis, A. A., Bollen, K. A., & Curran, P. J. (2004). The role of coding time in estimating and interpreting growth curve models. *Psychological Methods, 9*, 30–52.

Blozis, S. A., & Cho, Y. I. (2008). Coding and centering of time in latent curve models in the presence of interindividual time heterogeneity. *Structural Equation Modeling: A Multidisciplinary Journal, 15*, 413–433.

Blume, J. D., Greevy, R. A., Welty, V. F., Smith, J. R., & Dupont, W. D. (2019). An introduction to second-generation *p*-values. *The American Statistician, 73*(Supp. 1), 157–167.

Bollen, K. (1989). *Structural equations with latent variables*. Wiley.

Bollen, K. A., & Curran, P. J. (2006). *Latent curve models: A structural equation perspective*. Wiley.

Button, K. S., Ioannidis, J. P., Mokrysz, C., Nosek, B. A., Flint, J., Robinson, E. S., & Munafò, M. R. (2013). Power failure: Why small sample size undermines the reliability of neuroscience. *Nature Reviews Neuroscience, 14*, 365–376.

Byrne, B. M. (2013). *Structural equation modeling with Mplus: Basic concepts, applications, and programming*. Routledge.

Calin-Jageman, R. J., & Cumming, G. (2019). The new statistics for better science: Ask how much, how uncertain, and what else is known. *The American Statistician, 73*(Supp. 1), 271–280.

Carmody, J. K., Plevinsky, J., Peugh, J. L., Denson, L. A., Hyams, J. S., Lobato, D., et al. (2019). Longitudinal non-adherence predicts treatment escalation in paediatric ulcerative colitis. *Alimentary Pharmacology & Therapeutics, 50*, 911–918.

Cham, H., Reshetnyak, E., Rosenfeld, B., & Breitbart, W. (2017). Full information maximum likelihood estimation for latent variable interactions with incomplete indicators. *Multivariate Behavioral Research, 52*(1), 12–30.

Clark-Carter, D. (1997). The account taken of statistical power in research published in the British Journal of Psychology. *British Journal of Psychology, 88*, 71–83.

Cohen, J. (1962). The statistical power of abnormal-social psychological research: A review. *The Journal of Abnormal and Social Psychology, 65*, 145–153.

Cohen, J. (1992). A power primer. *Psychological Bulletin, 112*, 155–159.

Cole, D. A., & Maxwell, S. E. (2003). Testing mediational models with longitudinal data: Questions and tips in the use of structural equation modeling. *Journal of Abnormal Psychology, 112*, 558–577.

Cole, D. A., & Preacher, K. J. (2014). Manifest variable path analysis: Potentially serious and misleading consequences due to uncorrected measurement error. *Psychological Methods, 19*, 300–315.

Colquhoun, D. (2019). The false positive risk: A proposal concerning what to do about *p*-values. *The American Statistician, 73*(Supp. 1), 192–201.

Corona, R., Dvorsky, M. R., Romo, S., Parks, A. M., Bourchtein, E., & Smith, Z. R., et al. (2020). Integrating tobacco prevention skills into an evidence-based intervention for adolescents with ADHD: Results from a pilot efficacy randomized controlled trial. *Journal of Abnormal Child Psychology, 48*, 1439–1453.

Davis, D. A., Luecken, L. J., & Zautra, A. J. (2005). Are reports of childhood abuse related to the experience of chronic pain in adulthood?: A meta-analytic review of the literature. *The Clinical Journal of Pain, 21*, 398–405.

Davison, W. P. (1983). The third-person effect in communication. *Public Opinion Quarterly, 47*, 1–15.

Dumas-Mallet, E., Button, K. S., Boraud, T., Gonon, F., & Munafò, M. R. (2017). Low statistical power in biomedical science: A review of three human research domains. *Royal Society Open Science, 4*, 1–11.

Enders, C. K. (2010). *Applied missing data analysis.* Guilford Press.

Fairchild, A. J., & MacKinnon, D. P. (2009). A general model for testing mediation and moderation effects. *Prevention Science, 10*, 87–99.

Faul, F., Erdfelder, E., Buchner, A., & Lang, A.-G. (2009). Statistical power analyses using G*Power 3.1: Tests for correlation and regression analyses. *Behavior Research Methods, 41*, 1149–1160.

Faul, F., Erdfelder, E., Lang, A.-G., & Buchner, A. (2007). G*Power 3: A flexible statistical power analysis program for the social, behavioral, and biomedical sciences. *Behavior Research Methods, 39*, 175–191.

Feingold, A. (2021). Effect of parameterization on statistical power and effect size estimation in latent growth modeling. *Structural Equation Modeling: A Multidisciplinary Journal, 28*, 609–621.

Finch, H., & Bolin, J. (2017). *Multilevel modeling using Mplus.* CRC Press.

Fischer, S., Macare, C., & Cleare, A. J. (2017). Hypothalamic–pituitary–adrenal (HPA) axis functioning as predictor of antidepressant response–Meta-analysis. *Neuroscience & Biobehavioral Reviews, 83*, 200–211.

Fraley, R. C., & Vazire, S. (2014). The N-pact factor: Evaluating the quality of empirical journals with respect to sample size and statistical power. *PLOS One, 9*, e109019.

Fritz, M. S., Cox, M. G., & MacKinnon, D. P. (2015). Increasing statistical power in mediation models without increasing sample size. *Evaluation & the Health Professions, 38*, 343–366.

Gannon, M. A., de Bragança Pereira, C. A., & Polpo, A. (2019). Blending Bayesian and classical tools to define optimal sample-size-dependent significance levels. *The American Statistician, 73*(Supp. 1), 213–222.

Gaskin, C. J., & Happell, B. (2012). Power of mental health nursing research: A statistical analysis of studies in the International Journal of Mental Health Nursing. *International Journal of Mental Health Nursing, 22*, 69–75.

Geiser, C. (2012). *Data analysis with Mplus.* Guilford Press.

Geiser, C. (2020). *Longitudinal structural equation modeling with Mplus: A latent state–trait perspective.* Guilford Press.

Goodman, S. N. (2019). Why is getting rid of *p*-values so hard? Musings on science and statistics. *The American Statistician, 73*(Supp. 1), 26–30.

Goodman, W. M., Spruill, S. E., & Komaroff, E. (2019). A proposed hybrid effect size plus *p*-value criterion: Empirical evidence supporting its use. *The American Statistician, 73*(Supp. 1), 168–185.

Graham, J. W. (2003). Adding missing-data-relevant variables to FIML-based structural equation models. *Structural Equation Modeling, 10*(1), 80–100.

Graham, J. W. (2012). *Missing data: Analysis and design.* Springer Science & Business Media.

Greenland, S. (2019). Valid *p*-values behave exactly as they should: Some misleading criticisms of *p*-values and their resolution with *s*-values. *The American Statistician, 73*(Supp. 1), 106–114.

Grimm, K. J., Ram, N., & Estabrook, R. (2017). *Growth modeling: Structural equation and multilevel modeling approaches.* Guilford Press.

Halsey, L. G. (2019). The reign of the *p*-value is over: What alternative analyses could we employ to fill the power vacuum? *Biological Letters, 15*, 1–8.

Halsey, L. G., Curran-Everett, D., Vowler, S. L., & Drummond, G. B. (2016). Response to Lazzeroni et al. *Nature Methods, 13*(2), 108.

Hayduk, L. A. (1987). *Structural equation modeling with LISREL: Essentials and advances.* Johns Hopkins University Press.

Hayes, A. F. (2015). An index and test of linear moderated mediation. *Multivariate Behavioral Research, 50*, 1–22.

Hayes, A. F. (2017). *Introduction to mediation, moderation, and conditional process analysis: A regression-based approach.* Guilford Press.

Hayes, A. F., & Rockwood, N. J. (2017). Regression-based statistical mediation and moderation analysis in clinical research: Observations, recommendations, and implementation. *Behaviour Research and Therapy, 98,* 39–57.

Higginson, A. D., & Munafò, M. R. (2016). Current incentives for scientists lead to underpowered studies with erroneous conclusions. *PLOS Biology, 14,* e2000995.

Holmes, C. B. (1979). Sample size in psychological research. *Perceptual and Motor Skills, 49,* 283–288.

Holmes, C. B. (1983). Sample size in four areas of psychological research. *Transactions of the Kansas Academy of Science, 86,* 76–80.

Horn, S. R., Long, M. M., Nelson, B. W., Allen, N. B., Fisher, P. A., & Byrne, M. L. (2018). Replication and reproducibility issues in the relationship between C-reactive protein and depression: A systematic review and focused meta-analysis. *Brain, Behavior, and Immunity, 73,* 85–114.

Hosmer, D. W., Lemeshow, S., & May, S. (2008). *Applied survival analysis: Regression modeling of time-to-event data.* Wiley.

Hubbard, R. (2019). Will the ASA's efforts to improve statistical practice be successful? Some evidence to the contrary. *The American Statistician, 73*(Supp. 1), 31–35.

Ioannidis, J. P. (2005). Why most published research findings are false. *PLOS Medicine, 2*(8), e124.

Ioannidis, J. P. (2008). Why most discovered true associations are inflated. *Epidemiology, 19*(5), 640–648.

Ioannidis, J. P. (2018). The proposal to lower *P* value thresholds to .005. *Journal of the American Medical Association, 319,* 1429–1430.

Johnson, P. O., & Neyman, J. (1936). Tests of certain linear hypotheses and their application to some educational problems. *Statistical Research Memoirs, 1,* 57–93.

Johnson, V. E. (2019). Evidence from marginally significant *t* statistics. *The American Statistician, 73*(Supp. 1), 129–134.

Jorgensen, T. D., Pornprasertmanit, S., Schoemann, A. M., & Rosseel, Y. (2025). semTools: Useful tools for structural equation modeling. R package version 0.5-7. Retrieved from *https://CRAN.R-project.org/package=semTools*

Jóźwiak, K., & Moerbeek, M. (2012). Power analysis for trials with discrete-time survival endpoints. *Journal of Educational and Behavioral Statistics, 37,* 630–654.

Kahana, S., Drotar, D., & Frazier, T. (2008). Meta-analysis of psychological interventions to promote adherence to treatment in pediatric chronic health conditions. *Journal of Pediatric Psychology, 33,* 590–611.

Kelava, A., Werner, C. S., Schermelleh-Engel, K., Moosbrugger, H., Zapf, D., Ma, Y., et al. (2011). Advanced nonlinear latent variable modeling: Distribution analytic LMS and QML estimators of interaction and quadratic effects. *Structural Equation Modeling: A Multidisciplinary Journal, 18*(3), 465–491.

Kelloway, K. E. (2014). *Using Mplus for structural equation modeling.* SAGE.

Kennis, M., Gerritsen, L., van Dalen, M., Williams, A., Cuijpers, P., & Bockting, C. (2020). Prospective biomarkers of major depressive disorder: A systematic review and meta-analysis. *Molecular Psychiatry, 25,* 321–338.

Kosciulek, J. F., & Szymanski, E. M. (1993). Statistical power analysis of rehabilitation counseling research. *Rehabilitation Counseling Bulletin, 36,* 212–219.

Kraemer, H. C., Kiernan, M., Essex, M., & Kupfer, D. J. (2008). How and why criteria defining moderators and mediators differ between the Baron & Kenny and MacArthur approaches. *Health Psychology, 27*(2S), S101–S108.

Kraemer, H. C., Stice, E., Kazdin, A., & Kupfer, D. (2001). How do risk factors work together to produce an outcome? Mediators, moderators, independent, overlapping and proxy risk factors. *The American Journal of Psychiatry, 158,* 848–856.

Kraemer, H. C., Wilson, G. T., Fairburn, C. G., & Agras, W. S. (2002). Mediators and moderators of treatment effects in randomized clinical trials. *Archives of General Psychiatry, 59,* 877–883.

Krueger, J. I., & Heck, P. R. (2019). Putting the *p*-value in its place. *The American Statistician, 73*(Supp. 1), 122–128.

Kugler, K. C., Guastaferro, K., Shenk, C. E., Beal, S. J., Zadzora, K. M., & Noll, J. G. (2019). The effect of substantiated and unsubstantiated investigations of child maltreatment and subsequent adolescent health. *Child Abuse & Neglect, 87,* 112–119.

Kühberger, A., Fritz, A., & Scherndl, T. (2014). Publication bias in psychology: A diagnosis based on the correlation between effect size and sample size. *PLOS One, 9,* e105825.

Kuhlman, K. R., Chiang, J. J., Horn, S., & Bower, J. E. (2017). Developmental psychoneuroendocrine and psychoneuroimmune pathways from childhood adversity to disease. *Neuroscience & Biobehavioral Reviews, 80,* 166–184.

Kuhlman, K. R., Geiss, E. G., Vargas, I., & Lopez-Duran N. L. (2015). Differential associations between childhood trauma subtypes and adolescent HPA-axis functioning. *Psychoneuroendocrinology, 54,* 103–114.

Kuhlman, K. R., Horn, S. R., Chiang, J. J., & Bower, J. E. (2020). Early life adversity exposure and circulating markers of inflammation in children and adolescents: A systematic review and meta-analysis. *Brain, Behavior, and Immunity, 86,* 30–42.

Kuo, P. L., Huang, A. R., Ehrlich, J. R., Kasper, J., Lin, F. R., McKee, M. M., et al. (2021). Prevalence of concurrent functional vision and hearing impairment and association with dementia in community-dwelling Medicare beneficiaries. *JAMA Network Open, 4,* e211558.

Lamberink, H. J., Otte, W. M., Sinke, M. R., Lakens, D., Glasziou, P. P., Tijdink, J. K., & Vinkers, C. H. (2018). Statistical power of clinical trials increased while effect size remained stable: An empirical analysis of 136,212 clinical trials between 1975 and 2014. *Journal of Clinical Epidemiology, 102,* 123–128.

Lazzeroni, L. C., Lu, Y., & Belitskaya-Lévy, I. (2016). Solutions for quantifying *P*-value uncertainty and replication power. *Nature Methods, 13,* 107–108.

Lin, G. C., Wen, Z., Marsh, H. W., & Lin, H. S. (2010). Structural equation models of latent interactions: Clarification of orthogonalizing and double-mean-centering strategies. *Structural Equation Modeling, 17,* 374–391.

Little, R. J., & Rubin, D. B. (2019). *Statistical analysis with missing data* (Vol. 793). Wiley.

Little, T. D., Bovaird, J. A., & Widaman, K. F. (2006). On the merits of orthogonalizing powered and product terms: Implications for modeling interactions among latent variables. *Structural Equation Modeling, 13,* 497–519.

Liu, X., Spybrook, J., Congdon, R., Martinez, A., & Raudenbush, S. (2006). *Optimal Design for Multilevel and Longitudinal Research V. 1.77* [Computer software]. Ann Arbor, MI: University of Michigan, Survey Research Center of the Institute of Social Research.

Ma, Z. W., & Zeng, W. N. (2014). A multiple mediator model: Power analysis based on Monte Carlo simulation. *American Journal of Applied Psychology, 3,* 72–79.

Maddock, J. E., & Rossi, J. S. (2001). Statistical power of articles published in three health-psychology related journals. *Health Psychology, 20,* 76–78.

Marsh, H. W., Wen, Z., & Hau, K. T. (2004). Structural equation models of latent interactions: Evaluation of alternative estimation strategies and indicator construction. *Psychological Methods, 9,* 275–300.

Marszalek, J. M., Barber, C., Kohlhart, J., & Cooper, B. H. (2011). Sample size in psychological research over the past 30 years. *Perceptual and Motor Skills, 112,* 331–348.

Matthews, R. A. (2019). Moving towards the post $p < 0.05$ era via the analysis of credibility. *The American Statistician, 73*(Supp. 1), 202–212.

Maxwell, S. E. (2004). The persistence of underpowered studies in psychological research: Causes, consequences, and remedies. *Psychological Methods, 9,* 147–163.

Maxwell, S. E., & Cole, D. A. (2007). Bias in cross-sectional analyses of longitudinal mediation. *Psychological Methods, 12,* 23–44.

Maxwell, S. E., Cole, D. A., & Mitchell, M. A. (2011). Bias in cross-sectional analyses of longitudinal mediation: Partial and complete mediation under an autoregressive model. *Multivariate Behavioral Research, 46,* 816–841.

McDonald, J. A., & Clelland, D. A. (1984). Textile workers and union sentiment. *Social Forces, 63,* 502–521.

McDonald, R. P. (1999). *Test theory: A unified treatment.* Erlbaum.

McShane, B. B., Gal, D., Gelman, A., Robert, C., & Tackett, J. L. (2019). Abandon statistical significance. *The American Statistician, 73*(Supp. 1), 235–245.

Mehta, P. D., & West, S. G. (2000). Putting the individual back into individual growth curves. *Psychological Methods, 5*, 23–43.

Mone, M. A., Mueller, G. C., & Mauland, W. (1996). The perceptions and usage of statistical power in applied psychology and management research. *Personnel Psychology, 49,* 103–120.

Morris, T. P., White, I. R., & Crowther, M. J. (2019). Using simulation studies to evaluate statistical methods. *Statistics in Medicine, 38*, 2074–2102.

Mundform, D. J., Schaffer, J., Kim, M. J., Shaw, D., Thongteeraparp, A., & Supawan, P. (2011). Number of replications required in Monte Carlo simulation studies: A synthesis of four studies. *Journal of Modern Applied Statistical Methods, 10,* 19–28.

Muthén, B. O. (2016, May 23). *Mplus workshop, part 1: Highlights from Muthen, Muthen, & Asparouhov (2016). Regression and mediation analysis using Mplus.* Pre-conference workshop at the Modern Modeling Methods Conference, Storrs, CT.

Muthén, B., & Asparouhov, T. (2015). Causal effects in mediation modeling: An introduction with applications to latent variables. *Structural Equation Modeling: A Multidisciplinary Journal, 22*, 12–23.

Muthén, B., Asparouhov, T., Hunter, A. M., & Leuchter, A. F. (2011). Growth modeling with nonignorable dropout: Alternative analyses of the STAR* D antidepressant trial. *Psychological Methods, 16,* 17–33.

Muthén, L. K., & Muthén, B. O. (1998–2017). *Mplus user's guide* (8th ed.). Muthén & Muthén.

Muthén, L. K., & Muthén, B. O. (2002). How to use a Monte Carlo study to decide on sample size and determine power. *Structural Equation Modeling, 9*, 599–620.

Muthén, B. O., Muthén, L. K., & Asparouhov, T. (2017). *Regression and mediation analysis using Mplus.* Muthén & Muthén.

Nunnally, J., & Bernstein, I. (1994). *Psychometric theory* (3rd ed.). McGraw-Hill.

Nuzzo, R. (2014). Scientific method: Statistical errors. *Nature, 506*, 150–152.

Olson, A. E., Shenk, C. E., Noll, J. G., & Allen, B. (2022). Child maltreatment and substance use in emerging adulthood: Internalizing and externalizing behaviors at the transition to adolescence as indirect pathways. *Child Maltreatment, 27*(3), 490–500.

Open Science Collaboration. (2015). Estimating the reproducibility of psychological science. *Science, 349*, aac4716.

Palmos, A. B., Watson, S., Hughes, T., Finkelmeyer, A., McAllister-Williams, R. H., et al. (2019). Associations between childhood maltreatment and inflammatory markers. *British Journal of Psychiatry Open, 5,* 1–7.

Pearl, J. (2014). Interpretation and identification of causal mediation. *Psychological Methods, 19*(4), 459–481.

Peckins, M. K., Susman, E. J., Negriff, S., Noll, J., & Trickett, P. K. (2015). Cortisol profiles: A test for adaptive calibration of the stress response system in maltreated and nonmaltreated youth. *Development & Psychopathology, 27,* 1461–1470.

Perugini, M., Gallucci, M., & Costantini, G. (2018). A practical primer to power analysis for simple experimental designs. *International Review of Social Psychology, 31,* Article 20.

Peugh, J. L., Toland, M. D., & Harrison, H. (2023). A tutorial for handling suspected missing not at random data in longitudinal clinical trials. *The Quantitative Methods for Psychology, 19*(4), 347–367.

Pitharouli, M. C., Hagenaars, S. P., Glanville, K. P., Coleman, J. R., Hotopf, M., Lewis, C. M., & Pariante, C. M. (2022). Elevated C-reactive protein in patients with depression, independent of genetic, health, and psychosocial factors: Results from the UK Biobank. *American Journal of Psychiatry, 178*(6), 522–529.

Platt, A., Obala, A. A., MacIntyre, C., Otsyula, B, & O'Meara, W. P. (2018). Dynamic malaria hotspots in an open cohort in western Kenya. *Scientific Reports, 8,* 647–657.

Pogrow, S. (2019). How effect size (practical significance) misleads clinical practice: The case for switching to practical benefit to assess applied research findings. *The American Statistician, 73*(Supp. 1), 223–234.

Pornprasertmanit, S., Miller, P., Schoemann, A. M., & Jorgensen, T. D. (2025). simsem: SIMulated structural equation modeling. R package version 0.5-17. Retrieved from *https://CRAN.R-project.org/package=simsem*

Rivera, P. M., Bray, B. C., Guastaferro, K., Kugler, K., & Noll, J. G. (2018). Linking patterns of substance use with sexual risk-taking among female adolescents with and without histories of maltreatment. *Journal of Adolescent Health, 62,* 556–562.

Rosseel, Y. (2012). "lavaan: An R Package for Structural Equation Modeling." *Journal of Statistical Software, 48*(2), 1–36.

Rossi, J. S. (1990). Statistical power of psychological research: What have we gained in 20 years? *Journal of Consulting and Clinical Psychology, 58,* 646–656.

Rovine, M. J., & McDermott, P. A. (2018). Latent growth curve and repeated measures ANOVA contrasts: What the models are telling you. *Multivariate Behavioral Research, 53,* 90–101.

Rovine, M. J., & Molenaar, P. C. (1998). A LISREL model for the analysis of repeated measures with a patterned covariance matrix. *Structural Equation Modeling: A Multidisciplinary Journal, 5*(4), 318–343.

Rovine, M. J., & Molenaar, P. C. M. (2001). A structural equations modeling approach to the general linear mixed model. In L. M. Collins & A. G. Sayer (Eds.), *New methods for the analysis of change* (pp. 67–98). American Psychological Association.

Safarkhani, M., Jolani, S., & Moerbeek, M. (2014). Optimal number of accrual groups and accrual group sizes in longitudinal trials with discrete-time survival endpoints. *Statistica Neerlandica, 68,* 43–60.

Schimmack, U. (2012). The ironic effect of significant results on the credibility of multiple-study articles. *Psychological Methods, 17,* 551–566.

Schoemann, A. M., Boulton, A. J., & Short, S. D. (2017). Determining power and sample size for simple and complex mediation models. *Social Psychological and Personality Science, 8,* 379–386.

Schoemann, A. M., & Jorgensen, T. D. (2021). Testing and interpreting latent variable interactions using the semTools package. *Psych, 3*(3), 322–335.

Sedlmeier, P., & Gigerenzer, G. (1992). Do studies of statistical power have an effect on the power of studies? In A. E. Kazdin (Ed.), *Methodological issues and strategies in clinical research* (pp. 389–406). American Psychological Association.

Shen, W., Kiger, T. B., Davies, S. E., Rasch, R. L., Simon, K. M., & Ones, D. S. (2011). Samples in applied psychology: Over a decade of research in review. *Journal of Applied Psychology, 5,* 1055–1064.

Shenk, C. E., Noll, J. G., Peugh, J. L., Griffin, A. M., & Bensman, H. E. (2016). Contamination in the prospective study of child maltreatment and female adolescent health. *Journal of Pediatric Psychology, 41,* 37–45.

Sibley, M. H., Pelham, W., Derefinko, K., Kuriyan, A., Sanchez, F., & Graziano, P. (2013). A pilot trial of supporting teens' academic needs daily (STAND): A parent–adolescent collaborative intervention for ADHD. *Journal of Psychopathology and Behavioral Assessment, 35*(4), 436–449.

Sibley, M. H., Pelham, W., Molina, B. S., Coxe, S., Kipp, H., Gnagy, E. M., et al. (2014). The role of early childhood ADHD and subsequent CD in the initiation and escalation of adolescent cigarette, alcohol, and marijuana use. *Journal of Abnormal Psychology, 123*(2), 362–374.

Sim, M., Kim, S. Y., & Suh, Y. (2021). Sample size requirements for simple and complex mediation models. *Educational and Psychological Measurement, 82*(1), 76–106.

Singer, J. D., & Willett, J. B. (2003a). *Applied longitudinal data analysis: Modeling change and event occurrence.* Oxford University Press.

Singer, J. D., & Willett, J. B. (2003b). It's about time: Using discrete-time survival analysis to study duration and the timing of events. *Journal of Educational and Behavioral Statistics, 18,* 155–195.

Smaldino, P. E., & McElreath, R. (2016). The natural selection of bad science. *Royal Society Open Science, 3,* 1–17.

Spoth, R., Redmond, C., Mason, W. A., Schainker, L., & Borduin, L. (2015). Research on the strengthening families program for parents and youth 10–14: Long-term effects, mechanisms, translation to public health, PROSPER partnership scale up. In L. M. Scheier (Ed.), *Handbook of drug prevention.* American Psychological Association.

Spoth, R., Shin, C., Guyll, M., Redmond, C., & Azevedo, K. (2006). Universality of effects: An examination of the comparability of long-term family intervention effects on substance use across risk-related subgroups. *Prevention Science, 7,* 209–224.

Stubbs, B., Vancampfort, D., Veronese, N., Thompson, T., Fornaro, M., Schofield, P., et al. (2017). Depression and pain: Primary data and meta-analysis among 237,952 people across 47 low- and middle-income countries. *Psychological Medicine, 47,* 2906–2917.

Szucs, D., & Ioannidis, J. P. (2017a). Empirical assessment of published effect sizes and power in the recent cognitive neuroscience and psychology literature. *PLOS Biology, 15,* e2000797.

Szucs, D., & Ioannidis, J. (2017b). When null hypothesis significance testing is unsuitable for research: A reassessment. *Frontiers in Human Neuroscience, 11,* 390.

Tadikamalla, P. R, & Balakrishnan, N. (1996). Computer simulations. In N. Balakrishnan & A. P. Basu (Eds.), *The exponential distribution: Theory, methods, and applications* (pp. 547–558). CRC Press.

Tal-Or, N., Cohen, J., Tsfati, Y., & Gunther, A. C. (2010). Testing causal direction in the influence of presumed media influence. *Communication Research, 37,* 801–824.

Tauber, N. M., Zachariae, R., Jensen, A. B., Thewes, B., Skyt, I., Elkjaer, E., et al. (2021). ConquerFear-group: Feasibility study with pilot results of a psychological intervention for fear of cancer recurrence delivered in groups. *Psycho-Oncology, 31*(1), 30–38.

Thatcher, S. M., & Patel, P. C. (2012). Group faultlines: A review, integration, and guide to future research. *Journal of Management, 38,* 969–1009.

Thoemmes, F., MacKinnon, D. P., & Reiser, M. R. (2010). Power analysis for complex mediational designs using Monte Carlo methods. *Structural Equation Modeling, 17,* 510–534.

Trafimow, D. (2019). Five nonobvious changes in editorial practice for editors and reviewers to consider when evaluating submissions in a post $p < 0.05$ universe. *The American Statistician, 73*(Supp. 1), 340–345.

Vakhitova, Z. I., & Alston-Knox, C. L. (2018). Non-significant p-values? Strategies to understand and better determine the importance of effects and interactions in logistic regression. *PLOS One, 13,* e0205076.

Vakhitova, Z., Webster, J., Alston-Knox, C., Reynald, D., & Townsley, M. (2018). Offender–victim relationship and offender motivation in the context of indirect cyber abuse: A mixed-method exploratory analysis. *International Review of Victimology, 24,* 347–366.

Valeri, L., & VanderWeele, T. J. (2013). Mediation analysis allowing for exposure–mediator interactions and causal interpretation: Theoretical assumptions and implementation with SAS and SPSS macros. *Psychological Methods, 18,* 137–150.

Walson, J. L., Sangaré, L. R., Singa, B. O., Naulikha, J. M., Piper, B. K., Yuhas, K., et al. (2013). Evaluation of impact of long-lasting insecticide-treated bed nets and point-of-use water filters on HIV-1 disease progression in Kenya. *AIDS, 27,* 1493–1501.

Wang, Y. A., & Rhemtulla, M. (2021). Power analysis for parameter estimation in structural equation modeling: A discussion and tutorial. *Advances in Methods and Practices in Psychological Science, 4,* 1–17.

Wang, J., & Wang, X. (2019). *Structural equation modeling: Applications using Mplus* (2nd ed.). Wiley.

Wasserstein, R. L., & Lazar, N. A. (2016). The ASA statement on p-values: Context, process, and purpose. *The American Statistician, 70,* 129–133.

Wasserstein, R. L., Schirm, A. L., & Lazar, N. A. (2019). Moving to a world beyond "$p < 0.05$." *The American Statistician, 73*(Supp. 1), 1–19.

Wickham, H., & Grolemund, G. (2017). *R for data science: Import, tidy, transform, visualize, and model data.* O'Reilly Media.

Wickrama, K. K., Lee, T. K., O'Neal, C. W., & Lorenz, F. O. (2016). *Higher-order growth curves and mixture modeling with Mplus: A practical guide.* Routledge.

Wilkinson, L., & the Task Force on Statistical Inference. (1999). Statistical methods in psychology journals: Guidelines and explanations. *American Psychologist, 54,* 594–604.

Wright, S. (1921). Correlation and causation. *Journal of Agricultural Research, 20,* 557–580.

Wright, S. (1934). The method of path coefficients. *The Annals of Mathematical Statistics, 5,* 161–215.

Zickfeld, J. H., & Schubert, T. W. (2019). How to identify and how to conduct research that is informative and reproducible. In J. Valsiner (Ed.), *Social philosophy of science for the social sciences* (pp. 147–168). Springer International.

Author Index

E

F

G

H

I

J

K

L

M

Subject Index

Note. f or *t* following a page number indicates a figure or a table.

D

E

F

G

H

I

M

N

O

P

Q

R

U

W

About the Authors

James Peugh, PhD, is Director of Quantitative Services in the Division of Behavioral Medicine and Clinical Psychology, Cincinnati Children's Hospital Medical Center, and Research Professor in the Department of Pediatrics at the University of Cincinnati Medical School. His methodological interests focus on the use of Monte Carlo simulation techniques to test advanced statistical analyses. Dr. Peugh has also published pedagogical "how-to" papers demonstrating the application of statistical techniques. He has publications in a variety of quantitative, educational, and psychological journals.

Kaylee Litson, PhD, is Assistant Professor in the Department of Psychology at the University of Houston. As an interdisciplinary quantitative psychologist, they have a particular interest in the link between statistical model estimation and theory-driven interpretation, especially in the context of complex, multimethod, and longitudinal research design. Dr. Litson's work highlights the translation of quantitative psychology methods to applied research in fields such as cognition and educational psychology. Their publications have appeared in applied and quantitative journals.